Cystic Fibrosis in the Era of Highly Effective CFTR Modulator Therapy

Editors

CLEMENTE J. BRITTO
JENNIFER L. TAYLOR-COUSAR

CLINICS IN CHEST MEDICINE

www.chestmed.theclinics.com

December 2022 • Volume 43 • Number 4

ELSEVIER

1600 John F. Kennedy Boulevard • Suite 1800 • Philadelphia, Pennsylvania, 19103-2899

http://www.theclinics.com

CLINICS IN CHEST MEDICINE Volume 43, Number 4
December 2022 ISSN 0272-5231, ISBN-13: 978-0-323-84961-6

Editor: Joanna Collett
Developmental Editor: Karen Justine Solomon

Clinics in Chest Medicine (ISSN 0272-5231) is published quarterly by Elsevier Inc., 360 Park Avenue South, New York, NY 10010-1710. Months of issue are March, June, September, and December. Periodicals postage paid at New York, NY and additional mailing offices. Subscription prices are $408.00 per year (domestic individuals), $1049.00 per year (domestic institutions), $100.00 per year (domestic students/residents), $436.00 per year (Canadian individuals), $1091.00 per year (Canadian institutions), $499.00 per year (international individuals), $1091.00 per year (international institutions), $100.00 per year (Canadian Students), and $230.00 per year (International Students). International air speed delivery is included in all Clinics subscription prices. All prices are subject to change without notice. **POSTMASTER:** Send address changes to Clinics in Chest Medicine, Elsevier Health Sciences Division, Subscription Customer Service, 3251 Riverport Lane, Maryland Heights, MO 63043. **Customer Service: Telephone: 1-800-654-2452** (U.S. and Canada); **1-314-447-8871** (outside U.S. and Canada). **Fax: 1-314-447-8029. E-mail: journalscustomerservice-usa@elsevier.com (for print support); journalsonlinesupport-usa@elsevier.com (for online support).**

Reprints. For copies of 100 or more of articles in this publication, please contact the Commercial Reprints Department, Elsevier Inc., 360 Park Avenue South, New York, NY 10010-1710. Tel.: 212-633-3874; Fax: 212-633-3820; E-mail: reprints@elsevier.com.

Clinics in Chest Medicine is covered in *MEDLINE/PubMed (Index Medicus), Current Contents/Clinical Medicine, EMBASE/Excerpta Medica, Science Citation Index,* and *ISI/BIOMED.*

Contributors

EDITORS

CLEMENTE J. BRITTO, MD, ATSF
Associate Director, Adult Cystic Fibrosis Program, Assistant Professor of Medicine, Department of Internal Medicine, Division of Pulmonary, Critical Care, and Sleep Medicine, Yale School of Medicine, New Haven, Connecticut, USA

JENNIFER L. TAYLOR-COUSAR, MD, MSCS, ATSF
Co-Director and CF Therapeutics Development Center Director, Adult Cystic Fibrosis Program, Medical Director, Clinical Research Services, Professor, Departments of Internal Medicine and Pediatrics, Divisions of Pulmonary Sciences and Critical Care Medicine and Pediatric Pulmonology, National Jewish Medical Center, National Jewish Health, Denver, Colorado, USA

AUTHORS

KIMBERLY ALTMAN, MS, RD, CSP, CDN
Senior Nutritionist, Gunnar Esiason Adult Cystic Fibrosis and Lung Center, Columbia University Irving Medical Center, NewYork-Presbyterian Hospital, New York, New York, USA

DAVID N. ASSIS, MD
Section of Digestive Diseases, Yale School of Medicine, New Haven, Connecticut, USA

CHRISTINA JAYNE BATHGATE, PhD
Assistant Professor, Department of Medicine, National Jewish Health, Denver, Colorado, USA

TRACEY L. BONFIELD, PhD
Diplomate of the American Board of Medical Laboratory Immunologists; Associate Professor, Department of Genetics and Genome Sciences, Case Western Reserve University School of Medicine, Cleveland, Ohio, USA

JOHN J. BREWINGTON, MD, MS
Assistant Professor, Department of Pediatrics, University of Cincinnati College of Medicine, Division of Pulmonary Medicine, Cincinnati

Children's Hospital Medical Center, Cincinnati, Ohio, USA

CLEMENTE J. BRITTO, MD, ATSF
Associate Director, Adult Cystic Fibrosis Program, Assistant Professor of Medicine, Department of Internal Medicine, Division of Pulmonary, Critical Care, and Sleep Medicine, Yale School of Medicine, New Haven, Connecticut, USA

EMANUELA M. BRUSCIA, PhD
Associate Professor, Department of Pediatrics, Section of Pulmonology, Allergy, Immunology and Sleep Medicine, Yale School of Medicine, New Haven, Connecticut, USA

JENNIFER BUTCHER, PhD
Department of Pediatrics, Division of Pediatric Psychology, Mott Children's Hospital, University of Michigan Health, Ann Arbor, Michigan, USA

LINDSAY J. CAVERLY, MD
Assistant Professor, Department of Pediatrics, University of Michigan Medical School, Ann Arbor, Michigan, USA

JOHN P. CLANCY, MD
Vice President of Clinical Research, Cystic
Fibrosis Foundation, Bethesda, Maryland,
USA

GARRY R. CUTTING, MD
McKusick-Nathans Department of Genetic
Medicine, Johns Hopkins School of Medicine,
Baltimore, Maryland, USA

CHARLES L. DALEY, MD
Professor, Department of Medicine, National
Jewish Health, Denver, Colorado, USA;
University of Colorado Denver School of
Medicine, Aurora, Colorado, USA

**JANE C. DAVIES, MD, MB, ChB, MRCP,
MRCPCH**
National Heart and Lung Institute, Imperial
College London, Royal Brompton & Harefield
Hospital, Guys & St Thomas' Trust, London,
England, United Kingdom

PAMELA B. DAVIS, MD, PhD
The Arline H. and Curtis F. Garvin Research
Professor, Professor of General Medical
Sciences and Pediatrics, Center for
Community Health Integration, Case Western
Reserve University School of Medicine,
Cleveland, Ohio, USA

EUNICE M.M. DEFILIPPO, MD
Internal Medicine and Pediatrics, Yale School
of Medicine, New Haven, Connecticut, USA

MARIE E. EGAN, MD
Division of Pulmonary Allergy Immunology
Sleep Medicine, Professor of Pediatrics and
Cellular and Molecular Physiology, Vice Chair
of Research, Department of Pediatrics, Interim
Chief, Pediatric Pulmonary Allergy Immunology
and Sleep Medicine, Director, Yale Cystic
Fibrosis Center, School of Medicine, Yale
University, New Haven, Connecticut, USA

STEPHANIE S. FILIGNO, PhD
Professor of Pediatrics, University of Cincinnati
College of Medicine, Division of Behavioral
Medicine and Clinical Psychology, Cincinnati
Children's Hospital Medical Center, Cincinnati,
Ohio, USA

STEVEN D. FREEDMAN, MD, PhD
Beth Israel Medical Center, Harvard Medical
School, Boston, Massachusetts, USA

ANNA M. GEORGIOPOULOS, MD
Associate Professor of Psychiatry, Part-Time,
Harvard Medical School, Department of
Psychiatry, Massachusetts General Hospital,
Boston, Massachusetts, USA

ALEX H. GIFFORD, MD, FCCP
Pulmonary, Critical Care, and Sleep Medicine,
University Hospitals, Rainbow Babies and
Children's, Associate Professor of Medicine,
Division of Pulmonary, Critical Care, and Sleep
Medicine, University Hospitals Cleveland
Medical Center, Cleveland, Ohio, USA

JENNIFER S. GUIMBELLOT, MD, PhD
Associate Professor, Department of Pediatrics,
Division of Pulmonary and Sleep Medicine,
Associate Scientist, Gregory Fleming James
Cystic Fibrosis Research Center, The
University of Alabama at Birmingham,
Birmingham, Alabama, USA

ZACHARY M. HARRIS, MD
Yale Adult Cystic Fibrosis Program, Section of
Pulmonary, Critical Care, and Sleep Medicine,
Yale School of Medicine, New Haven,
Connecticut, USA

KATHERINE B. HISERT, MD, PhD
Assistant Professor, Department of Medicine,
National Jewish Health, Denver, Colorado,
USA

MICHELLE HJELM, MD
Assistant Professor of Pediatrics, University of
Cincinnati College of Medicine, Division of
Pulmonary Medicine, Cincinnati Children's
Hospital Medical Center, Cincinnati, Ohio, USA

RAKSHA JAIN, MD, MSCI
Department of Medicine, The University of
Texas Southwestern Medical Center, Dallas,
Texas, USA

ANYA T. JOYNT, PhD
McKusick-Nathans Department of Genetic
Medicine, Johns Hopkins School of Medicine,
Baltimore, Maryland, USA

TRACI M. KAZMERSKI, MD, MS
Department of Pediatrics, University of
Pittsburgh School of Medicine, Center for
Innovative Research on Gender Health Equity
(CONVERGE), University of Pittsburgh,
Pittsburgh, Pennsylvania, USA

ANDREA KELLY, MD, MSCE
Attending Physician, Division of Endocrinology and Diabetes, Children's Hospital of Philadelphia, Professor of Pediatrics, CE, University of Pennsylvania Perelman School of Medicine, Philadelphia, Pennsylvania, USA

JONATHAN L. KOFF, MD
Director, Adult Cystic Fibrosis Program, Yale University Center for Phage Biology and Therapy, Associate Professor, Department of Internal Medicine, Section of Pulmonary, Critical Care and Sleep Medicine, Yale School of Medicine, New Haven, Connecticut, USA

BRYNN E. MARKS, MD, MSHPED
Attending Physician, Director of Technology of the Diabetes Center, Division of Endocrinology and Diabetes, Assistant Professor of Pediatrics, University of Pennsylvania Perelman School of Medicine, Children's Hospital of Philadelphia, Philadelphia, Pennsylvania, USA

STACEY L. MARTINIANO, MD
Associate Professor, Department of Pediatrics, Children's Hospital Colorado, University of Colorado Denver School of Medicine, Aurora, Colorado, USA

KIMBERLY A. MCBENNETT, MD, PhD, FACP
Associate Professor, Medicine and Pediatrics, Case Western Reserve University School of Medicine, LeRoy W. Matthews Cystic Fibrosis Center, University Hospitals, Rainbow Babies and Children's, Cleveland, Ohio, USA

PAUL MCNALLY, MD, MB, BCh, BAO
Department of Paediatrics, RCSI University of Medicine and Health Sciences, Cystic Fibrosis Center, Children's Health Ireland, Dublin, Ireland

LAUREN N. MEISS, MD, MS
Department of Obstetrics, Gynecology, and Reproductive Sciences, Yale School of Medicine, New Haven, Connecticut, USA

THOMAS S. MURRAY, MD, PhD
Associate Professor, Department of Pediatrics, Section of Infectious Diseases and Global Health, Yale School of Medicine, New Haven, Connecticut, USA

SAMYA Z. NASR, MD
Department of Pediatrics, Division of Pediatric Pulmonology, Mott Children's Hospital, University of Michigan Health, Ann Arbor, Michigan, USA

DAVID P. NICHOLS, MD
Associate Professor, Department of Pediatrics, Division of Pulmonary Medicine, Seattle Children's Hospital, University of Washington School of Medicine, Seattle, Washington, USA

JERRY A. NICK, MD
Professor, Department of Medicine, National Jewish Health, Denver, Colorado, USA; University of Colorado Denver School of Medicine, Aurora, Colorado, USA

JOSEPH M. PILEWSKI, MD
Associate Chief for Clinical Affairs, Medical Director, Lung Transplant Program, Pulmonary, Allergy, and Critical Care Medicine Division, University of Pittsburgh Medical Center, Co-Director, Cystic Fibrosis Center, Associate Professor of Medicine, Pediatrics, Cell Biology, and Clinical and Translational Science, University of Pittsburgh, UPMC Children's Hospital of Pittsburgh, Pittsburgh, Pennsylvania, USA

FELIX RATJEN, MD, PhD, FRCP(C) FERS
Professor, University of Toronto, Head, Division of Respiratory Medicine, Program Head, Translational Medicine, University of Toronto Hospital for Sick Children, Toronto, Ontario, Canada

SEBASTIÁN A. RIQUELME, PhD
Assistant Professor, Department of Pediatrics, College of Physicians and Surgeons, Columbia University, Columbia University Irving Medical Center, New York, New York, USA

TERRI SCHINDLER, MS, RDN
Nutritionist, Pediatric Pulmonology, University Hospitals Cleveland Medical Center, Rainbow Babies and Children's, Cleveland, Ohio, USA

SARAH JANE SCHWARZENBERG, MD
Professor, Department of Pediatrics, University of Minnesota Masonic Children's Hospital, Academ, Minneapolis, Minnesota, USA

NEERAJ SHARMA, DVM, PhD
McKusick-Nathans Department of Genetic Medicine, Johns Hopkins School of Medicine, Baltimore, Maryland, USA

BETH A. SMITH, MD
Professor of Psychiatry and Pediatrics, Jacobs School of Medicine and Biomedical Sciences, Children's Psychiatry Clinic, Buffalo, New York, USA

MICHAEL S. STALVEY, MD
Associate Professor of Pediatrics, Departments of Pediatrics and Medicine, Gregory Fleming James Cystic Fibrosis Research Center, The University of Alabama at Birmingham, Children's of Alabama, Birmingham, Alabama, USA

GAIL STANLEY, MD
Clinical Fellow, Department of Internal Medicine, Section of Pulmonary, Critical Care and Sleep Medicine, Yale School of Medicine, Adult Cystic Fibrosis Program, Yale University Center for Phage Biology and Therapy, New Haven, Connecticut, USA

JAIDEEP S. TALWALKAR, MD
Internal Medicine and Pediatrics, Yale Adult Cystic Fibrosis Program, Section of Pulmonary, Critical Care, and Sleep Medicine, Yale School of Medicine, New Haven, Connecticut, USA

JENNIFER L. TAYLOR-COUSAR, MD, MSCS, ATSF
Co-Director and CF Therapeutics Development Center Director, Adult Cystic Fibrosis Program, Medical Director, Clinical Research Services, Professor, Departments of Internal Medicine and Pediatrics, Divisions of Pulmonary Sciences and Critical Care Medicine and Pediatric Pulmonology, National Jewish Medical Center, National Jewish Health, Denver, Colorado, USA

CHRISTOPHER VÉLEZ, MD
Division of Gastroenterology, Department of Medicine, Center for Neurointestinal Health, Massachusetts General Hospital, Harvard Medical School, Boston, Massachusetts, USA

ALEXANDRA WILSON, MS, RDN, CDCES
Manager, Cystic Fibrosis Clinical Research, Clinical Research Services, National Jewish Health, Denver, Colorado, USA

Contents

Toward a Broader Understanding of Cystic Fibrosis Epidemiology and Its Impact on Clinical Manifestations 579

Kimberly A. McBennett and Pamela B. Davis

The incidence of cystic fibrosis remains constant in North America and Western Europe is 1 in 3500 live births, but survival and quality of life have improved. The cystic fibrosis population has shifted toward the adult age range with a concomitant shift in the spectrum of complications. Survival increased because of aggressive symptomatic therapy, earlier diagnosis by newborn screening, and the introduction of modulators of the cystic fibrosis transmembrane conductance regulator, so that predicted median survival age is now about 50 years. In the United States, members of low socioeconomic status populations or members of racial or ethnic minorities have benefitted less from these advances.

Genetics of Cystic Fibrosis: Clinical Implications 591

Anya T. Joynt, Garry R. Cutting, and Neeraj Sharma

Cystic fibrosis (CF) is a multiorgan disease caused by a wide variety of mutations in the cystic fibrosis transmembrane conductance regulator gene. As treatment has progressed from symptom mitigation to targeting of specific molecular defects, genetics has played an important role in identifying the proper precision therapies for each individual. Novel therapeutic approaches are focused on expanding treatment to a greater number of individuals as well as working toward a cure. This review discusses the role of genetics in our understanding of CF with a particular emphasis on how genetics informs the exciting landscape of current and novel CF therapies.

Update on Innate and Adaptive Immunity in Cystic Fibrosis 603

Emanuela M. Bruscia and Tracey L. Bonfield

Cystic fibrosis (CF) pathophysiology is hallmarked by excessive inflammation and the inability to resolve lung infections, contributing to morbidity and eventually mortality. Paradoxically, despite a robust inflammatory response, CF lungs fail to clear bacteria and are susceptible to chronic infections. Impaired mucociliary transport plays a critical role in chronic infection but the immune mechanisms contributing to the adaptation of bacteria to the lung microenvironment is not clear. CFTR modulator therapy has advanced CF life expectancy opening up the need to understand changes in immunity as CF patients age. Here, we have summarized the current understanding of immune dysregulation in CF.

Novel Applications of Biomarkers and Personalized Medicine in Cystic Fibrosis 617

Jennifer S. Guimbellot, David P. Nichols, and John J. Brewington

As routine care in cystic fibrosis (CF) becomes increasingly personalized, new opportunities to further focus care on the individual have emerged. These opportunities are increasingly filled through research in tools aiding drug selection, drug monitoring and titration, disease-relevant biomarkers, and evaluation of therapeutic benefits. Herein, we will discuss such research tools presently being translated into the clinic to improve the personalization of care in CF.

As we characterize the clinical benefits of highly effective modulator therapy (HEMT) in the cystic fibrosis (CF) population, our paradigm for treating and monitoring disease continues to evolve. More sensitive approaches are necessary to detect early disease and clinical progression. This article reviews evolving strategies to assess disease control and progression in the HEMT era. This article also explores developments in pulmonary function monitoring, advanced respiratory imaging, tools for the collection of patient-reported outcomes, and their application to profile individual responses, guide therapeutic decisions, and improve the quality of life of people with CF.

Highly effective cystic fibrosis (CF) transmembrane conductance regulator (CFTR) modulator therapy (HEMT) corrects the underlying molecular defect causing CF disease. HEMT decreases symptom burden and improves clinical metrics and quality of life for most people with CF (PwCF) and eligible cftr mutations. Improvements in measures of pulmonary health suggest that restoration of function of defective CFTR anion channels by HEMT not only enhances airway mucociliary clearance, but also reduces chronic pulmonary infection and inflammation. This article reviews the evidence for how HEMT influences the dynamic and interdependent processes of infection and inflammation in the CF airway, and what questions remain unanswered.

Patients with cystic fibrosis (CF) often develop respiratory tract infections with pathogenic multidrug-resistant organisms (MDROs) such as methicillin-resistant Staphylococcus aureus, and a variety of gram-negative organisms that include Pseudomonas aeruginosa, Burkholderia sp., Stenotrophomonas maltophilia, Achromobacter xylosoxidans, and nontuberculous mycobacteria (NTM). Despite the introduction of new therapies to address underlying cystic fibrosis transmembrane conductance regulator (CFTR) dysfunction, MDRO infections remain a problem and novel antimicrobial interventions are still needed. Therapeutic approaches include improving the efficacy of existing drugs by adjusting the dose based on differences in CF patient pharmacokinetics/pharmacodynamics, the development of inhaled formulations to reduce systemic adverse events, and the use of newer beta-lactam/beta-lactamase combinations. Alternative innovative therapeutic approaches include the use of gallium and bacteriophages to treat MDRO pulmonary infections including those with extreme antibiotic resistance. However, additional clinical trials are required to determine the optimal dosing and efficacy of these different strategies and to identify patients with CF most likely to benefit from these new treatment options.

Based on the cystic fibrosis transmembrane conductance regulator (CFTR) genotype, approximately 90% of people with cystic fibrosis (CF) are candidates for highly effective modulator therapy (HEMT). Clinical trials conducted over the last 11 years have shown that these oral therapies substantially restore CFTR function, leading to improvements in lung function, nutritional status, and health-related quality of life.

Here, we review safety and efficacy data from phase 3 clinical trials and observational studies which support the use of HEMT in most adults and children with CF. We also discuss opportunities for additional investigation in groups underrepresented or excluded from phase 3 clinical trials, and challenges in the evaluation of the safety and efficacy of HEMT at increasingly earlier stages of CFTR-mediated pathophysiology.

Nontuberculous mycobacteria (NTM) are important pathogens, with a longitudinal prevalence of up to 20% within the cystic fibrosis (CF) population. Diagnosis of NTM pulmonary disease in people with CF (pwCF) is challenging, as a majority have NTM infection that is transient or indolent, without evidence of clinical consequence. In addition, the radiographic and clinical manifestations of chronic coinfections with typical CF pathogens can overlap those of NTM, making diagnosis difficult. Comprehensive care of pwCF must be optimized to assess the true clinical impact of NTM and to improve response to treatment. Treatment requires prolonged, multidrug therapy that varies depending on NTM species, resistance pattern, and extent of disease. With a widespread use of highly effective modulator therapy (HEMT), clinical signs and symptoms of NTM disease may be less apparent, and sensitivity of sputum cultures further reduced. The development of a disease-specific approach to the diagnosis and treatment of NTM infection in pwCF is a research priority, as a lifelong strategy is needed for this high-risk population.

Cystic fibrosis transmembrane conductance regulator (CFTR) modulator therapy brings hope to most patients with cystic fibrosis (CF), but not all. For approximately 12% of CF patients with premature termination codon mutations, large deletions, insertions, and frameshifts, the CFTR modulator therapy is not effective. Many believe that genetic-based therapies such as RNA therapies, DNA therapies, and gene editing technologies will be needed to treat mutations that are not responsive to modulator therapy. Delivery of these therapeutic agents to affected cells is the major challenge that will need to be overcome if we are to harness the power of these emerging therapies for the treatment of CF.

Attainment and maintenance of good nutrition has been an important aspect of management in cystic fibrosis (CF) for decades. In the era of highly effective modulator therapy for CF, the quality of the nutrients we recommend is increasingly important. Our therapy must support our patients' health for many years beyond what we previously thought. Preventing cardiovascular disease, reducing hyperlipidemia, and optimizing lean body mass for active, longer lives now join the long-standing goal of promoting lung function through nutrition. This chapter summarizes recent developments in nutrition in people with CF, with an eye to the evolution of our practice.

Clinical complications of cystic fibrosis (CF) include a variety of gastrointestinal (GI) and hepatobiliary manifestations. Recent years have witnessed several advances in the understanding and management of these complications, in addition to opportunities for therapeutic innovations. Herein we review the current understanding of these disorders and also discuss the management of the GI and hepatobiliary complications experienced by persons with CF.

The development of formal transition models emerged to reduce variability in care, including cystic fibrosis (CF) responsibility, independence, self-care, and education (RISE), which provides a standardized transition program, including knowledge assessments, self-management checklists, and milestones for people with CF. Despite these interventions, the current landscape of health care transition (HCT) remains suboptimal, and additional focused attention on HCT is necessary. Standardization of assessment tools to gauge the efficacy of transfer from pediatric to adult care is a high priority. Such tools should incorporate both clinical and patient-centered outcomes to provide a comprehensive picture of progress and deficiencies of the HCT process.

Endocrine comorbidities have become increasingly important medical considerations as improving cystic fibrosis (CF) care increases life expectancy. Although the underlying pathophysiology of CF-related diabetes remains elusive, the use of novel technologies and therapeutics seeks to improve both CF-related outcomes and quality of life. Improvements in the overall health of those with CF have tempered concerns about pubertal delay and short stature; however, other comorbidities such as hypogonadism and bone disease are increasingly recognized. Following the introduction of highly effective modulator therapies there are many lessons to be learned about their long-term impact on endocrine comorbidities.

This article is intended for use among all cystic fibrosis care team members. It covers common mental health concerns and their unique presentations in persons with cystic fibrosis (pwCF) in areas such as depression, anxiety, trauma, behavioral disorders emerging in childhood, sleep, problematic eating patterns, and the impact of substance use. Furthermore, the authors address ways to manage these mental health symptoms through risk assessment, psychological interventions, and/or psychotropic medications. Quick reference tables are provided for evidence-based psychological interventions and medications often used for mental health conditions in pwCF.

Family planning in cystic fibrosis (CF) is an increasingly important aspect of care, as improvements in care and outcomes lead to a rise in the number of pregnancies and parenthood in people with CF. This article highlights: (1) Health considerations for people with CF related to pregnancy, contraception, and parenthood. (2) Facets of reproductive planning, fertility, and preconception counseling. (3) Relationship-centered reproductive health discussions.

Lung transplantation provides a treatment option for many individuals with advanced lung disease due to cystic fibrosis (CF). Since the first transplants for CF in the 1980s, survival has improved and the opportunity for transplant has expanded to include individuals who previously were not considered candidates for transplant. Criteria to be a transplant candidate vary significantly among transplant programs, highlighting that the engagement in more than one transplant program may be necessary. Individuals with highly resistant CF pathogens, malnutrition, osteoporosis, CF liver disease, and other comorbidities may be suitable candidates for lung transplant, or if needed, multi-organ transplant. The transplant process involves several phases, from discussion of prognosis and referral to a transplant center, to transplant evaluation, to listing, transplant surgery, and care after transplant. While the availability of highly effective CF transmembrane conductance regulator (CFTR) modulators for many individuals with CF has improved lung function and slowed progression to respiratory failure, early discussion regarding transplant as a treatment option and referral to a transplant program are critical to maximizing opportunity and optimizing patient and family experience. The decision to be evaluated for transplant and to list for transplant are distinct, and early referral may provide a treatment option that can be urgently executed if needed. Survival after transplant for CF is improving, to a median survival of approximately 10 years, and most transplant survivors enjoy significant improvement in quality of life.

CLINICS IN CHEST MEDICINE

SERIES OF RELATED INTEREST

Critical Care Clinics
Available at: https://www.criticalcare.theclinics.com/

THE CLINICS ARE AVAILABLE ONLINE!
Access your subscription at:
www.theclinics.com

Preface

Cystic Fibrosis in the Era of Highly Effective CFTR Modulators

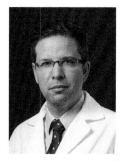
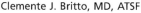
Clemente J. Britto, MD, ATSF

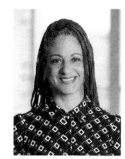
Jennifer L. Taylor-Cousar, MD, MSCS, ATSF

Editors

Cystic fibrosis (CF) was described as a clinical entity more than eighty years ago.[1–3] With the development of comprehensive care centers and therapies directed at the signs and symptoms of the disease, survival improved.[4] What once was a disease only of children has become a chronic disease of adults for whom the median predicted survival is fifty years of age.[5,6] As the natural history of CF has evolved, so has the recognition of previously underdiagnosed populations of people with CF, contributing to its rising prevalence around the world.[7–10]

We are in the midst of a new era in CF care ushered in by the advent of cystic fibrosis transmembrane conductance regulator (CFTR) modulators, small molecules that significantly restore CFTR protein function. People with CF are experiencing marked rapid and sustained improvements in lung function, nutritional state, and quality of life.[11–13] With the approval of the first triple-modulator combination, elexacaftor/tezacaftor/ivacaftor, for people with CF with at least one copy of the most common CF mutations in those of European ancestry, *Phe508del* (*F508del*), approximately 90% of the CF population is now eligible for highly effective modulator therapy

(HEMT) and its associated transformational health benefits.[13]

Since the previous CF-focused issue of *Clinics in Chest Medicine*,[14] there have been broad advances in our understanding of the immunopathogenesis of CF and the remarkable impact of modulators on immune cell function, inflammation, and repair mechanisms.[15–17] Indeed, the CFTR correction afforded by HEMT is increasingly recognized as a modifying factor in the microbiome and airway inflammatory response of people with CF.[18–22]

Advances have also emerged in animal models, cell-based assays, and approaches to measure and titrate functional responses to modulators in human tissues and cells.[23–26] Emerging tools, such as novel pulmonary function measures, pulmonary imaging, patient-reported outcomes, and new molecular biomarkers, will become increasingly important in understanding CF pathogenesis and treatment response.[27–34]

Apart from the well-documented impact of HEMT on lung function and nutritional outcomes, HEMT promises to have extensive effects in multiple areas of clinical care. Emerging reports of effects range from changes in airway microbial

Clin Chest Med 43 (2022) xiii–xvi
https://doi.org/10.1016/j.ccm.2022.07.003
0272-5231/22/© 2022 Published by Elsevier Inc.

communities with associated opportunities for developing novel antimicrobial therapies, evolving knowledge regarding the surveillance and management of long-term endocrine and gastrointestinal complications, and new opportunities in family planning and reproductive health.[35–41]

HEMT has had a transformative effect on the lives of many people with CF. However, some questions remain to be answered. For example, there are ongoing efforts to develop safe and effective readthrough agents and the next generation of modulators and immunomodulatory drugs for those ineligible for or intolerant of currently approved HEMT. Ultimately, gene replacement or editing will be necessary to cure CF.[42–47] We speculate that one day we will be able to turn back the clock on the development of clinical disease through very early intervention; such intervention is currently being investigated in animal models of CF and in trials of HEMT administration in infants and toddlers.[48,49] Finally, although we anticipate that recent advances will result in a smaller proportion of people with CF requiring lung transplantation or end-of-life care,[50] the CF community remains committed to optimizing care for each individual with CF.

In this issue of *Clinics in Chest Medicine*, we take stock of the gains enabled by the development of HEMT and consider the remaining challenges to assessing and improving the quantity and quality of life for all people with CF. As the clinical course and management of CF evolve in this new therapeutic era, we look forward to a promising and bright future in which CF-related morbidity is rare, health is maintained, and CF finally becomes a curable disease.

Clemente J. Britto, MD, ATSF
Department of Internal Medicine
Division of Pulmonary, Critical Care
and Sleep Medicine
Yale University School of Medicine
300 Cedar Street, TAC-S419
New Haven, CT 06520, USA

Jennifer L. Taylor-Cousar, MD, MSCS, ATSF
Departments of Medicine and Pediatrics
Divisions of Pulmonary Sciences and
Critical Care Medicine and Pediatric Pulmonology
University of Colorado
Anschutz Medical Campus
1400 Jackson Street, J318
Denver, CO 80206, USA

E-mail addresses:
clemente.britto@yale.edu (C.J. Britto)
taylorcousarj@njhealth.org (J.L. Taylor-Cousar)

REFERENCES

1. Riordan JR, Rommens JM, Kerem B, et al. Identification of the cystic fibrosis gene: cloning and characterization of complementary DNA. Science 1989; 245(4922):1066–73.

2. Davis PB. Cystic fibrosis since 1938. Am J Respir Crit Care Med 2006;173(5):475–82.

3. Andersen DH. Cystic fibrosis of the pancreas and its relation to celiac disease: a clinical and pathologic study. Am J Dis Child 1938;56(2):344–99.

4. Patient Registry. Cystic Fibrosis Foundation. Available at: https://www.cff.org/medical-professionals/patient-registry. Accessed March 29, 2022.

5. McKone EF, Ariti C, Jackson A, et al. Survival estimates in European cystic fibrosis patients and the impact of socioeconomic factors: a retrospective registry cohort study. Eur Respir J 2021;58(3). https://doi.org/10.1183/13993003.02288-2020.

6. Stephenson AL, Sykes J, Stanojevic S, et al. Survival Comparison of Patients With Cystic Fibrosis in Canada and the United States: A Population-Based Cohort Study. Ann Intern Med 2017;166(8): 537–46.

7. Hamosh A, FitzSimmons SC, Macek M Jr, et al. Comparison of the clinical manifestations of cystic fibrosis in black and white patients. J Pediatr 1998; 132(2):255–9.

8. Powers CA, Potter EM, Wessel HU, et al. Cystic fibrosis in Asian Indians. Arch Pediatr Adolesc Med 1996;150(5):554–5.

9. Yamashiro Y, Shimizu T, Oguchi S, et al. The estimated incidence of cystic fibrosis in Japan. J Pediatr Gastroenterol Nutr 1997;24(5):544–7.

10. Stafler P, Mei-Zahav M, Wilschanski M, et al. The impact of a national population carrier screening program on cystic fibrosis birth rate and age at diagnosis: Implications for newborn screening. J Cyst Fibros 2016;15(4):460–6.

11. Ramsey BW, Davies J, McElvaney NG, et al. A CFTR potentiator in patients with cystic fibrosis and the G551D mutation. N Engl J Med 2011;365(18): 1663–72.

12. Taylor-Cousar JL, Munck A, McKone EF, et al. Tezacaftor–Ivacaftor in Patients with Cystic Fibrosis Homozygous for Phe508del. N Engl J Med 2017; 377(21):2013–23.

13. Middleton PG, Mall MA, Dřevínek P, et al. Elexacaftor–Tezacaftor–Ivacaftor for Cystic Fibrosis with a Single Phe508del Allele. N Engl J Med 2019; 381(19):1809–19.

14. Koff J. Cystic Fibrosis, an Issue of Clinics in chest medicine. Elsevier Health Sciences; 2016.

15. Gillan JL, Davidson DJ, Gray RD. Targeting cystic fibrosis inflammation in the age of CFTR modulators: focus on macrophages. Eur Respir J 2021;57(6). https://doi.org/10.1183/13993003.03502-2020.

16. Hisert KB, Birkland TP, Schoenfelt KQ, et al. Ivacaftor decreases monocyte sensitivity to interferon-γ in people with cystic fibrosis. ERJ Open Res 2020;6(2). https://doi.org/10.1183/23120541.00318-2019.

17. Jarosz-Griffiths HH, Scambler T, Wong CH, et al. Different CFTR modulator combinations downregulate inflammation differently in cystic fibrosis. Elife 2020;9. https://doi.org/10.7554/eLife.54556.

18. Harris JK, Wagner BD, Zemanick ET, et al. Changes in Airway Microbiome and Inflammation with Ivacaftor Treatment in Patients with Cystic Fibrosis and the G551D Mutation. Ann Am Thorac Soc 2020;17(2):212–20.

19. Grasemann H, Gonska T, Avolio J, et al. Effect of ivacaftor therapy on exhaled nitric oxide in patients with cystic fibrosis. J Cyst Fibros 2015;14(6):727–32.

20. Green M, Lindgren N, Henderson A, et al. Ivacaftor partially corrects airway inflammation in a humanized G551D rat. Am J Physiol Lung Cell Mol Physiol 2021;320(6):L1093–100.

21. Barnaby R, Koeppen K, Nymon A, et al. Lumacaftor (VX-809) restores the ability of CF macrophages to phagocytose and kill Pseudomonas aeruginosa. Am J Physiol Lung Cell Mol Physiol 2018;314(3):L432–8.

22. Ruffin M, Roussel L, Maillé É, et al. Vx-809/Vx-770 treatment reduces inflammatory response to Pseudomonas aeruginosa in primary differentiated cystic fibrosis bronchial epithelial cells. Am J Physiol Lung Cell Mol Physiol 2018;314(4):L635–41.

23. Clancy JP, Cotton CU, Donaldson SH, et al. CFTR modulator theratyping: Current status, gaps and future directions. J Cyst Fibros 2019;18(1):22–34.

24. Pedemonte N, Zegarra-Moran O, Galietta LJV. High-throughput screening of libraries of compounds to identify CFTR modulators. Methods Mol Biol 2011;741:13–21.

25. Sui J, Cotard S, Andersen J, et al. Optimization of a Yellow fluorescent protein-based iodide influx high-throughput screening assay for cystic fibrosis transmembrane conductance regulator (CFTR) modulators. Assay Drug Dev Technol 2010;8(6):656–68.

26. Liang F, Shang H, Jordan NJ, et al. High-Throughput Screening for Readthrough Modulators of CFTR PTC Mutations. SLAS Technol 2017;22(3):315–24.

27. Horsley AR, Belcher J, Bayfield K, et al. Longitudinal assessment of lung clearance index to monitor disease progression in children and adults with cystic fibrosis. Thorax 2021. https://doi.org/10.1136/thoraxjnl-2021-216928.

28. Smith L, Aldag I, Hughes P, et al. Longitudinal monitoring of disease progression in children with mild CF using hyperpolarised gas MRI and LCI. Eur Respir J 2016;48(suppl 60). https://doi.org/10.1183/13993003.congress-2016.OA284.

29. Szczesniak R, Turkovic L, Andrinopoulou ER, et al. Chest imaging in cystic fibrosis studies: What counts, and can be counted? J Cyst Fibros 2017;16(2):175–85.

30. Dournes G, Walkup LL, Benlala I, et al. The Clinical Use of Lung MRI in Cystic Fibrosis: What, Now, How? Chest 2021;159(6):2205–17.

31. Beswick DM, Humphries SM, Balkissoon CD, et al. Impact of CFTR Therapy on Chronic Rhinosinusitis and Health Status: Deep Learning CT Analysis and Patient Reported Outcomes. Ann Am Thorac Soc 2021. https://doi.org/10.1513/AnnalsATS.202101-057OC.

32. Sathe M, Moshiree B, Vu PT, et al. Utilization of electronic patient-reported outcome measures in cystic fibrosis research: Application to the GALAXY study. J Cyst Fibros 2021;20(4):605–11.

33. Ishak A, Stick SM, Turkovic L, et al. BAL Inflammatory Markers Can Predict Pulmonary Exacerbations in Children With Cystic Fibrosis. Chest 2020;158(6):2314–22.

34. Khanal S, Webster M, Niu N, et al. SPLUNC1: a novel marker of cystic fibrosis exacerbations. Eur Respir J 2021. https://doi.org/10.1183/13993003.00507-2020.

35. Payne JE, Dubois AV, Ingram RJ, et al. Activity of innate antimicrobial peptides and ivacaftor against clinical cystic fibrosis respiratory pathogens. Int J Antimicrob Agents 2017;50(3):427–35.

36. Volkova N, Moy K, Evans J, et al. Disease progression in patients with cystic fibrosis treated with ivacaftor: Data from national US and UK registries. J Cyst Fibros 2020;19(1):68–79.

37. Shteinberg M, Taylor-Cousar JL, Durieu I, et al. Fertility and Pregnancy in Cystic Fibrosis. Chest 2021. https://doi.org/10.1016/j.chest.2021.07.024.

38. Freeman AJ, Sathe M, Aliaj E, et al. Designing the GALAXY study: Partnering with the cystic fibrosis community to optimize assessment of gastrointestinal symptoms. J Cyst Fibros 2021;20(4):598–604.

39. Smith S, Rowbotham NJ, Regan KH. Inhaled antipseudomonal antibiotics for long-term therapy in cystic fibrosis. Cochrane Database Syst Rev 2018;3(3):CD001021.

40. Abdalla MY, Switzer BL, Goss CH, et al. Gallium Compounds Exhibit Potential as New Therapeutic Agents against Mycobacterium abscessus. Antimicrob Agents Chemother 2015;59(8):4826–34.

41. Chan BK, Stanley G, Modak M, et al. Bacteriophage therapy for infections in CF. Pediatr Pulmonol 2021;56(Suppl 1):S4–9.

42. Christopher Boyd A, Guo S, Huang L, et al. New approaches to genetic therapies for cystic fibrosis. J Cyst Fibros 2020;19:S54–9.

43. Pranke I, Golec A, Hinzpeter A, et al. Emerging Therapeutic Approaches for Cystic Fibrosis. From Gene Editing to Personalized Medicine. Front Pharmacol 2019;10:121.

44. Lueck JD, Yoon JS, Perales-Puchalt A, et al. Engineered transfer RNAs for suppression of premature termination codons. Nat Commun 2019; 10(1):822.

45. Crane AM, Kramer P, Bui JH, et al. Targeted correction and restored function of the CFTR gene in cystic fibrosis induced pluripotent stem cells. Stem Cell Rep 2015;4(4):569–77.

46. Xia E, Zhang Y, Cao H, et al. TALEN-Mediated Gene Targeting for Cystic Fibrosis-Gene Therapy. Genes 2019;10(1). https://doi.org/10.3390/genes10010039.

47. King NE, Suzuki S, Barillà C, et al. Correction of Airway Stem Cells: Genome Editing Approaches for the Treatment of Cystic Fibrosis. Hum Gene Ther 2020;31(17–18):956–72.

48. Egan ME. Cystic fibrosis transmembrane conductance receptor modulator therapy in cystic fibrosis, an update. Curr Opin Pediatr 2020;32(3):384–8.

49. Guimbellot JS, Taylor-Cousar JL. Combination CFTR modulator therapy in children and adults with cystic fibrosis. The Lancet Respir Med 2021;9(7):677–9.

50. Lehr CJ, Pilewski JM. Cystic fibrosis: candidate selection and impact of the cystic fibrosis transmembrane conductance regulator therapy. Curr Opin Organ Transpl 2022. https://doi.org/10.1097/MOT.0000000000000975.

Toward a Broader Understanding of Cystic Fibrosis Epidemiology and Its Impact on Clinical Manifestations

Kimberly A. McBennett, MD, PhD[a], Pamela B. Davis, MD, PhD[b],*

KEYWORDS

- Cystic fibrosis • Cystic fibrosis epidemiology • Cystic fibrosis incidence • Cystic • Fibrosis survival

KEY POINTS

- Although the incidence of cystic fibrosis in North America and Western Europe remains steady at about 1 in 3500 live births, prevalence is increasing due to early diagnosis by newborn screening and longer patient survival, with the median survival age now predicted to be about 50 years.
- There is increasing recognition of cystic fibrosis in countries and ethnic groups in which previously it had been thought to be rare.
- Survival of patients with cystic fibrosis, as well as quality of life, has improved because of comprehensive care in centers, aggressive application of and improvements in symptomatic therapy, earlier diagnosis due to newborn screening allowing earlier institution of therapy, and the development of small molecule therapeutics aimed directly at the basic defect in the cystic fibrosis transmembrane conductance regulator.
- Survival of patients with cystic fibrosis in the United States lags in racial and ethnic minorities and in those of lower socioeconomic status despite comparable access to center care and comparable prescription of drugs.
- The population of patients with cystic fibrosis has shifted more to the adult age range, and the spectrum of complications has changed, with less nutritional deficiency and more complications of aging.

INTRODUCTION

Cystic fibrosis (CF) arises from the mutation of a single gene encoding the cystic fibrosis transmembrane conductance regulator (CFTR),[1] a chloride channel that is widely distributed on epithelial surfaces. Epithelia in the airway, paranasal sinuses, pancreas, gut, biliary tree, vas deferens, and sweat ducts express CFTR. Dysfunction of this protein leads to lung infection and bronchiectasis, pancreatic insufficiency with malabsorption, episodic intestinal obstruction, liver disease, and male infertility.[2] Failure of CFTR-mediated chloride transport in the sweat ducts leads to a markedly elevated concentration of chloride in sweat, which is the basis for the definitive diagnostic test for CF.[3]

When the disease was initially described in 1938, children with CF were severely

[a] Medicine and Pediatrics, Case Western Reserve University School of Medicine, LeRoy W. Matthews Cystic Fibrosis Center, University Hospitals Rainbow Babies & Children's, 11100 Euclid Avenue, RBC 3001, Cleveland, OH 44106, USA; [b] Center for Community Health Integration, Case Western Reserve University School of Medicine, 10900 Euclid Avenue, Suite T-402, Cleveland, OH 44106-4922, USA
* Corresponding author.
E-mail address: pbd@case.edu

Clin Chest Med 43 (2022) 579–590
https://doi.org/10.1016/j.ccm.2022.06.002
0272-5231/22/© 2022 Elsevier Inc. All rights reserved.

malnourished and died of malnutrition or pneumonia by the age of 2 years.[2] Since that time, vast improvements have been made in both scientific understanding of the underlying defect, and the clinical care of those living with the disease. Advances in the treatment of the symptoms of CF, followed by the discovery of the gene coding for CFTR, and ultimately the development of small molecule therapy directed at correction of CFTR defects, have revolutionized how the disease is identified and treated. Currently, the predicted median survival age (the predicted age to which 50% of the infants born this year will survive) for children with CF born in developed countries is about 50 years (**Table 1**,[4–20] **Fig. 1**). This article will describe the changing demographics and epidemiology of CF and the scientific discoveries and the changes in care that produced them.

DIAGNOSIS

The epidemiology and incidence of CF depend upon clear diagnostic criteria. Diagnosis rests upon the clinical manifestations, genetic testing, and the sweat test, which is a simple measure of CFTR function. The key observations of Paul Di Sant'Agnese[21] that infants with CF had extraordinary salt losses in their sweat during a New York heat wave led ultimately to the diagnostic "sweat test." Sweat is stimulated in a circumscribed area by iontophoresis of pilocarpine into the skin, and the sweat is collected for measurement of chloride concentration. This test remains the gold standard for demonstrating CFTR dysfunction and making the diagnosis of CF, however, It is important to note that those with residual CFTR function (eg, adults with Class III-VI mutations) may have nondiagnostic sweat chloride values, making CF diagnosis confirmation challenging.

In areas in which CF is prevalent, most diagnoses today are made from newborn screening. Screening was instituted because the outcome is improved by early treatment, and there are inexpensive methods of detection on a small blood spot. Usually, initial screening tests for immunoreactive trypsin (IRT). An elevated value prompts screening for 23 to 40 known CF mutations.[22] A child with an elevated IRT and 1 or 2 CFTR mutations is referred to a CF center for sweat testing. A double-blind study in Wisconsin showed that infants diagnosed by screening had superior height and weight 13 years later compared with those diagnosed based on symptoms.[23] Some other studies, but not all, also demonstrated improved pulmonary function in the screened group.[23,24]

Today, although the specific testing strategy varies, all 50 of the United States, 22 countries in Europe, Russia, Australia, New Zealand, Canada, and several South American countries offer newborn screening for CF.[6] To address the diagnostic dilemmas that arose in screening, the Cystic Fibrosis Foundation convened an international committee of experts, which published consensus guidelines on the diagnosis of CF in 2017.[25] The diagnosis of CF is based on a sweat chloride concentration $\geq$60 mEq/L in the setting of a positive newborn screen, a positive family history, compatible symptoms, or 2 known disease-causing mutations. Individuals with sweat chloride concentration of less than 30 mEq/L usually will not have CF unless certain rare genotypes are present, such as c.3717 + 12191C > T (legacy: 3849 + 10 kb C- > T). For those with intermediate sweat chloride concentration, CFTR physiologic testing such as nasal or intestinal potential difference measurements may clarify the function of CFTR. Babies with a positive newborn screen but less than 2 identified disease-causing mutations in CFTR may receive a diagnosis of cystic fibrosis related metabolic syndrome (CRMS) or the European term, cystic fibrosis screen positive, inconclusive diagnosis (CFSPID).[25] Sometimes, when decreased CFTR function is not severe enough to meet diagnostic criteria at birth, it may worsen over time, so a child with CRMS may be diagnosed with CF as they age. Persons with symptoms related to CF who may have a CF mutation (often heterozygotes) but do not meet criteria for CF or CRMS may be labeled as CFTR related disorder (CFRD). In 2019 in the US CF Data Registry, of 970 diagnoses, 12.1% were CRMS and 8.9% were of CFRD, so these designations are not rare.[8] This consensus on nomenclature will affect determination of the incidence of CF.

INCIDENCE

The incidence and prevalence of CF vary widely throughout the world (see **Table 1**). The reliability of the estimates of incidence also are variable. As CF is among the most common serious genetic diseases in Caucasians and its course can be modified by treatment, many areas of Europe, North America, and Australia provide newborn screening programs and collect registry data, which have improved the accuracy of these estimates. On the other hand, where CF has been thought to be less common, mechanisms of data collection are less robust. In Europe, North America, and Australia, the overall incidence is about 1 in 3500 live births, with considerable national variation.[5] Within the United States, various diverse ethnic groups vary widely in incidence. In the Middle East, also with a very diverse population,

Table 1
Incidence of CF around the world

Country/region	Incidence	Reference	Median Predicted Survival Age	Reference
Ireland	1/1353	4	45.7	18
Europe	1/3500	5	51.7	19
Russia	1/10,000	6		
Canada	1/3300	7	50.9	20
United States	1/4000	8	48.4	8
Black Americans	1/15,000	9		
Asian Americans	1/35,000	10		
Native Americans	1/10,900	9		
Ohio Amish	1/569	11		
Jordan	1/2560	12		
Israel	1/16,000	13		
Argentina	1/6100	6		
Costa Rica	1/1500	6		
India	1/10,000–1/100,000	14–16		
Japan	1/350,000	17		

estimates range from 1/2560 in Jordan[12] to 1/16,000 in Israel.[13] In areas where CF is thought to be less common, such as Central and South America, more comprehensive data collection will be required for more accurate estimates. In India, estimates of incidence vary widely.[14–16] The disease is rare in Japan.[17] Few data are available in African populations.

The observed incidence of CF in a given region may change over time due to institution of newborn screening, improved data collection and registry information, or implementation of heterozygote screening programs. In the United States, for example, Hale and colleagues[26] reported a significant decrease in the number of CF diagnoses in Massachusetts following the publication of the US

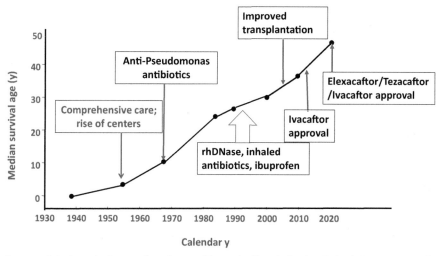

Fig. 1. Median predicted survival age of patients with cystic fibrosis in the United States. Data after 1980 are taken from the US CF Data Registry. Earlier data are estimates taken from the literature. Arrows indicate clinically relevant advances that affect survival in CF. (*Adapted from* Davis PB. Cystic fibrosis since 1938. Am J Respir Crit Care Med. 2006 Mar 1;173(5):475 to 82. Copyright © 2021 American Thoracic Society. All rights reserved. The American Journal of Respiratory and Critical Care Medicine is an official journal of the American Thoracic Society. Readers are encouraged to read the entire article for the correct context at https://doi.org/10.1164/rccm.200505-840OE. The authors, editors, and The American Thoracic Society are not responsible for errors or omissions in adaptations.)

recommendations for population carrier screening in 2003, but in Colorado, there was no decline in incidence from 1983 to 2006,[27] nor in Wisconsin, from 1994 to 2011.[28] In Italy[29] and Israel,[13] decreased incidence aligns temporally with population screening. On the other hand, it has been suggested that the identified population with CF is increasing in South America, Africa, Turkey, the Middle East, and Asia,[30] likely due to better identification in newborn screening programs, migration, and intermarriage.

PREVALENCE

In 2019, 31,199 patients diagnosed with CF (not CFMS or CFRD) who were seen in a center in that calendar year and who consented to contribute their data were included in the US CF Foundation's Data Registry.[8] Of these, 56% are over the age of 18 years. Over the last 30 years, the number of children with CF has remained stable, but the number of adults has increased because of longer survival and increased awareness and diagnostic screening in previously underappreciated segments of the CF population (ie, older age groups, people with single-organ manifestations, underrepresented minorities, etc., **Table 2**)[8,31,32] The prevalence of CF depends on the incidence of CF at birth, patient ascertainment, and patient survival. Although the birth of children with CF can be prevented by heterozygote identification, prenatal testing combined with the willingness to terminate the pregnancy, and in vitro fertilization with embryo selection can be chosen, these measures are not extensively used in the United States, and initial incidence remains stable. With a stable incidence, the overall prevalence of CF is increasing (see **Table 2**) because newborn screening identifies most affected children early in life and the survival of patients with CF has been markedly extended. The adult population with CF is growing, and that improvement is expected to continue, so prevalence may continue to increase.

VARIABILITY IN PHENOTYPE

More than 2000 disease-causing mutations have been identified in the CF gene. Patients who harbor 2 "severe" mutations with very little CFTR activity usually manifest pancreatic insufficiency, CF sinus and lung disease (eg, airflow obstruction, bronchiectasis, recurrent infections), elevated sweat chloride concentration, congenital bilateral absence of the vas deferens in males, and sometimes liver disease and intestinal obstruction. Individuals with at least 1 "mild" allele, with some residual CFTR function, may retain some pancreatic function but be subject to recurrent bouts of pancreatitis, and have statistically significantly lower, but still abnormal, sweat chloride concentration.[33] A third group may include others with 2 mild CF-causing mutations, who may experience minimal, if any, symptoms at all until later in life. Clinical manifestations of CF and their severity vary from patient to patient, even for individuals with identical mutations in the CFTR gene. The phenotype depends not only on the CFTR mutations but also on the environment in which the patient is born and develops, and the presence of other genes that may modulate the impact of the CFTR mutation, either exacerbating or mitigating its effect. Modifier genes may be organ specific, so that a gene variant that exacerbates disease in one organ may have little impact on another. Strategies to identify potential genetic modifiers include candidate gene investigations, twin studies (monozygotic vs dizygotic), family studies, and genome-wide association studies, which vary in their power and sensitivity.

About 50% to 80% of the variation in lung disease appears to be accounted for by modifier genes, but the specific mechanism by which they exert their influence is often unclear.[34,35] Therapy adherence, socioeconomic factors, and environmental influences, such as exposure to cigarette smoke or air pollution, also influence severity of lung disease. Variants of genes apart from CFTR that modify the course of the disease may help explain gender, racial, or ethnic variations in the disease. Moreover, determining their mechanism of action may suggest useful therapeutic interventions.

SURVIVAL
Improved Symptomatic Treatment

Centers for the care of patients with CF were founded in the mid-1950s. They emphasized comprehensive, vigorous symptomatic care as well as the associated basic and clinical research. The Cystic Fibrosis Foundation created a national data registry and supported research relevant to clinical care. This infrastructure advanced symptomatic care and permitted development of clinical care guidelines that were widely disseminated. Vigorous airway clearance was a cornerstone of therapy. The techniques advanced from manual postural drainage to include the percussion vest and devices that use both air and sound to mobilize secretions. To liquefy secretions, patients inhaled recombinant human DNase to lyse the DNA from neutrophils, which contributed to the adherent secretions, or hypertonic saline to induce water secretion. Improved pancreatic enzyme supplements led

Table 2
Demographics reported in the United States Cystic Fibrosis Foundation patient registry

	1999[a]	2009[c]	2019[c]
Number with CF (n)	20,679	26,112	31,199
New diagnoses in calendar year(n)	896	1148	766
Detected by Newborn Screen (%)	7.1	50.7	62.4
Adults >18 y (% of total)	37.9	47.2	56.0
Race/Ethnicity (% of total)			
White (Caucasian)	95.5	94.6	93.4
African American	3.7	4.3	4.7
Other	Not reported	2.6	3.8
Hispanic (black or white)	5.3	6.9	9.4
Median Predicted Survival (years)	29.1	37.9	46.2
Median Age at Death (years)	23	26.3	32.4
Number of pregnancies (n)	137[c]	230	310
Lung transplant per year (n)	114	207[b]	241

[a] Cystic Fibrosis Foundation Patient Registry Annual Data Report, 1999, except as noted.
[b] Cystic Fibrosis Foundation Patient Registry Annual Data Report, 2009.
[c] Cystic Fibrosis Foundation Patient Registry Annual Data Report, 2019, including updates for prior years

to aggressive nutritional repletion with high fat, high calorie diets along with supplemental fat-soluble vitamins. Antistaphylococcal and antipseudomonal therapy had profound effects, and new drug development usually kept up with the acquisition of resistance by the chronic bacterial flora. Intravenous antibiotics to treat pulmonary exacerbations protected the lung against infection-related damage and inflammation, and soon inhaled antibiotics were given regularly to reduce the bacterial load. Infection provoked inflammation, and it became clear that the inflammatory response in CF is excessive. High-dose ibuprofen slowed the rate of decline of lung function and improved life expectancy[36,37] if administered in childhood. Later, chronic azithromycin was administered, in part for its anti-inflammatory effect.[38] New therapies were introduced after clear evidence of benefit, clinical guidelines were drawn up and issued, and the results of therapeutic recommendations were followed in the CF Data Registry. Survival improved dramatically, even with no knowledge of the basic defect. Newborn screening allowed therapy to be instituted earlier with better results. Respiratory failure remains the leading cause of death in CF (see **Fig. 1**).

Transplantation

Patients with CF become candidates for transplantation once the forced expiratory volume in one second (FEV$_1$) falls to about 30% predicted. Initially, the extension of life was not great compared with patients who did not receive a transplant, but steady improvement in patient selection, surgical technique, and postoperative care has greatly extended post-transplant survival and improved quality of life. For adults who underwent primary lung transplantation for any indication from 2009 to June 2016, the median survival was 6.5 years, but the median survival for recipients with CF was 9.5 years.[39] Meanwhile, median transplant free survival after FEV1 <30% was 6.6 years in a recent study[40] suggesting that transplantation affords a life-extending option. Complications of transplantation have become the second leading cause of death in CF.[8]

CFTR Modulators

Although improvements in symptomatic treatments and early diagnosis led to steady improvements in survival, correction of CFTR malfunction has been a crucial goal. Although the goal of restoring an entirely normal CFTR protein has been elusive, small molecules that restore partial function of CFTR have revolutionized therapy for CF.

The production, proper cell positioning, and achievement of functional conformation of CFTR is a complex, multistep process, and the 1480 amino acids of CFTR, participate in this molecular program at different steps, so CF-causing point

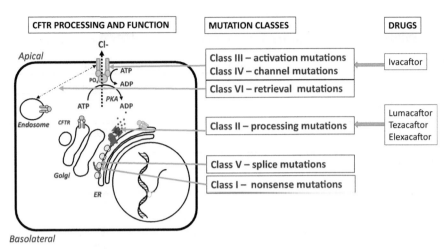

Fig. 2. Processing of CFTR in epithelial cells, mutation classes, and drugs that target these steps. The CF gene is transcribed in the nucleus and the mRNA is translated by ribosomes in the endoplasmic reticulum (ER). The completed protein chain is folded, reaches the Golgi apparatus where it is glycosylated, and the protein then arrives at the apical cell membrane. The chloride channel opens after phosphorylation by protein kinase A (PKA) and binding and hydrolysis of ATP in the nucleotide binding domain(s). CFTR is recycled from the apical membrane by endocytosis and exocytosis (*dotted line*). Class I mutations produce premature protein chain termination and nonfunctional proteins. Class II mutations produce misfolding of CFTR, which is then degraded, so that little reaches the cell surface. Class III and IV mutations reach the apical surface but fail to be activated (class III) or to transmit the chloride ion through the channel (class IV). A few mutations with errors at splice sites produce misassembled mRNA and nonfunctional protein (Class V). A very few mutations accelerate the retrieval of CFTR from the apical cell membrane (Class VI). Ivacaftor promotes passage of the chloride ion through channels that reach the cell surface (especially Classes III and IV, but it can contribute to greater activity in Classes II, V, and VI for the channels that reach the apical surface). Elexacaftor, Lumacaftor, and Tezacaftor act upon the folding or processing of CFTR, presumably at different steps in folding, so that more of it assumes a configuration that reaches the cell surface.

mutations affect the process in different ways. Besides point mutations, other genetic lesions in CFTR are reported, such as larger deletions, translocations or duplications, but most CF-causing mutations fall into 1 of 6 categories (**Fig. 2**). Small molecules known as CFTR "modulators" restore some CFTR function by correcting the steps of folding and/or channel opening of CFTR.

The development of these modulators is a remarkable milestone for people with CF. The first such drug, the CFTR potentiator ivacaftor (IVA), which acts to increase channel opening in the apical membrane, was approved by the Food and Drug Administration (FDA) in 2012 for patients with at least 1 copy of the c.1652 G > A (legacy: G551D) allele based on the demonstration of significant improvement in lung function and body weight, a decrease in sweat chloride (often <60 mEq/L), improved quality of life, and fewer pulmonary exacerbations.[41] Unfortunately, these patients comprise less than 5% of US CF patients. However, the strong correlation between modulator-induced in vitro CFTR function and the classic outcome measures for CF clinical trials (sweat chloride, FEV_1) allowed the FDA to expand the approved use of IVA to CF patients

with additional mutations, most of which were so rare that it would be difficult to conduct a clinical trial. Based on the well-known pathophysiology of CF, a documented excellent risk–benefit profile from those already treated, and a standardized in vitro assay (stimulation of over 10% wild-type CFTR activity by the drug after variant CFTR cDNA expression from a standard construct in Fisher rat thyroid cells), the FDA reasoned that IVA could be approved for use in such patients without a specific clinical trial.[42,43] Indications have since been expanded to over 90 rare CFTR mutations. This approach, dubbed "theratyping", has emerged as an alternative mechanism to assess drug effect on rare mutations. Improvement in CFTR activity in response to modulator drugs in bronchial or nasal epithelial cells grown in culture or in rectal organoids also correlates well with in vivo improvements in FEV_1 and sweat chloride seen in modulator clinical trials.[43] Theratyping to extend indications for the CFTR modulators is important not only for CF patients, but also for other diseases for which the small number of patients limits the ability to conduct clinical trials but for which robust in vitro surrogate markers are available.

The most common CF mutation is c.1521_1523del (legacy: Phe508del), a class II mutation. This mutation prevents normal folding and trafficking of CFTR, and the few proteins that do reach the surface do not open to the same extent as normal CFTR and also are retrieved from the surface more rapidly than in normal CFTR (see **Fig. 2**). Therefore, modulators initially developed for c.1521_1523del combine a potentiator such as IVA with corrector(s) of CFTR folding and transport lumacaftor (LUM) or tezacaftor (TEZ). These combination drugs made CFTR modulation available to an additional 45% of patients with CF homozygous c.1521_1523del although their clinical impact was not as profound as IVA was on patients with gating mutations,[44,45] and adverse events were limiting for some patients. There are multiple steps in CFTR folding, and later efforts to include two correctors of CFTR folding, presumably working at different steps, were highly successful. In 2019, the FDA approved the triple combination of CFTR potentiator IVA with two CFTR correctors TEZ and elexacaftor (ELX). This combination was found, even in people with a single c.1521_1523del allele, to result in significant improvement in CFTR function as measured by sweat chloride, FEV_1, BMI, and patient reported quality of life, as well as a significantly lower rate of pulmonary exacerbations relative to placebo.[46] IVA/TEZ/ELX can provide a highly effective modulator treatment regimen for more than 85% of the people living with CF world-wide.

The full impact of modulators on the health and longevity of those with CF is only now becoming clear. People taking IVA,[47,48] LUM/IVA [49] and TEZ/IVA[50] have reduced rate of decline of lung function, but decline is not halted. More time is needed to evaluate the ultimate benefit of IVA/TEZ/ELX on lung disease progression and survival. This initial experience suggests that the CFTR modulators may be a historic inflection point on the upward trajectory of improved survival and quality of life for patients with CF. The mutant c.1521_1523del accounts for approximately 66% of mutations worldwide,[51] and 85% of those living with CF in the United States have at least 1 copy of this mutant.[8] These patients can be treated with triple drug therapy with the expectation of excellent benefit.

Challenges to Improved Survival in CF

The impressive improvements in survival and quality of life in CF have been limited by several potentially modifiable factors.

Disparities Due to Socioeconomic Status

Outcomes in CF patients in the United States are profoundly affected by socioeconomic status (SES). People with CF and low SES have increased mortality, worse nutritional status and pulmonary function, more frequent exacerbations, are more likely to be infected with *Pseudomonas aeruginosa*, and are accepted less often for lung transplantation.[52] For the most part, these results occur despite center care, comparable number of clinic visits, and comparable prescription of medications important for treatment of CF. To realize the full benefit of the improvements in therapeutics for CF patients in the United States, this disparity must be addressed.

Disparities Due to Race/ethnicity

Minorities with CF suffer worse health outcomes: even after adjustment for SES, Hispanic patients have higher mortality than non-Hispanic white patients.[53] Both Hispanic and black patients with CF have worse pulmonary function than non-Hispanic white patients despite the Hispanic population having a higher BMI, higher likelihood of pancreatic sufficiency, and a higher proportion of "mild" mutations.[52,54,55]

One possible contributor to worse outcomes in minorities is the higher likelihood of missing CF on the newborn screen. The CFTR mutations included in most newborn screens do not include some of the alleles that are more common in patients of African, Hispanic, Asian, and Middle Eastern ancestry.[56] Review of the genotypes of people included in the US CF demonstrated that 13% to 16% of Hispanic, 15% to 18% of Black, 23% to 28% of Asian, and 7% to 8% of Native Americans would not be identified compared with only 3% of non-Hispanic Whites.[56] Children diagnosed from symptoms rather than by newborn screening are diagnosed later and have increased complications including hospitalization, *Pseudomonas* colonization, and decreased lung function.[57,58] Adjusting the screening tests to include more of the mutations more frequent in minority populations would reduce this disparity.

In addition, patients from minority ethnic groups are less likely to have a mutation that qualifies for CFTR modulator therapy. Although c.1521_1523del is the most common mutation in all groups, patients of a minority group are less likely to have a copy of c.1521_1523del and are more likely to have a deletion or duplication mutation. Based on CFTR genotype alone, 92.4% of non-Hispanic white patients, 69.7% of Black/African American patients, 75.6% of Hispanic patients, and 80.5% of other race patients have a CFTR genotype eligible for at least one CFTR modulator therapy.[59] Mutation-agnostic therapies, which are being actively sought in many laboratories, would address these disparities.

New Infections/Environmental Challenges/ COVID

CF patients may have severe lung disease and are more susceptible to colonization or infection with new pathogens. For example, in the early 1980s a new pathogen, *Burkholderia cepacia,* devastated CF patients at several centers, causing high initial mortality and prompting upgraded infection control protocols.[60] More recently, atypical mycobacteria have emerged as problematic for CF patients.[61] The COVID pandemic raised alarm among patients with CF, but several small studies suggested that outcomes may not be as poor as feared.[62] A later report compared the outcomes of people with CF to a propensity score matched cohort of people without CF found that the CF patients had higher hospitalization rates, critical care needs, and acute renal injury as compared with patients without CF, and 5.2% of these patients died within 1 month of COVID-19 diagnosis.[63] Other pathogens may emerge to threaten the improving survival of patients with CF. Continued clinical vigilance and the maintenance of registry data may allow early warning and early action.

CHANGING OUTCOMES AND CLINICAL MANIFESTATIONS

Concomitant with the steady improvement in predicted survival in CF (see **Fig. 1**), health and quality of life has improved and changed the clinical picture of h CF.

Pulmonary Outcomes

Respiratory failure remains the primary cause of death in people with CF, and lung disease is a major cause of morbidity. The proportion of children with CF who reach 18 years of age with lung function in the normal/mild lung disease category (FEV1 $\geq$70% predicted) has increased from 33.8% in 1989 to 78.3% in 2019.[8] Conversely, the proportion of 18-year-old patients in the severe lung disease category (FEV1 <40%) decreased from 24.0% in 1988 to 2.6% in 2019.[8] Most of the children now reach adulthood with only mild lung disease or normal pulmonary function (**Table 3**).[8,31,32,64]

Growth and Nutrition

Weight[65] and height[66,67] are independent predictors of survival in CF. The goal established by the CF Foundation nutrition guidelines for children age 2 to 19 years is a BMI percentile at or above 50% using Centers for Disease Control growth curves. The median BMI percentile in 2019 was

Table 3
Clinical outcomes reported in the United States Cystic Fibrosis Foundation patient registry

	2009	2019
Pulmonary outcomes		
Median FEV1% predicted ages 6–17 y	93.6[a]	95.2[c]
Median FEV1% predicted age >18 y	65.3[a]	71.1[c]
% 18 year old with FEV1 >70% predicted	65[a]	78.3[c]
% 18 year old with FEV1 <40% predicted	8[a]	2.6[c]
Nutrition Outcomes		
Median BMI %ile in children ages 2–19 y	48.7[c]	58.4[c]
Median weight %ile in children ages 2–19 y	38.2[b]	49.3[c]
Median height %ile in children ages 2–19 y	30.6[b]	38.4[c]
Median BMI in adults > 20 y	22.0[c]	23.0[c]
Adults with BMI >25 (%)		31.4[c]

[a] Cystic Fibrosis Foundation Patient Registry Annual Data Report, 2009.
[b] Cystic Fibrosis Foundation Patient Registry Center Specific Annual Report, 2016. National median data obtained from center specific report.
[c] Cystic Fibrosis Foundation Patient Registry Annual Data Report, 2019, including updates for prior years

58.4%, thus achieving that goal. On the other hand, height percentile remains well below that of the general population at a median of 38.4%. For adults, consensus guidelines recommend a BMI of greater than 22 to 23, and in 2019 it reached 23.0[8] (see **Table 3**). Better nutrition probably contributes to improved lung function and improved digestion reduces gastrointestinal symptoms.

Pregnancy

Although studies of women with CF suggest they are less fertile than age-matched women without CF, with improved nutrition and lung function and the advent of modulator therapy, pregnancies in women with CF are becoming more common[68] (see **Table 2**). Initial reports suggest modulators may be safe in both pregnancy and breastfeeding[69] and, if the infant has CF, may inhibit early organ destruction in utero.[70]

Spectrum of Complications in the Aging CF Population

Historically, because children with CF rarely survived beyond childhood, the care of patients with

CF fell to pediatric specialists. Now that 56% of the CF population in the United States is over 18 years of age (see **Table 2**), physicians with expertise in the care of adults are needed to manage these patients. For example, frequent and prolonged courses of antibiotics needed to preserve lung function have caused a rising incidence of renal insufficiency,[71] hearing loss from ototoxic antibiotics,[72] and superior vena cava syndrome[73] from years of indwelling vascular catheter use. Additionally, the 6-fold higher incidence of GI cancers in adults with CF is a more pressing problem as the number of adults increases.[74]

As the CF population grows older, we need to better understand aging in this population. Although children with CF have historically been underweight and sarcopenic, increasing numbers of overweight and even obese people with CF are being recognized (see **Table 3**). This trend, along with studies showing unusually stiff blood vessels in people with CF[75,76] may presage risk for cardiovascular disease. In addition, basic research suggests that CF cells undergo an accelerated aging process, also known as cellular senescence, which is associated with inflammation, tissue damage, and the development of cancer.[77] The consequences of this accelerated aging process are not known. Much work is needed as we enter the new era of the aging person with CF.

SUMMARY

The incidence of CF remains highest in Caucasian populations, particularly those in Western Europe, Australia, and North America, about 1 in 3500 live births, but there is increasing recognition of CF in other populations, though the spectrum of recognized mutations is different. As the incidence has remained steady but case ascertainment has increased and survival has markedly improved over the last several decades, the prevalence of CF in the population is increasing. Survival improvement has occurred because of aggressive symptomatic care in centers, improvements in new drugs and devices to assist symptomatic therapies, early recognition of the disease which allows earlier institution of therapy, and recently, small molecule treatments directed at the basic defect in CFTR that have been highly effective in restoring function. These therapeutic improvements have produced a patient population that is better nourished and living longer, and assumes the responsibilities and risks of adulthood. However, there exist substantial racial, ethnic, and socioeconomic disparities in the outcomes of CF in the United States. Further efforts toward health equity and continued pursuit of definitive genetic

therapies can be expected to further alter the demographics and epidemiology of CF.

CLINICS CARE POINTS

- Survival among patients with cystic fibrosis is increasing due to aggressive symptomatic therapy, early diagnosis from newborn screening, and the introduction of modulators that increase function of CFTR itself, so that median predicted survival age in North America and Western Europe is now about 50 years.

- Despite these improvements, decline in pulmonary function has slowed but not stopped, so symptomatic therapy is still important.

- The incidence of cystic fibrosis is about 1 in 3500 live births in the United States and is less frequent among black persons and those of Asian ancestry.

- Most patients are now diagnosed by newborn screening, but many mutations are not tested, and these untested mutations are more frequent in racial and ethnic minority populations.

- In the United States, survival lags in those of lower socioeconomic status and those in minority populations.

DISCLOSURE

PBD gratefully acknowledges support from NIH grant UL1TR002548.

REFERENCES

1. Riordan JR, Rommens JM, Kerem B, et al. Identification of the cystic fibrosis gene: cloning and characterization of complementary DNA. Science 1989; 245(4922):1066–73.

2. Davis PB. Cystic fibrosis since 1938. Am J Respir Crit Care Med 2006;173(5):475–82.

3. LeGrys VA, Yankaskas JR, Quittell LM, et al. Diagnostic sweat testing: the cystic fibrosis foundation guidelines. J Pediatr 2007;151(1):85–9.

4. Farrell P, Joffe S, Foley L, et al. Diagnosis of cystic fibrosis in the republic of Ireland: epidemiology and costs. Ir Med J 2007;100(8):557–60.

5. Southern KW, Munck A, Pollitt R, et al. A survey of newborn screening for cystic fibrosis in Europe. J Cyst Fibros 2007;6(1):57–65.

6. Scotet V, Gutierrez H, Farrell PM. Newborn screening for CF across the Globe—where is it worthwhile? Int J Neonatal Screen 2020;6(1):18.

7. Lilley M, Christian S, Hume S, et al. Newborn screening for cystic fibrosis in Alberta: two years of experience. Paediatr Child Health 2010;15(9):590–4.

8. 2019 Annual data report. cystic fibrosis foundation patient registry. Available at: https://www.cff.org/medical-professionals/patient-registry. Accessed November 21, 2021.

9. Hamosh A, FitzSimmons SC, Macek M Jr, et al. Comparison of the clinical manifestations of cystic fibrosis in black and white patients. J Pediatr 1998; 132(2):225–59.

10. Palomaki GE, FitzSimmons SC, Haddow JE. Clinical sensitivity of prenatal screening for cystic fibrosis via CFTR carrier testing in a United States panethnic population. Genet Med 2004;6(5):405–14.

11. Klinger KW. Cystic fibrosis in the Ohio amish: gene frequency and founder effect. Hum Genet 1983;65: 94–8.

12. Nazer HM. Early diagnosis of cystic fibrosis in jordanian children. J Trop Pediatr 1992;38(3):113–5.

13. Stafler P, Mei-Zahav M, Wilschanski M, et al. The impact of a national population carrier screening program on cystic fibrosis birth rate and age at diagnosis: implications for newborn screening. J Cyst Fibros 2016;15(4):460–6.

14. Powers CA, Potter EM, Wessel HU, et al. Cystic fibrosis in Asian Indians. Arch Pediatr Adolesc Med 1996;150(5):554–5.

15. Kapoor V, Shastri SS, Kabra M, et al. Carrier frequency of F508del mutation of cystic fibrosis in Indian population. J Cyst Fibros 2006;5(1):43–6.

16. Kabra SK, Kabra M, Lodha R, et al. Cystic fibrosis in India. Pediatr Pulmonol 2007;42(12):1087–94.

17. Yamashiro Y, Shimizu T, Oguchi S, et al. The estimated incidence of cystic fibrosis in Japan. J Pediatr Gastroenterol Nutr 1997;24(5):544–7.

18. 2019 annual data report. the cystic fibrosis registry of Ireland. Available at: https://cfri.ie/annual-reports/. Accessed November 17, 2021.

19. McKone EF, Ariti C, Jackson A, et al. Survival estimates in European cystic fibrosis patients and the impact of socioeconomic factors: a retrospective registry cohort study. Eur Respir J 2021;58(3):2002288.

20. Stephenson AL, Sykes J, Stanojevic S, et al. Survival comparison of patients with cystic fibrosis in Canada and the United States: a population-based cohort study. Ann Intern Med 2017;166(8):537–46.

21. Di Sant'Agnese PA, Darling RC, Perera GA, et al. Abnormal electrolyte composition of sweat in cystic fibrosis of the pancreas; clinical significance and relationship to the disease. Pediatrics 1953;12(5): 549–63.

22. Gregg RG, Wilfond BS, Farrell PM, et al. Application of DNA analysis in a population-screening program for neonatal diagnosis of cystic fibrosis (CF): comparison of screening protocols. Am J Hum Genet 1993;52(3):616–26.

23. Farrell PM, Kosorok MR, Rock MJ, et al. Early diagnosis of cystic fibrosis through neonatal screening prevents severe malnutrition and improves long-term growth. Pediatrics 2001;107(1):1–13.

24. Grosse S, Boyle C, Botkin J, et al. Newborn screening for cystic fibrosis: evaluation of benefits and risks and recommendations for state newborn screening programs. MMWR Recomm Rep 2004; 53(RR-13):1–36.

25. Farrell PM, White TB, Ren CL, et al. Diagnosis of cystic fibrosis: consensus guidelines from the cystic fibrosis foundation. J Pediatr 2017;181S:S4–15.

26. Hale JE, Parad RB, Comeau AM. Newborn screening showing decreasing incidence of cystic fibrosis. N Engl J Med 2008;358(9):973–4.

27. Sontag MK, Wagener JS, Accurso F, et al. Consistent incidence of cystic fibrosis in a long-term newborn screen population. Pediatr Pulmonol 2008;43(suppl 31):272.

28. Parker-McGill K, Nugent M, Bersie R, et al. Changing incidence of cystic fibrosis in Wisconsin, USA. Pediatr Pulmonol 2015;50(11):1065–72.

29. Castellani C, Picci L, Tamanini A, et al. Association between carrier screening and incidence of cystic fibrosis. JAMA 2009;302(23):2573.

30. De Boeck K. Cystic fibrosis in the year 2020: a disease with a new face. Acta Paediatr 2020;109(5): 892–9.

31. Cystic Fibrosis Foundation Patient Registry. 1999 annual data report. Bethesda, Maryland: Cystic Fibrosis Foundation; 2000.

32. Cystic Fibrosis Foundation Patient Registry. 2009 annual data report. Bethesda, Maryland: Cystic Fibrosis Foundation; 2010.

33. Davis PB, Schluchter MD, Konstan MW. Relation of sweat chloride concentration to severity of lung disease in cystic fibrosis. Pediatr Pulmonol 2004;38(3): 204–9.

34. Cutting GR. Modifier genetics: cystic fibrosis. Annu Rev Genomics Hum Genet 2005;6(1):237–60.

35. O'Neal WK, Knowles MR. Cystic fibrosis disease modifiers: complex genetics defines the phenotypic diversity in a monogenic disease. Annu Rev Genomics Hum Genet 2018;19(1):201–22.

36. Konstan MW, Schluchter MD, Xue W, et al. Clinical use of Ibuprofen is associated with slower FEV1 decline in children with cystic fibrosis. Am J Respir Crit Care Med 2007;176(11):1084–9.

37. Konstan MW, VanDevanter DR, Sawicki GS, et al. Association of high-dose ibuprofen use, lung function decline, and long-term survival in children with cystic fibrosis. Ann Am Thorac Soc 2018;15(4): 485–93.

38. Saiman L, Marshall BC, Mayer-Hamblett N, et al. Azithromycin in patients with cystic fibrosis chronically infected with Pseudomonas aeruginosa. JAMA 2003;290(13):1749.

39. Chambers DC, Cherikh WS, Goldfarb SB, et al. The international thoracic organ transplant registry of the international society for heart and lung transplantation: thirty-fifth adult lung and heart-lung transplant report—2018; focus theme: multi-organ transplantation. J Heart Lung Transplant 2018;37(10):1169–83.

40. Ramos KJ, Quon BS, Heltshe SL, et al. Heterogeneity in survival in adult patients with cystic fibrosis with FEV1 < 30% of predicted in the United States. Chest 2017;151(6):1320–8.

41. Ramsey BW, Davies J, McElvaney NG, et al. A CFTR potentiator in patients with cystic fibrosis and the G551D mutation. N Engl J Med 2011;365(18):1663–72.

42. Durmowicz T, Pacanowski M. Novel approach allows expansion of indication for cystic fibrosis drug. In: Spotlight on center for drug evaluation and research science. Available at: https://www.fda.gov/drugs/news-events-human-drugs/novel-approach-allows-expansion-indication-cystic-fibrosis-drug. Content current as of 5/18/2017. Accessed: November 27, 2021.

43. Clancy J, Cotton C, Donaldson S, et al. CFTR modulator theratyping: current status, gaps and future directions. J Cyst Fibros 2019;18(1):22–34.

44. Wainwright CE, Elborn JS, Ramsey BW, et al. Lumacaftor–Ivacaftor in patients with cystic fibrosis homozygous for Phe508del CFTR. N Engl J Med 2015; 373(3):220–31.

45. Taylor-Cousar JL, Munck A, McKone EF, et al. Tezacaftor–Ivacaftor in Patients with Cystic Fibrosis Homozygous for Phe508del. N Engl J Med 2017; 377(21):2013–23.

46. Middleton PG, Mall MA, Dřevínek P, et al. Elexacaftor–Tezacaftor–Ivacaftor for Cystic Fibrosis with a Single Phe508del Allele. N Engl J Med 2019; 381(19):1809–19.

47. Sawicki GS, McKone EF, Pasta DJ, et al. Sustained benefit from ivacaftor demonstrated by combining clinical trial and cystic fibrosis patient registry data. Am J Respir Crit Care Med 2015;192(7): 836–42.

48. Guimbellot JS, Baines A, Paynter A, et al. Long term clinical effectiveness of ivacaftor in people with the G551D CFTR mutation. J Cyst Fibros 2021;20(2): 213–9.

49. Konstan MW, McKone EF, Moss RB, et al. Assessment of safety and efficacy of long-term treatment with combination lumacaftor and ivacaftor therapy in patients with cystic fibrosis homozygous for the F508del-CFTR mutation (PROGRESS): a phase 3, extension study. Lancet Respir Med 2017;5(2): 107–18.

50. Flume PA, Biner RF, Downey DG, et al. Long-term safety and efficacy of tezacaftor–ivacaftor in individuals with cystic fibrosis aged 12 years or older who are homozygous or heterozygous for Phe508del CFTR (EXTEND): an open-label extension study. Lancet Respir Med 2021;9(7):733–46.

51. Bobadilla JL, Macek M, Fine JP, et al. Cystic Fibrosis: a worldwide analysis of CFTR mutations – correlation with incidence data and application to screening. Hum Mutat 2002;19(6):575–606.

52. McGarry ME, Williams WA 2nd, McColley SA. The demographics of adverse outcomes in cystic fibrosis. Pediatr Pulmonol 2019;54(Suppl 3): S74–83.

53. Rho J, Ahn C, Gao A, et al. Disparities in mortality of hispanic patients with cystic fibrosis in the United States. A national and regional cohort study. Am J Respir Crit Care Med 2018;198(8):1055–63.

54. McGarry ME, Neuhaus JM, Nielson DW, et al. Pulmonary function disparities exist and persist in Hispanic patients with cystic fibrosis: a longitudinal analysis. Pediatr Pulmonol 2017;52(12):1550–7.

55. McGarry ME, Neuhaus JM, Nielson DW, et al. Regional variations in longitudinal pulmonary function: a comparison of Hispanic and non-Hispanic subjects with cystic fibrosis in the United States. Pediatr Pulmonol 2019;54(9):1382–90.

56. Pique L, Graham S, Pearl M, et al. Cystic fibrosis newborn screening programs: implications of the CFTR variant spectrum in nonwhite patients. Genet Med 2016;19(1):36–44.

57. Accurso FJ, Sontag MK, Wagener JS. Complications associated with symptomatic diagnosis in infants with cystic fibrosis. J Pediatr 2005;147(3): S37–41.

58. Campbell PW, White TB. Newborn screening for cystic fibrosis: an opportunity to improve care and outcomes. J Pediatr 2005;147(3):S2–5.

59. McGarry ME, McColley SA. Cystic fibrosis patients of minority race and ethnicity less likely eligible for CFTR modulators based on CFTR genotype. Pediatr Pulmonol 2021;56(6):1496–503.

60. Thomassen MJ, Demko CA, Klinger JD, et al. Pseudomonas cepacia colonization among patients with cystic fibrosis. Am Rev Respir Dis 1985;131:791–6.

61. Floto RA, Olivier KN, Saiman L, et al. US Cystic Fibrosis Foundation and European Cystic Fibrosis Society consensus recommendations for the management of non-tuberculous mycobacteria in individuals with cystic fibrosis. Thorax 2016;71(Suppl 1):i1–22.

62. McClenaghan E, Cosgriff R, Brownlee K, et al. The global impact of SARS-CoV-2 in 181 people with cystic fibrosis. J Cyst Fibros 2020;19(6):868–71.

63. Hadi YB, Lakhani DA, Naqvi SF, et al. Outcomes of SARS-CoV-2 infection in patients with cystic fibrosis: a multicenter retrospective research network study. Respir Med 2021;188:106606.

64. Cystic Fibrosis Foundation Patient Registry. 2016 center specific data report. Bethesda, Maryland: Cystic Fibrosis Foundation; 2017.

65. Sharma R. Wasting as an independent predictor of mortality in patients with cystic fibrosis. Thorax 2001;56(10):746–50.

66. Beker LT, Russek-Cohen E, Fink RJ. Stature as a prognostic factor in cystic fibrosis survival. J Am Diet Assoc 2001;101(4):438–42.

67. Vieni G, Faraci S, Collura M, et al. Stunting is an independent predictor of mortality in patients with cystic fibrosis. Clin Nutr 2013;32(3):382–5.

68. Taylor-Cousar JL. CFTR modulators: impact on fertility, pregnancy, and lactation in women with cystic fibrosis. J Clin Med 2020;9(9):2706.

69. Nash EF, Middleton PG, Taylor-Cousar JL. Outcomes of pregnancy in women with cystic fibrosis (CF) taking CFTR modulators – an international survey. J Cyst Fibros 2020;19(4):521–6.

70. Fortner CN, Seguin JM, Kay DM. Normal pancreatic function and false-negative CF newborn screen in a child born to a mother taking CFTR modulator therapy during pregnancy. J Cyst Fibros 2021;20(5): 835–6.

71. Lai S, Mazzaferro S, Mitterhofer AP, et al. Renal involvement and metabolic alterations in adults patients affected by cystic fibrosis. J Transl Med 2019;17(1):388.

72. Tarshish Y, Huang L, Jackson FI, et al. Risk factors for hearing loss in patients with cystic fibrosis. J Am Acad Audiol 2016;27(1):6–12.

73. Garwood S, Flume PA, Ravenel J. Superior vena cava syndrome related to indwelling intravenous catheters in patients with cystic fibrosis. Pediatr Pulmonol 2006;41(7):683–7.

74. Hadjiliadis D, Khoruts A, Zauber AG, et al. Cystic fibrosis colorectal cancer screening consensus recommendations. Gastroenterology 2018;154(3): 736–45.

75. Hull JH, Garrod R, Ho TB, et al. Increased augmentation index in patients with cystic fibrosis. Eur Respir J 2009;34(6):1322–8.

76. Macnee W. Premature vascular ageing in cystic fibrosis. Eur Respir J 2009;34(6):1217–8.

77. Bezzerri V, Piacenza F, Caporelli N, et al. Is cellular senescence involved in cystic fibrosis? Respir Res 2019;20(1):32.

Genetics of Cystic Fibrosis
Clinical Implications

Anya T. Joynt, PhD, Garry R. Cutting, MD, Neeraj Sharma, DVM, PhD*

KEYWORDS

- Cystic fibrosis transmembrane conductance regulator • Allelic heterogeneity • Precision therapies
- Genotype agnostic

KEY POINTS

- Understanding the diversity of cystic fibrosis (CF) causing cystic fibrosis transmembrane conductance regulator variants is critical for accurate diagnosis, prediction of disease progression, and identification of appropriate treatments for each individual.
- Expanding effective treatment to all individuals with CF will require continued development of alternative therapies beyond modulators.
- Therapeutic approaches that can address the underlying cause of all cases of CF could provide a genotype agnostic approach.
- Gene editing technology represents a possible curative approach for the treatment of CF.

INTRODUCTION

Cystic fibrosis (CF) is an autosomal recessive condition that is estimated to affect ~ 80,000 individuals worldwide. It is the most common life-limiting single-gene disorder among individuals of European descent; however, prevalence varies widely across different populations. CF is caused by mutations in the cystic fibrosis transmembrane conductance regulator (*CFTR*) gene, which encodes a chloride channel that facilitates ion and fluid transport across epithelial mucosal layers throughout the body. A key genetic feature of CF is allelic heterogeneity, with more than 2000 reported variants in the *CFTR* gene with varying disease liability. Although the well-known c.1521_1523delCTT (legacy F508del) mutation is the most commonly reported disease-causing allele in individuals of European descent, variants that are rarer overall have been observed at a higher rate in individuals of African or Asian descent.

CLASSIFICATION OF CYSTIC FIBROSIS TRANSMEMBRANE CONDUCTANCE REGULATOR VARIANTS BY MOLECULAR MECHANISM

The wide array of *CFTR* variants are typically divided into 6 or 7 "classes" based on the primary molecular mechanism (**Fig. 1**). Class I variants produce no CFTR protein (e.g., c.1624G>T, legacy G542X); Class II variants allow for protein to be produced but not successfully trafficked to the cell membrane (e.g., F508del); Class III variants produce protein but with a defect in channel gating (e.g., c.1652G>A, legacy G551D); Class IV variants produce protein with a defect in channel conductance (e.g., c.350G>A, legacy R117H); Class V variants produce reduced levels of protein (e.g., c.3717+12191C>T, legacy 3849+10kbC>T); and Class VI are those variants that produce functional protein but it is turned over quickly due to a stability defect (e.g., c.4147_4148insA, legacy 4279insA). Classification of variants by this system provides

The authors have nothing to disclose.
McKusick-Nathans Department of Genetic Medicine, Johns Hopkins University School of Medicine, Baltimore, MD, USA
* Corresponding author.
E-mail address: nsharma5@jhmi.edu

chestmed.theclinics.com

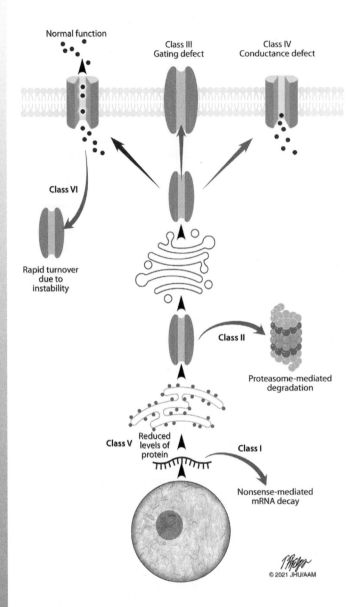

Fig. 1. *Classification of CFTR variants by molecular mechanism of disease.* Figure showing the steps from *CFTR* DNA to functional CFTR protein and the points at which a problem can occur designated as classes I–VI. Class I variants allow for no production of CFTR protein; Class II variants result in protein that is not trafficked to the cell membrane; Class III variants produce protein with a defect in channel gating; Class IV variants produce protein with a defect in channel conductance; Class V variants have reduced levels of protein; and Class VI variants make protein with reduced stability. (Illustrations: Tim Phelps © 2021 JHU AAM Department of Art as Applied to Medicine The Johns Hopkins University School of Medicine.)

a useful method for breaking down the breadth of different *CFTR* alleles when considering how to approach treatment of individuals. However, one limitation of this classification system is that some variants may fall into more than one class. For example, F508del primarily results in a trafficking defect, however when this is corrected, it becomes evident that this protein isoform is not fully functional at the cell surface and, therefore, also has characteristics of class III. Similarly, this classification system can erroneously group variants that would require different treatment approaches (**Table 1**). This is exemplified by class I variants. Although all variants in this class do indeed result in no production of CFTR protein, this encompasses nonsense, frameshifts, and some splice

variants. Treatment approaches for these 3 types of variants will likely be different, and this is one reason why class I is sometimes broken into 2 classes, class I and class VII, with class I remaining "no protein" and class VII being "no mRNA."[1,2]

GENOTYPE–PHENOTYPE CORRELATION

The diversity of *CFTR* variants is reflected in a wide range of disease presentations. The classical presentation of CF includes high sweat chloride (>60 mmol/L), reduced lung function with frequent lung infections, exocrine pancreatic insufficiency, meconium ileus at birth, earlier onset of CF-related diabetes (CFRD), nutritional deficiencies and difficulty maintaining BMI, and congenital

Table 1
Treatment approaches for cystic fibrosis based on genotype

Target	Treatment Type	Molecular Defects	Treatment Approach	Examples of *CFTR* Variants Tested[a]
DNA	Gene editing	Any G>A or C>T point mutations	CRISPR/Cas9 adenine base editing	W1282X, R553X, R785X[49–51]
		Any T>C or A>G point mutations	CRISPR/Cas9 cytosine base editing	711+3A>G[b,47]
		Any C>G or G>C point mutations	CRISPR/Cas9 C·G to G·C base editing	S1196X, G970R[b]
		Any point mutations and indels	CRISPR/Cas9 prime editing	F508del[54]
			CRISPR/Cas NHEJ or HDR	3849+10kb, 3272–26A>G, F508del, W1282X[43–46]
			Triplex forming Peptide Nucleic Acids (PNAs)	F508del[41]
	Gene replacement	All	Superexons	F508del[41]
			Gene delivery	F508del[39]
			mRNA delivery	F508del[38]
RNA	Splice modulation	Splice variants outside the 5'GT or 3'AG	Antisense oligonucleotides to direct splicing	3849+10kbC>T, 2789+5A>G[16–18]
			Chemical compounds (BPN-15477, CaNDY)	3120G>A, 3849+10kbC>T[20,21]
			Exon Specific U1s (ExSpeU1s)	1863C > T, 1898+3A>G, 2789+5A>G[19]
	NMD inhibition	Nonsense	Antisense oligonucleotides to knockdown NMD machinery, NMD inhibitor (NMDI-14)	W1282X[23,24]
	Readthrough		Pseudouridylation recoding	R1162X, R553X[b,31]
			Readthrough compounds[c] (G418, PTC-124, ELX-02, SRI-41315)	G542X, W1282X[26–29]
			Nonsense suppressor tRNAs	G542X, W1282X[33]
Protein	CFTR modulators	Reduced levels of protein	Amplifiers (PTI-CH)	F508del[14]
		Misfolded protein or reduced levels of protein	Correctors (tezacaftor, elexacaftor)	F508del[12,13]
		Non-functional protein or reduced levels of protein	Potentiators (ivacaftor, elexacaftor)	G551D[12,13]

(continued on next page)

Table 1
(continued)

Target	Treatment Type	Molecular Defects	Treatment Approach	Examples of *CFTR* Variants Tested[a]
Non-CFTR	Alternative targets	All	ENaC inhibition TMEM 16A potentiation	F508del[34] F508del/F508del and F508del + "minimal function"[35]

[a] Variant names are given using legacy nomenclature for simplicity.
[b] Use of these treatment strategies for CFTR have not been reported in the literature. Variants given are examples of those that might benefit from these approaches.
[c] Readthrough has a direct action on protein but may indirectly regulate RNA stability.

bilateral absence of the vas deferens (CBAVD) in the case of men. The more severe manifestations and rapid progression of disease are typically seen in individuals who harbor 2 *CFTR* variants falling into classes I–III. Those with only variants in classes IV–VI are more likely to present with a milder phenotype, which can include pancreatic sufficiency, increased lung function, decreased sweat chloride, and later onset of CFRD. Even mild dysfunction in CFTR has been shown to result in some phenotype, often referred to as CFTR-related disease. For example, *CFTR* variants that are not necessarily pathogenic in terms of CF have been shown to be sufficient to cause CBAVD.[3] Characterization of the CFTR function of heterologous cell lines expressing individual *CFTR* variants has allowed for a better understanding of the correlation between *CFTR* genotype and clinical presentation. By comparing *in vitro* results against clinical data, we have learned that individuals harboring variants with residual function have milder phenotypes and are more likely to respond to modulator therapies.[4–6]

Although this correlation is helpful, there are a variety of factors that can complicate interpretation of a variant. For instance, some alleles are "complex" meaning that 2 *CFTR* variants exist *in cis* on one allele and a third variant *in trans* on the other allele.[7] A classic example of this is the class IV variant R117H. On its own, R117H is not sufficient for a definitive diagnosis of CF and is classified as a variant of varying clinical consequences (www.cftr2.org). However, this variant is often found *in cis* with an intron 9 variant, "5T," which results in exon skipping and decreased abundance of full-length *CFTR* transcript. The combination of reduced transcript brought on by the intronic variant and the conductance defect caused by the R117H amino acid substitution is sufficient to reduce CFTR channel function to the point of causing CF. An additional factor that

complicates accurate genotype–phenotype correlation is modifier genes. These are genes outside of the *CFTR* locus that contain variants that can influence disease severity, manifestation, progression, and so forth. Several genome-wide association studies have allowed for the identification of loci that modify different CF phenotypes. For example, loci have been identified that include variants that modify the age of onset of CFRD and fall within annotated protein-coding genes (e.g., *SLC26A9, TCF7L2*).[8,9]

DIAGNOSTICS

Being one of the more common single gene disorders, CF is routinely tested for in Newborn Screening programs. Immunoreactive trypsinogen is the first-line screen, which identifies babies with pancreatic insufficiency, one of the hallmarks of CF. Although this is a useful screening approach, a final diagnosis of CF is not given without a second positive sweat test and/or identification of 2 pathogenic *CFTR* variants. Individuals may be classified as CF screen positive indeterminate diagnosis/CF-related metabolic syndrome, if they do not meet the full diagnostic criteria for CF.[10] One major challenge in proper diagnosis of CF is identification of the 2 disease causing alleles. Given the allelic heterogeneity in the *CFTR* gene identifying which variants are disease causing can be difficult because some individuals harbor rare variants that are not routinely included on genotyping panels. Luckily, because DNA and RNA sequencing technology has continued to improve and become more cost effective, it has become easier to identify genetic variants although this comes with the caveat of overidentification. In a given individual with CF, there may be more than 2 variants present but 2 *in trans* pathogenic alleles need to be identified for a definitive CF diagnosis. Publicly available databases, such as CFTR2,

CFTR-France, and ClinVar have improved variant interpretation through aggregation of genotype and phenotype data. However, interpretation of ultrarare variants remains a challenge. Another class of variants that can be difficult to identify are large insertions, deletions, or rearrangements. Identification of these genetic lesions requires more advanced and expensive sequencing approaches, such as long-read sequencing. A new and exciting method for identifying *CFTR* mutations and their disease liability simultaneously is mRNA sequencing, which allows for identification of amino acid substitutions as well as deviations from expected transcript abundance and splicing patterns.[11]

TREATMENT
Precision Therapies

Although initial treatments for CF focused on mitigating symptoms and minimizing exacerbations, the era of CFTR-targeted modulator therapies has allowed for focus on treatment of specific molecular defects, thus providing more substantial relief and lengthening the expected life span for individuals with CF. With recent advancements in combination modulator therapies, more than 90% of individuals with CF are currently eligible for treatment. The remaining ~10% will necessitate continued innovation and development of novel precision therapies to address more complex molecular defects. Here, we provide a brief synopsis of current and future precision therapy approaches and the role of genetics in their continued development and refinement.

Modulators
Since the initial Food and Drug Administration (FDA) approval in 2015, modulator therapies have revolutionized treatment of CF. These drugs fall into 3 classes: correctors, which help to facilitate proper folding and trafficking of the protein; potentiators, which increase the open probability of the CFTR channel; and amplifiers, which increase the efficiency of translation of CFTR. The ground-breaking triple combination therapy, Trikafta,[12,13] consisting of 2 correctors (tezacaftor, elexacaftor) and 2 potentiators (ivacaftor, elexacaftor) was FDA-approved in 2019 for individuals harboring at least one F508del allele, which accounts for ~90% of the CF population.[12] During the following 2 years, the label has expanded to include an additional 100+ variants.[13] However, there are additional individuals who are not eligible for treatment with these drugs due to rare variants that have not undergone *in vitro* or *in vivo* testing or characterization. In addition, individual responses

vary even among those with the same genotype. Genetics will play a key role in understanding this variation and allowing for a more nuanced approach to dosing based on individual differences in drug metabolism. Primary cell model systems, such as nasal and bronchial epithelial cultures and intestinal organoids[13] will be critical to understanding the effect of genetic background on response to modulators. For those individuals that produce reduced levels of protein (i.e. those with class VI variants), a new class of modulator therapy, amplifiers, could be promising in increasing the available substrate for targeting by correctors and potentiators.[14]

Splice modulation
CFTR variants that affect mRNA splicing account for ~10% of all reported alleles. Treatment approaches for these variants depend on the mechanism of missplicing and the mRNA and protein isoforms produced. Variants that allow for the production of some normally spliced transcript are likely to respond to modulator therapies.[15] For the remaining variants, current treatment approaches include antisense oligonucleotides (ASOs) and direct modulation of splicing. ASOs work by base pairing with the mRNA to preclude access to regions of the transcript to facilitate a particular splicing pattern. For example, ASOs have been shown to successfully prevent the inclusion of pseudoexons, specifically in the case of deep intronic variants (e.g., 3849+10kbC>T).[16,17] ASOs can also be designed to increase exon inclusion, as demonstrated by correction of missplicing caused by c.2657+5G>A (legacy 2789+5G>A).[18] Another approach for modulation of splicing is the treatment with exogenous components of the splicing machinery modified to target the mutated splice site. These approaches have shown mixed results depending on the sequence context of the variant of interest.[19] Recently, modulation with chemical compounds has been shown to be effective in correction of missplicing for specific *CFTR* variants. The chemical compound BPN-15477 was identified through a high-throughput screen and shown to reduce exon skipping caused by c.2988G>A (legacy 3120G>A).[20] Separately, the compound CaNDY was shown to promote pseudoexon exclusion in 3849+10kbC>T cells.[21] To date, none of these approaches has proven successful in restoring normal splicing in variants affecting the critical 5'GT or 3'AG of the splice site.

Nonsense-mediated mRNA decay inhibition and readthrough
Another "difficult to treat" class of *CFTR* variants are those that result in the introduction of a

premature termination codon (PTC) either through a single nucleotide change, a frameshift, or an aberrant splice isoform. These variants are particularly challenging because they engage two mechanisms of cellular quality control. First, they can result in nonsense-mediated mRNA decay (NMD), which leads to a loss of CFTR transcript. Second, even if NMD is escaped, these variants result in the production of truncated CFTR protein, which is often unstable and will undergo proteasome-mediated degradation. Thus, a treatment approach for these variants would need to address both of these problems.[22]

The process of NMD is complex and plays a critical role in transcriptome quality control. Current NMD inhibition approaches focus on targeting of NMD factors, such as siRNA targeting UPF1[2] or inhibition of SMG1 by targeting with ASOs.[23] Although these approaches are effective in vitro, the potential to cause global dysregulation of the transcriptome remains a major pitfall. Thus, a crucial barrier to making NMD-inhibition a viable treatment is increasing specificity. Naturally occurring variation in NMD efficiency among individuals and understanding the genetic factors that drive this variability, may provide insight into improving these therapies.[24,25]

A second class of treatments targeting PTCs are readthrough drugs, which allow translation to continue despite the presence of a PTC in the open reading frame. These include a variety of chemical compounds that function by acting on different components of the translational machinery. Such compounds used in vitro include the aminoglycoside G418, which allows for readthrough, but has a high rate of cytotoxicity[26] and PTC-124, which has shown limited success in the treatment of CF in vivo.[27] Recently, 2 new readthrough agents have been reported for the treatment of CF. These are ELX-02,[28] an aminoglycoside analog, and SRI-41315,[29] a novel compound that promotes readthrough by depletion of eRF1. Similar to NMD-inhibitors, one limitation of readthrough reagents is lack of specificity. Although recent studies of naturally occurring stop codons throughout the genome show that the translational machinery may be able to distinguish native termination codons (NTCs) based on sequence context, there is still the potential for aberrant readthrough of NTCs in therapies meant for PTC readthrough.[26] Additionally, insertion of a random amino acid at the PTC site could lead to misfolded protein,[30] although this may be rescued by modulator therapies. An alternative, more targeted approach to induce readthrough is pseudouridylation of the PTC. This method uses naturally occurring box H/ACA RNPs, which target specific uridine residues of the mRNA and isomerize to pseudouridine, resulting in readthrough of the PTC.[31] Finally, an approach that acts directly at the translation step is nonsense suppressor tRNAs, which are modified tRNAs that recognize stop codons but are charged with amino acids and thus facilitate readthrough.[32,33]

Assignment of precision therapies

When treating a genetic disease such as CF, we have to consider the myriad of molecular processes that generate a disease phenotype from a DNA-level change. The treatment approaches described above all share the common feature of targeting one of these intermediate steps rather than the primary genetic defect. Therefore, accurately assigning which individuals will benefit from which treatment, or combination of treatments, requires careful assessment of the RNA and protein-level consequences of a particular variant (**Fig. 2**). For example, some nonsense variants allow for escape from NMD (i.e. N-terminal variants) and thus could respond to modulator therapies alone.[2] Similarly, C-terminal nonsense variants that would result in only slightly shortened protein could be treated with a combination of NMD-inhibition and modulators.[2] Although splice variants that allow for residual normally spliced transcript could respond to modulators,[15] those that result in out-of-frame insertions or deletions will prove more difficult to treat. Similarly, frameshift variants remain a difficult to treat category because every amino acid downstream of the PTC will be read incorrectly, thus even if NMD is evaded readthrough therapy is not a viable approach. Given this complexity, a large subset of nonsense variants, most canonical splice site variants, and all frameshift variants will require alternative treatments.

Gene Therapy and Genotype Agnostic Approaches

Within the subset of CFTR variants that are not currently or likely to be modulator eligible, the options for feasible alternative treatment approaches vary widely depending on the specific mechanism of the variants. Given that the most common CFTR variant (F508del) accounts for both alleles in ∼50% of individuals, the rare nature of many of the remaining variants makes it difficult to identify and test treatment approaches for all individuals. Thus, there is incentive for the development of "genotype agnostic" treatment approaches. These include some promising approaches, such as targeting of alternative ion channels to compensate for the CFTR channel defect or gene replacement therapy either through delivery of CFTR DNA

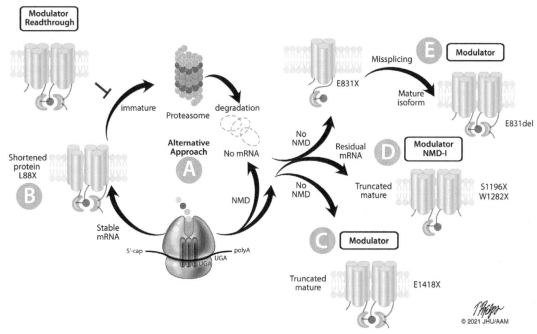

Fig. 2. *Heterogeneity informs assignment of precision therapies for nonsense variants.* (A) Variants that undergo severe mRNA decay need alternative treatments (e.g. gene editing). (B) N-terminal nonsense variants that evade NMD are ideal targets for readthrough drugs and modulators. (C) C-terminal nonsense variants that evade NMD and produce fully processed protein are targets for modulators alone. (D) Nonsense variants that result in protein isoforms lacking NBD2 are fully processed and may benefit from modulators when NMD is inhibited. (E) Variants that result in misspliced isoforms that produce fully processed protein are modulator responsive. MSD1 and MSD2 denote 6 membrane-spanning domains each. NBD1 and NBD2 denote nucleotide-binding domains. R denotes regulatory domain. (Illustrations: Tim Phelps © 2021 JHU AAM Department of Art as Applied to Medicine The Johns Hopkins University School of Medicine.)

or mRNA. Additionally, gene editing offers a highly targeted approach that can be used in both a genotype agnostic and genotype-specific manner and has the potential to offer a truly curative therapy to all individuals with CF.

Targeting alternative ion channels
Targeting of alternative channels typically focuses on either inhibition or activation of naturally occurring epithelial transporters where ion flow can be harnessed to compensate for defective CFTR transport. Both inhibition of the epithelial sodium channel (ENaC) and potentiation of a calcium-gated chloride channel (TMEM16 A) have been shown to modulate CFTR function.[34,35]

Gene replacement
Gene replacement has been under development since 1990, shortly after the *CFTR* gene was identified.[36] However, these approaches have been greatly limited by the large size of the *CFTR* gene, which exceeds the capacity of standard delivery approaches. In fact, effective delivery is a major barrier to clinical translation of many

nonmodulator treatment approaches. Finding a delivery approach that can shuttle large nucleic acids to not only different affected tissues throughout the body but more specifically to the *CFTR* expressing cells within those tissues will be critical to the success of these approaches. Current methods under development include viral vectors that allow for splitting of the construct between viral particles and recombination within the cell[37] and nanoparticles,[38] which have greater cargo capacities.

Attempts have been made to work around the large size of the *CFTR* gene by delivering only the open-reading frame either in the form of *CFTR* cDNA or mRNA.[38,39] However, even the *CFTR* cDNA alone is 4.4kb, which exceeds the packaging capacity of standard adeno-associated viral vectors.[39] One approach that has been taken to circumvent this issue is delivery of CFTR-delR, which is a cDNA construct encoding the *CFTR* reading frame with the omission of 156-nucleotides from the region corresponding to the R domain.[39] This deletion yields no functional defect, and allows for a smaller overall construct size, which expands options for packaging.[39]

Gene editing

The recent rapid development of gene editing technology now makes direct targeting of CFTR at the DNA-level feasible. In the last several years, these technologies have become more efficient and more precise. Gene editing strategies have the potential to be a curative treatment because corrections made to the genome may be passed through cell divisions and differentiation.

Targeted insertion into the endogenous locus

One approach that sits at the confluence of gene replacement and gene editing is the integration of the complete CFTR cDNA into the endogenous locus.[40] Although this method maintains the advantage of being genotype agnostic, it could also be curative by creating a permanent insertion in the genome. A variation on this approach is the targeting of "superexons" to the endogenous CFTR locus. These constructs replace a large region of the gene, typically several exons[41] and could be used to correct many variants with the same treatment, while also maintaining a larger portion of the endogenous CFTR.

Triplex-forming peptide nucleic acids

Peptide nucleic acids (PNAs) function by disrupting the DNA double helix in a targeted region through interaction of the PNA, a nucleotide analog, with one strand of the DNA to form a PNA/DNA/PNA triplex. A DNA donor is also delivered containing the desired edit and this will then be used as a template for repair of the targeted region. This strategy has been shown to successfully correct the F508del mutation in immortalized cells and CF mice.[42]

Clustered regularly interspersed palindromic repeats/Cas-mediated editing approaches

CRISPR/Cas-mediated editing approaches CRISPR/Cas (clustered regularly interspersed palindromic repeats/CRISPR-associated proteins) technology takes advantage of the naturally occurring bacterial Cas endonucleases, which complex with a structured RNA to target the enzyme to DNA in a sequence-specific manner. This simple system has been used to create a variety of technologies, which rely on engineered single-guide RNAs (sgRNAs), to bring enzymes into proximity with a particular region of the genome. "Traditional" CRISPR/Cas approaches introduce a double-strand break to the target region. Repair of the break can occur either by nonhomologous end joining (NHEJ) or homology-directed repair (HDR; **Fig. 3**A). NHEJ introduces random insertions and deletions (indels), which can facilitate knockout of a certain region (e.g. this has been used to disrupt the pseudoexon introduced by 3849+10kbC>T).[43,44] Alternatively, by delivering an exogenous repair template, a targeted edit can be made when the template is used for HDR as has been shown for correction of F508del and c.3846G>A (legacy W1282X).[45,46] One limitation of the CRISPR/Cas HDR approach, however, is that it has a relatively low efficiency and a relatively high chance of off-targets.

To address this issue, a new type of gene editing known as CRISPR/Cas-mediated base editing has been developed. The first iteration of this technology was cytosine base editing (CBE), which uses an sgRNA to target a Cas/cytidine deaminase fusion protein to a particular region of the genome where cytidines falling within a ~5 nt window will be deaminated to uracil, which is corrected to thymine by the cellular DNA repair machinery (**Fig. 3**B). This results in C>T editing as well as G>A editing by targeting of the opposite strand. This approach proved to be substantially more efficient than HDR and uses a Cas protein that is altered to introduce only a single-strand break, or nick, which reduces the rate of indels and off-targets.[47] Adenine base editing (ABE, **Fig. 3**C) was the next approach introduced, which allows for A>G edits and T>C edits.[48] In this case, adenosine is deaminated to inosine, which is converted to guanine.[48] ABEs have already proven successful in targeting of otherwise difficult-to-treat CFTR variants, such as W1282X, c.1567C>T (legacy R553X), and c.2353C>T (legacy R785X).[49–51] Recently, a third base-editing approach has been developed, C • G to G • C base editing (CGBE), which can convert G>C and C>G.[52] CBE and CGBE have not been reported for use in correction of CFTR variants; however, many could benefit from application of these tools to CF.

Despite the success of base editing, variants that induce an A>C/C>A, A>T/T>A, or G>T/T>G as well as insertions and deletions cannot be corrected by these approaches. Although CRISPR/Cas-mediated HDR would be a viable option, the low efficiency of this approach has led to the development of an alternative gene editing technology called prime editing.[53] Prime editing fuses a reverse transcriptase to a Cas and uses a special prime editing guide RNA (pegRNA) to both target the fusion protein to a region of the genome and act as a primer and template for the reverse transcription (**Fig. 3**D). The template portion of the pegRNA allows for introduction of any point mutation desired as well as insertions up to 44 bp or deletions up to 80 bp.[53] This approach has already been tested for correction of the most common CFTR variant, F508del.[54]

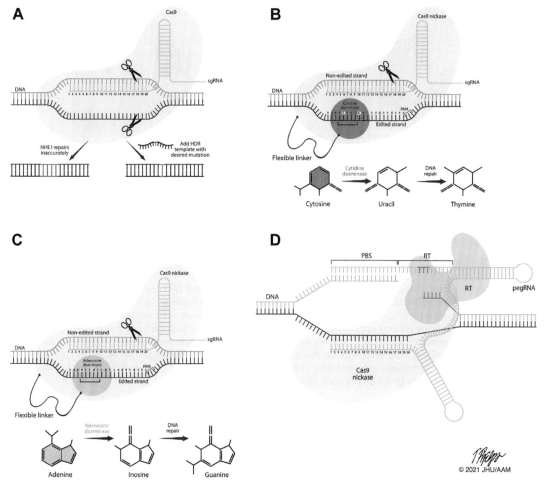

Fig. 3. *Mechanisms of different CRISPR/Cas-mediated editing technologies.* (*A*) "Traditional" CRISPR/Cas editing results in a double-strand break, which is repaired either by NHEJ, thus introducing random insertions and deletions, or HDR, allowing for generation of a specific point mutation, insertion, or deletion. (*B*) Cytosine base editing converts C > T without the need for a double-strand break. (*C*) Adenine base editing converts A > G. (*D*) Prime editing uses a reverse transcriptase and desired template to introduce any point mutation at a target site in the genome as well as insertions and deletions. (Illustrations: Tim Phelps © 2021 JHU AAM Department of Art as Applied to Medicine The Johns Hopkins University School of Medicine.)

Advantages and limitations of gene therapies

Because gene replacement and gene editing approaches either circumvent the primary defect or correct it entirely, these therapies could in theory be applicable to any *CFTR* variant. However, there are several major limitations to these approaches becoming widely available. The first is delivery and the second is targeting the correct cell types (**Fig. 4**). In addition to delivery approaches being limited depending on the size of the construct, thickened mucus in the CF airways provides a physical barrier and delivery of reagents to the necessary cell type will also require an understanding of cell-type specific markers and receptors. Genetics, specifically single-cell transcriptomics, has and will continue to play a powerful role in elucidating the cell types that need to be targeted and where they are located.[39] Gene replacement approaches will

need to specifically target cell types where *CFTR* is known to be expressed endogenously (e.g. goblet cells and ionocytes in the case of airway epithelia).[39] For gene editing therapies to be truly curative, they will need to target progenitor cells (e.g., basal cells in the airway epithelia[39]) so that the genetic correction can be propagated through cell divisions and differentiation.

SUMMARY

Genetics and our understanding of the role it plays in interindividual variability will continue to be important in moving toward more individualized and precise treatment. In the age of highly effective CFTR modulator therapies, understanding the unique genetic context of each individual is key to identifying who can receive the benefits of

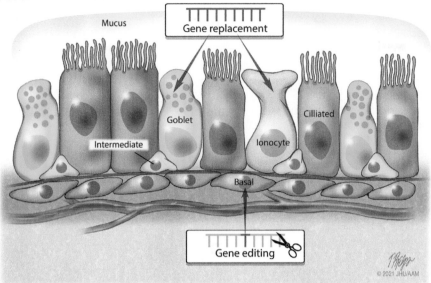

Fig. 4. *Different treatment approaches will require targeting of specific cell types present in the airway epithelia.* Basal cells differentiate into goblet cells and ionocytes, which have high levels of *CFTR* expression. Gene replacement should be targeted specifically to *CFTR* expressing cells to avoid unintended consequences from delivery to non-native cell types. Gene editing approaches will need to target basal cells in order to permanently correct the *CFTR* gene in future generations of cells. Delivery remains a challenge because mucous on the apical surface poses a barrier to aerosol delivery, and receptors on the apical and basolateral sides differ, necessitating different approaches for the systemic delivery. (Illustrations: Tim Phelps © 2021 JHU AAM Department of Art as Applied to Medicine The Johns Hopkins University School of Medicine.)

these life-changing drugs. Novel therapeutic approaches that could be applicable to all genotypes remain promising, if major barriers to translation can be overcome. Ultimately, truly curative treatments will have to act at the DNA-level and correct the primary genetic defect in order to mitigate the need for life-long treatment.

CLINICS CARE POINTS

- Improvements in accuracy and cost efficiency of sequencing technologies allow for more accurate cystic fibrosis transmembrane conductance regulator variant detection and increased diagnostic yield.

- Functional characterization of rare variants, as well as the use of primary tissue models, will increase access to modulator therapies to a more diverse population.

- Genotype agnostic approaches may provide more equitable treatment, whereas gene editing approaches offer a potential cure.

- Translation of novel treatment approaches to individuals with cystic fibrosis will rely on continued improvement of delivery technologies for targeting these treatments to the correct organs and cell types.

ACKNOWLEDGMENTS

The authors thank Tim Phelps at the Johns Hopkins Department of Art as Applied to Medicine for preparation of figures. The authors are supported by the following grants: Vertex Research and Innovation Award to NS; RO1DK044003, CUTTIN13A1, and CUTTIN20G0 to GRC.

REFERENCES

1. De Boeck K, Amaral MD. Progress in therapies for cystic fibrosis. Lancet Respir Med 2016;4(8): 662–74.
2. Sharma N, Evans TA, Pellicore MJ, et al. Capitalizing on the heterogeneous effects of CFTR nonsense and frameshift variants to inform therapeutic strategy for cystic fibrosis. PLoS Genet 2018;14(11):e1007723.
3. Fedder J, Jørgensen MW, Engvad B. Prevalence of CBAVD in azoospermic men carrying pathogenic CFTR mutations - evaluated in a cohort of 639 non-vasectomized azoospermic men. Andrology 2021; 9(2):588–98.
4. Raraigh KS, Han ST, Davis E, et al. Functional assays are essential for interpretation of missense variants associated with variable expressivity. Am J Hum Genet 2018;102(6):1062–77.
5. Han ST, Rab A, Pellicore MJ, et al. Residual function of cystic fibrosis mutants predicts response to small molecule CFTR modulators. JCI Insight 2018;3(14): 121159.

6. McCague AF, Raraigh KS, Pellicore MJ, et al. Correlating cystic fibrosis transmembrane conductance regulator function with clinical features to inform precision treatment of cystic fibrosis. Am J Respir Crit Care Med 2019;199(9):1116–26.

7. Chevalier B, Hinzpeter A. The influence of CFTR complex alleles on precision therapy of cystic fibrosis. J Cyst Fibros 2020;19(Suppl 1):S15–8.

8. Aksit MA, Pace RG, Vecchio-Pagán B, et al. Genetic Modifiers of cystic fibrosis-related diabetes have extensive overlap with type 2 diabetes and related traits. J Clin Endocrinol Metab 2020;105(5):dgz102.

9. Paranjapye A, Ruffin M, Harris A, et al. Genetic variation in CFTR and modifier loci may modulate cystic fibrosis disease severity. J Cyst Fibros 2020; 19(Suppl 1):S10–4.

10. Barben J, Castellani C, Munck A, et al. Updated guidance on the management of children with cystic fibrosis transmembrane conductance regulator-related metabolic syndrome/cystic fibrosis screen positive, inconclusive diagnosis (CRMS/CFSPID). J Cyst Fibros 2021;20(5):810–9.

11. Felício V, Ramalho AS, Igreja S, et al. mRNA-based detection of rare CFTR mutations improves genetic diagnosis of cystic fibrosis in populations with high genetic heterogeneity. Clin Genet 2017;91(3):476–81.

12. Middleton PG, Mall MA, Dřevínek P, et al. Elexacaftor-tezacaftor-ivacaftor for cystic fibrosis with a single Phe508del allele. N Engl J Med 2019;381(19): 1809–19.

13. Lopes-Pacheco M, Pedemonte N, Veit G. Discovery of CFTR modulators for the treatment of cystic fibrosis. Expert Opin Drug Discov 2021;16(8): 897–913.

14. Dukovski D, Villella A, Bastos C, et al. Amplifiers co-translationally enhance CFTR biosynthesis via PCBP1-mediated regulation of CFTR mRNA. J Cyst Fibros 2020;19(5):733–41.

15. Joynt AT, Evans TA, Pellicore MJ, et al. Evaluation of both exonic and intronic variants for effects on RNA splicing allows for accurate assessment of the effectiveness of precision therapies. PLoS Genet 2020; 16(10):e1009100.

16. Michaels WE, Bridges RJ, Hastings ML. Antisense oligonucleotide-mediated correction of CFTR splicing improves chloride secretion in cystic fibrosis patient-derived bronchial epithelial cells. Nucleic Acids Res 2020;48(13):7454–67.

17. Oren YS, Irony-Tur Sinai M, Golec A, et al. Antisense oligonucleotide-based drug development for Cystic Fibrosis patients carrying the 3849+10 kb C-to-T splicing mutation. J Cyst Fibros 2021;20(5):865–75.

18. Igreja S, Clarke LA, Botelho HM, et al. Correction of a cystic fibrosis splicing mutation by antisense oligonucleotides. Hum Mutat 2016;37(2):209–15.

19. Donegà S, Rogalska ME, Pianigiani G, et al. Rescue of common exon-skipping mutations in cystic fibrosis with modified U1 snRNAs. Hum Mutat 2020;41(12):2143–54.

20. Gao D, Morini E, Salani M, et al. A deep learning approach to identify gene targets of a therapeutic for human splicing disorders. Nat Commun 2021; 12(1):3332.

21. Shibata S, Ajiro M, Hagiwara M. Mechanism-based personalized medicine for cystic fibrosis by suppressing pseudo exon inclusion. Cell Chem Biol 2020;27(12):1472–82.e6.

22. Dyle MC, Kolakada D, Cortazar MA, et al. How to get away with nonsense: mechanisms and consequences of escape from nonsense-mediated RNA decay. Wiley Interdiscip Rev RNA 2020;11(1):e1560.

23. Keenan MM, Huang L, Jordan NJ, et al. Nonsense-mediated RNA decay pathway inhibition restores expression and function of W1282X CFTR. Am J Respir Cell Mol Biol 2019;61(3):290–300.

24. Aksit MA, Bowling AD, Evans TA, et al. Decreased mRNA and protein stability of W1282X limits response to modulator therapy. J Cyst Fibros 2019; 18(5):606–13.

25. Clarke LA, Awatade NT, Felício VM, et al. The effect of premature termination codon mutations on CFTR mRNA abundance in human nasal epithelium and intestinal organoids: a basis for read-through therapies in cystic fibrosis. Hum Mutat 2019;40(3): 326–34.

26. Wangen JR, Green R. Stop codon context influences genome-wide stimulation of termination codon read-through by aminoglycosides. eLife 2020;9:e52611.

27. Kerem E, Konstan MW, De Boeck K, et al. Ataluren for the treatment of nonsense-mutation cystic fibrosis: a randomised, double-blind, placebo-controlled phase 3 trial. Lancet Respir Med 2014; 2(7):539–47.

28. Crawford DK, Mullenders J, Pott J, et al. Targeting G542X CFTR nonsense alleles with ELX-02 restores CFTR function in human-derived intestinal organoids. J Cyst Fibros 2021;20(3):436–42.

29. Sharma J, Du M, Wong E, et al. A small molecule that induces translational readthrough of CFTR nonsense mutations by eRF1 depletion. Nat Commun 2021;12(1):4358.

30. Dietz HC. New therapeutic approaches to mendelian disorders. N Engl J Med 2010;363(9):852–63.

31. Adachi H, Yu YT. Pseudouridine-mediated stop codon readthrough in S. cerevisiae is sequence context–independent. RNA 2020;26(9):1247–56.

32. Porter JJ, Heil CS, Lueck JD. Therapeutic promise of engineered nonsense suppressor tRNAs. Wiley Interdiscip Rev RNA 2021;12(4):e1641.

33. Lueck JD, Yoon JS, Perales-Puchalt A, et al. Engineered transfer RNAs for suppression of premature termination codons. Nat Commun 2019;10(1):822.

34. Nickolaus P, Jung B, Sabater J, et al. Preclinical evaluation of the epithelial sodium channel inhibitor

BI 1265162 for treatment of cystic fibrosis. ERJ Open Res 2020;6(4):00429–2020.

35. Danahay HL, Lilley S, Fox R, et al. TMEM16A potentiation: a novel therapeutic approach for the treatment of cystic fibrosis. Am J Respir Crit Care Med 2020;201(8):946–54.

36. Cooney AL, McCray PB, Sinn PL. Cystic fibrosis gene therapy: looking back, looking forward. Genes 2018;9(11):E538.

37. Yan Z, Sun X, Feng Z, et al. Optimization of recombinant adeno-associated virus-mediated expression for large transgenes, using a synthetic promoter and tandem array enhancers. Hum Gene Ther 2015; 26(6):334–46.

38. Robinson E, MacDonald KD, Slaughter K, et al. Lipid nanoparticle-delivered chemically modified mRNA restores chloride secretion in cystic fibrosis. Mol Ther J Am Soc Gene Ther 2018;26(8):2034–46.

39. Tang Y, Yan Z, Engelhardt JF. Viral vectors, animal models, and cellular targets for gene therapy of cystic fibrosis lung disease. Hum Gene Ther 2020; 31(9–10):524–37.

40. Vaidyanathan S, Baik R, Chen L, et al. Targeted replacement of full-length CFTR in human airway stem cells by CRISPR-Cas9 for pan-mutation correction in the endogenous locus. Mol Ther J Am Soc Gene Ther 2021. https://doi.org/10.1016/j.ymthe. 2021.03.023.

41. Bednarski C, Tomczak K, Vom Hövel B, et al. Targeted integration of a super-exon into the CFTR locus leads to functional correction of a cystic fibrosis cell line model. PLoS One 2016;11(8): e0161072.

42. McNeer NA, Anandalingam K, Fields RJ, et al. Nanoparticles that deliver triplex-forming peptide nucleic acid molecules correct F508del CFTR in airway epithelium. Nat Commun 2015;6:6952.

43. Maule G, Casini A, Montagna C, et al. Allele specific repair of splicing mutations in cystic fibrosis through AsCas12a genome editing. Nat Commun 2019; 10(1):3556.

44. Sanz DJ, Hollywood JA, Scallan MF, et al. Cas9/gRNA targeted excision of cystic fibrosis-causing deep-intronic splicing mutations restores normal splicing of CFTR mRNA. PLoS One 2017;12(9): e0184009.

45. Vaidyanathan S, Salahudeen AA, Sellers ZM, et al. High-Efficiency, selection-free gene repair in airway stem cells from cystic fibrosis patients rescues CFTR function in differentiated epithelia. Cell Stem Cell 2020;26(2):161–71.e4.

46. Santos L, Mention K, Cavusoglu-Doran K, et al. Comparison of Cas9 and Cas12a CRISPR editing methods to correct the W1282X-CFTR mutation. J Cyst Fibros 2021. https://doi.org/10.1016/j.jcf. 2021.05.014.

47. Komor AC, Kim YB, Packer MS, et al. Programmable editing of a target base in genomic DNA without double-stranded DNA cleavage. Nature 2016; 533(7603):420–4.

48. Gaudelli NM, Komor AC, Rees HA, et al. Programmable base editing of A•T to G•C in genomic DNA without DNA cleavage. Nature 2017;551(7681): 464–71.

49. Krishnamurthy S, Traore S, Cooney AL, et al. Functional correction of *CFTR* mutations in human airway epithelial cells using adenine base. Nucleic Acids Res 2021;gkab788. https://doi.org/10.1093/nar/gkab788.

50. Geurts MH, de Poel E, Amatngalim GD, et al. CRISPR-based adenine editors correct nonsense mutations in a cystic fibrosis organoid biobank. Cell Stem Cell 2020;26(4):503–10.e7.

51. Jiang T, Henderson JM, Coote K, et al. Chemical modifications of adenine base editor mRNA and guide RNA expand its application scope. Nat Commun 2020;11(1):1979.

52. Koblan LW, Arbab M, Shen MW, et al. Efficient C•G-to-G•C base editors developed using CRISPRi screens, target-library analysis, and machine learning. Nat Biotechnol 2021. https://doi.org/10. 1038/s41587-021-00938-z.

53. Anzalone AV, Randolph PB, Davis JR, et al. Search-and-replace genome editing without double-strand breaks or donor DNA. Nature 2019;576(7785): 149–57.

54. Geurts MH, de Poel E, Pleguezuelos-Manzano C, et al. Evaluating CRISPR-based prime editing for cancer modeling and CFTR repair in organoids. Life Sci Alliance 2021;4(10):e202000940. https://doi.org/10.26508/lsa.202000940.

Update on Innate and Adaptive Immunity in Cystic Fibrosis

Emanuela M. Bruscia, PhD[a,1,]*, Tracey L. Bonfield, PhD, D(ABMLI)[b,1,]*

KEYWORDS

- Innate immunity • Adaptive immunity • Inflammation • Infections • Cystic fibrosis

KEY POINTS

- Innate and adaptive immunity are dysregulated in cystic fibrosis (CF).
- Inherited and acquired factors contribute to immune dysregulation in CF.
- Therapies regulating immunity are required to attenuate CF lung disease.

IMMUNE BARRIER FUNCTION AND HOST DEFENSE IN CYSTIC FIBROSIS LUNGS

The primary barrier between the external environment and internal structures is the airway epithelium. The integrity of this barrier is disrupted in cystic fibrosis (CF), playing a central role in the altered immune response to lung infections.

Mucociliary Clearance

Mucociliary clearance removes pathogens from the airways.[1] The airway mucus is composed of organized gel-forming mucins secreted by both submucosal glands and secretory cells of the airway epithelium. An optimal mucus viscosity is needed for efficient transport and release. Loss of the cystic fibrosis transmembrane conductance regulator (CFTR) function leads to defective epithelial chloride and bicarbonate transport, causing dehydration of the airway surface liquid (ASL), and abnormal mucin release and folding. As a consequence, mucus secretions in CF airways are desiccated, adherent, and difficult to clear by periciliary transport and cough. Airway mucus obstruction fosters a hypoxic environment that alters airway epithelial cell gene expression, enhancing mucins production and activating airway macrophages (MΦ) to secrete pro-inflammatory mediators.[2–4] The reduced bicarbonate transport also typical of CF airways, creates an acidic airway environment that alters mucus elasticity and adherence, impacting its release from the submucosal gland ducts and impairing removal.[5] These stagnant secretions provide an optimal milieu for pathogen colonization and retention, perpetuating lung inflammation in CF.

Drugs that have been used to improve ASL hydration and mucociliary clearance include dornase alfa, hypertonic saline, and inhaled mannitol.[6] OligoG that decreases mucus thickness was found to be safe in a recent phase 2b clinical trial in adults with CF.[7] Modulation of alternative epithelial ion channel activity (eg, TMEM16 A and βENaC) may also be a strategy to improve mucociliary transport in CF.[8]

Airway Surface Liquid and Airway Secretion Composition in Cystic Fibrosis

Airway surface liquid antimicrobial composition

The acidic pH of the CF ASL neutralizes the activity of several enzymes/antimicrobial peptides (eg, β-defensin-3 and cathelicidin) that normally protect against pathogens.[9] lactoferrin, the iron chelator, is lower in CF lungs relative to healthy individuals, altering efficient pathogen management.[10,11]

[a] Department of Pediatrics, Section of Pulmonology, Allergy, Immunology and Sleep Medicine, Yale University School of Medicine, New Haven, CT, USA; [b] Department of Genetics and Genome Sciences, Case Western Reserve University School of Medicine, Cleveland, OH, USA
[1] Equal contributors.
* Corresponding authors.
E-mail addresses: emanuela.bruscia@yale.edu (E.M.B.); tracey.bonfield@case.edu (T.L.B.)

Clin Chest Med 43 (2022) 603–615
https://doi.org/10.1016/j.ccm.2022.06.004

Hypothiocyanite (OSCN-), a potent antimicrobial molecule on the airway mucosal surfaces,[12] is also defective in CF. CF secretions have defective levels of the secreted protein short palate lung and nasal epithelial Clone 1 (SPLUNC1) that contributes to the host response by binding bacterial products and inhibiting sodium absorption.[13] The CF ASL also exhibits impaired antiviral activity against several enveloped and encapsulated viruses (eg, respiratory syncytial virus and influenza A).[14] Therapeutically, a drug that combines OSCN- and lactoferrin (ALX-009), a SPLUNC1 mimetic peptide (SPX-101), and formulations of metal gallium to sequester iron are under clinical evaluations.[15–17]

Protease activity

Lung neutrophilia is a hallmark of CF disease. In the normal lung, neutrophils migrate to the airways in response to chemokines, followed by apoptosis and removal by MΦs or expectoration. Elevated neutrophil numbers increase the amount and activity of neutrophil elastase (NE),[18] with concentrations correlating with CF lung damage and function.[19] NE remains active because of low pH, degrading structural airway matrix proteins (eg, collagen), cleaving plasma membrane (PM) proteins involved in immune signaling, and altering the complement. Active neutrophil-derived cathepsin G,[18] cathepsin S,[20] and proteinase 3[21] are also elevated in CF sputum, neutralizing antimicrobial protein function.[20] The zinc-metalloproteinase family (eg, MMP-9) that normally promotes tissue repair is abundantly recovered in CF sputum. The combined activity of MMPs and prolyn endopeptidases generates collagen products [for example, proline–glycine–proline (PGP)] by degrading lung collagen that further promotes inflammation and neutrophil chemotaxis in the lungs.[22] Longitudinal studies with CFTR modular therapies in CF suggest a lack of improvement in the levels of sputum NE.[23] Several drugs designed to block neutrophil proteases are being tested in people with CF.[24–27]

Nitric oxide content

Nitric oxide (NO) is produced from the amino acid L-arginine by the enzymatic action of nitric oxide synthase proteins (NOS). NO is essential for controlling inflammation and infection, and for modulating ciliary activity, vasodilatation, and bronchodilatation.[28] It is decreased in the exhaled breath of CF patients with severe disease. Further, low NO levels may be because of low expression of NOS and/or low availability of the NO substrate—arginine.[29–31] Importantly, treatment with ivacaftor resulted in increased NO in CF airways.[32]

Clinical trials are ongoing to determine the safety and effectiveness of controlled inhalation of NO on lung inflammation.[33]

Oxidative environment

The CF ASL contains high levels of reactive oxygen species (ROS) derived from the immune and airway epithelial cells. The increased oxidative stress is exacerbated by diminished antioxidant activity, including reduced glutathione, vitamin E, carotenoids, and coenzyme Q-10, as well as blunted antioxidant responses.[34] Further, oxidative stress exacerbates inflammation, tissue damage, and affects multiple bioactive lipid metabolic pathways that likely play a role in CF lung disease progression.[34,35]

Abnormal Cell–Cell Connections

The airway barrier function is maintained by cell junctions (tight, adherent, and gap) that provide contact and adhesion of airway epithelial cells.[36] Loss of CFTR results in altered levels and positioning of airway epithelial junction proteins creating weak connections, compromising epithelial paracellular permeability to ions, metabolites, immune mediators, and bacterial products. Thus, it contributes to altered ASL content and inflammation.[37–39] Further studies are required to correlate changes in epithelial paracellular permeability observed in experimental models to CF disease. Interestingly, azithromycin, a macrolide-type antibiotic with anti-inflammatory properties commonly used to treat infection in patients with CF, augments airway epithelial integrity.[40]

In summary, defects in immune barriers in CF dysregulate immunity by

- Altering ASL and fostering hyper-inflammation in early stages of the disease;
- Disrupting mucociliary clearance that favors bacterial trapping and adaptation, perpetuating inflammation; and
- Increasing protease activity, inflammatory mediators, and ROS that interfere with efficient bacterial clearance and compromise CF lung tissue integrity.

ALTERED INNATE IMMUNE RESPONSES AND HYPER-INFLAMMATION IN CYSTIC FIBROSIS
Pattern Recognition Receptor Signaling

The innate immune system senses microorganisms through pattern recognition receptors (PRRs) (**Table 1**) that recognize specific pathogen-associated molecular patterns (PAMPs) and damage-associated molecular patterns (DAMPs). PRRs are expressed on immune and

Table 1
PRRs

Types of PRRs	Cellular Locations	Major PAMPs
TLRs	Plasma or intracellular organelle membranes	Lipopolysaccharide, flagellin, peptidoglycans, lipoteichoic acid, glycosylphosphatidylinositol, microbial nucleic acids, porins, N-formylmethionine, etc.
Nucleotide-binding domain and leucine-rich repeat containing receptors	Cytosol	Ligands present in the cytosol and induce the inflammasome
RIG-I (retinoic acid-inducible gene I)-like receptors and cGAS (cyclic guanosine monophosphate-adenosine monophosphate)/STING (stimulator of interferon genes)	Cytosol	Nucleic acid sensors

structural cells that include the airway epithelium. Once activated, PRRs activate tightly regulated signal transduction mechanisms to initiate the inflammatory response. This results in the production of inflammatory mediators that lead to pathogen elimination, followed by a return to tissue homeostasis. Regulation of the PRRs by abundance, location, turnover, and signal transduction determines the quality, intensity, and duration of the immune response.[41] The PRRs in CF cells are continuously activated by microorganisms and the CF lung milieu reaches DAMPs (eg, ROS, PGP, adenosine triphosphate, and high mobility group box 1), perpetuating activation of pro-inflammatory pathways, and enhancing poor pathogen management and lung damage.[42–44] Sensing of viral PAMPs altered in in CF, and viral infections are frequently associated with exacerbation of lung disease. Interestingly, severe acute respiratory syndrome coronavirus 2 (SARS-CoV2) infections are not more frequent or more severe in the CF population compared with the general population.[45] Potentially, this can be explained by intensive self-care practiced by patients with CF. In addition, long-term use of azithromycin antibiotics[46], CFTR modulator therapy[136] and the potential decrease of ACE2 expression due to lung damage, may minimize CF susceptibility to SARS-CoV2.[47]

activating the inflammasome pathway.[44,48] Elevated interleukin-1β (IL-1β) following inflammasome activation further augments mucin production and the T helper 17 cells response (Th17 response).[3,49] Autophagy is also dysfunctional in CF, resulting in the accumulation of damaged organelles and malformed, nonfunctional proteins in lysosomes. Further, inefficient autophagy also contributes to the lack of efficient intracellular pathogen killing (eg, Burkholderia cepacia, Pseudomonas aeruginosa), perpetuating infections and inflammation.[50]

The altered lipid metabolism in CF also contributes to dysregulated immunity.[51] Pro-inflammatory lipid metabolites, such as arachidonic acid, prostaglandins, and neutrophil chemoattractant leukotriene B4 (LTB4), are elevated in CF. In contrast, levels of the anti-inflammatory omega-3 polyunsaturated fatty acid (eg, docosahexaenoic acid) and pro-resolving lipid mediators (eg, lipoxin A4, 15-lipoxygenase 2) that are necessary for the resolution of the inflammatory response, are reduced in CF.[52–54] The level and cellular distribution of sphingolipids and cholesterol, key components of the cellular plasma membrane (PM), are also altered in CF.[55,56] Changes in PM lipid composition impact the localization and activation of PM immune receptors, with consequences on downstream immune signaling regulation.[42,43]

Dysregulated Immune Pathways

Dysfunctional control of mitochondrial metabolism in response to infection leads to immune dysfunction in CF-affected cells by increasing pro-inflammatory metabolites (eg, succinate) and

Anti-inflammatory Therapeutic Development

The CF Foundation therapeutic development pipeline has targeted the CF-altered immune response. High-dose ibuprofen is highly effective in attenuating inflammation, although dosing and side effects complicate utilization in patients.[57] LAU-7b is considered because of its ability to normalize ceramide imbalance in CF cells[58] and to inhibit the inflammasome/IL-1 pathway.[59] Boosting anti-inflammatory responses through stimulating NO production via L-arginine administration,[60] increasing nuclear factor erythroid 2–related factor 2 activity,[61] pro-resolving lipid mediator treatment,[52] and the use of human mesenchymal stem cells (hMSCs) have also been explored in CF.[62,63] It is important to note that recently approved CFTR modulator therapies that improve mutation-specific function may not suppress CF hyper-inflammation long-term[23] (see Lindsay J. Caverly and colleagues' article, "The Impact of Highly Effective Modulator Therapy on Cystic Fibrosis Microbiology and Inflammation," in this issue).

In summary

- Pathways involved in recognition and killing of pathogens and promotion of inflammation resolution are disrupted in CF, promoting hyper-inflammation.
- 1) Treatment of infection and inflammation in CF may require a multi-tiered approach, integrating immune-modulatory interventions for optimal inflammation and infection resolution.

PHAGOCYTE FUNCTION AND HOST DEFENSE IN CYSTIC FIBROSIS
Neutrophils

Neutrophils are the most abundant immune cells recovered from the bronchoalveolar fluid in the sputum of CF patients (**Fig. 1**). Excessive migration of neutrophils into CF lungs is attributed to a massive increase in chemokines and chemoattractant molecules (eg, IL-8, LTB4, C-X-C motif chemokine ligand 10, IL-17, and PGP). Yet, the

elevated numbers of neutrophils do not efficiently clear infections and, at the same time, secrete high levels of proteases, pro-inflammatory cytokines, ROS, and neutrophil extracellular traps (NETs), amplifying lung hyper-inflammation and damage.[43] Dysregulated NETosis, a controlled release of nuclear DNA coated with proteases that normally help to capture and kill bacteria, is a major contributor to the high DNA content observed in CF lungs.[64] Enhanced neutrophil numbers, impaired degranulation, and delayed apoptosis contribute to NETs accumulation in CF airways. The failure of neutrophils to phagocytize bacteria is augmented by the shielding effect of the viscous mucus in the CF airways, and by P aeruginosa's exopolysaccharide secretions and biofilm formation.[65] Loss of CFTR also directly contributes to neutrophil dysfunction by impairing their ability to generate intraphagosomally hypochlorous acid[66] and to efficiently release secondary and tertiary granules[67] that contain antimicrobial molecules. In addition, neutrophils from patients with CF acquire an altered activated state when exposed to the CF lung microenvironment. They retain sustained viability, primary granule exocytosis (release of proteases, ROS), and activation of the inflammasome, while down-regulating antimicrobial functions.[68,69]

Despite the clear contributions of neutrophils in CF lung disease progression, clinical interventions targeting neutrophil recruitment have not provided clinical benefits. A study using an LTB4 inhibitor (BIIL4) resulted in an increased incidence of pulmonary exacerbations because of its excessive inhibitory anti-inflammatory effects.[70] A clinical trial using a new LTB4 inhibitor (acebilustat), shows that this drug, while safe, does not improve lung function. However, a trend toward reduced pulmonary exacerbations in subjects with an earlier stage of CF lung disease has been observed.[71]

Macrophages/Monocytes

Macrophages (MΦs) and monocytes (MOs) are regulators of inflammation and host immunity. They are instrumental in maintaining tissue homeostasis, and their dysfunction contributes to the pathogenesis of several diseases, including CF.

Altered MΦ immune pathways in cystic fibrosis
Many key pathways are dysregulated in CF MΦ/MO leading to failures in properly controlling inflammatory triggers, resolving inflammation, and clearing bacteria. Uncontrolled activation of toll-like receptors (TLRs) and PTEN-AKT immune signaling, autophagy, the unfolded protein response, and inflammasome activation contribute to CF MΦ

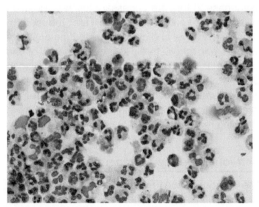

Fig. 1. Cytospin of cells recovered from bronchoalveolar fluid of a CF patient.

dysfunction. Current therapeutics aimed at controlling inflammation or restoring CFTR function modulate MΦ/MO function.[42–44,72]

MO and monocyte-derived MΦ in the chronically infected cystic fibrosis lung

The lung contains resident MΦs that can be classified as alveolar MΦ (AMs), and interstitial MΦs (IMs). In response to infection or injury, lungs are populated by circulating pro-inflammatory MOs that acquire a tissue-resident phenotype on interfacing with the lung microenviroment.[73] MΦ numbers are elevated in the airways of fetuses and young CF children before chronic infection, suggesting sterile inflammation in early CF.[74,75] These MΦs display altered expression of immune receptors [for example, TLR4, TLR5, CD11b, and the major histocompatibility complex (MHC) class II] and of scavenger receptors involved in phagocytosis.[42] A single-cell-RNAseq study on immune cells isolated from CF and non-CF airway secretions has shown that most of the MΦs in the CF airways originate from circulating MOs.[76] Increased numbers of blood-derived MΦ/MO can impede the resolution of inflammation, promote pathogen colonization, and participate in CF lung remodeling.[73]

Proinflammatory circulating monocyte in cystic fibrosis

MOs recruited into the infected CF lungs are pre-primed to respond to the unique CF lung microenvironment. Chronic lung infections provide a constant presence of lipopolysaccharide in CF, promoting a state of tolerance in circulating MOs.[77,78] They also display altered adhesion and chemotaxis into the lung in response to chemoattractants.[79] MO isolated from patients before and after starting CFTR modulator therapy suggests that restoration of CFTR function causes increased expression of genes that positively regulate the inflammatory response.[80] In disagreement with a "tolerance" state, MOs from CF patients produce high IL-1β and IL-18 levels[81] and have an active IFNγ/STAT1 signaling[82] that is decreased by CFTR modulators.

MΦ function is altered by the cystic fibrosis environment, enhancing the metabolic adaptation of microorganisms

As with neutrophils, MΦ function is altered by the CF lung microenvironment that impacts the ability to regulate inflammation and infection. The elevated levels of proteases in CF lungs cleave MΦs phosphatidylserine receptors[83] and other PM-associated molecules,[84] decreasing the effectiveness of MΦ/MO airway clearance of apoptotic cells and impeding re-establishment of tissue homeostasis. Moreover, CF MΦ's produce high

levels of succinate, itaconate, and ROS due to alteration of PTEN-PI3K-AKT signaling and mitochondrial metabolism. Succinate favors *P aeruginosa* colonization, and itaconate perpetuates their conversion toward a mucoid phenotype, promoting the persistence of the infection by evading host immunity.[44]

In summary

- Inefficient neutrophil and MO/MΦ functions contribute to the overall pathophysiology in CF.
- An effective treatment aimed to control inflammation, infection, and reduce lung tissue damage will need to control pathologic responses of these immune cells.

ADAPTIVE IMMUNITY IN CYSTIC FIBROSIS
Communication Between the Innate and Adaptive Immune Systems

The immune system involves a collaborative interaction between the MHC on MΦ, dendritic cells (DCs), and T-cells. DCs as the primary antigen-presenting cells, are central to the integration of innate and adaptive immunity and are located throughout the respiratory mucosa and alveolar epithelium where they sense and process antigens. Peripheral blood DCs from CF patients have lower levels of MHC Class II receptors when compared with healthy controls[85] suggesting altered antigen presentation.[86] In addition, DC maturation and function may be compromised by NE cleavage of CD86 in CF airway fluids.[87]

T Lymphocytes and Adaptive Immune Activation in Cystic Fibrosis

CFTR-deficient T lymphocytes have aberrant cytokine secretion and are hyper-inflammatory due to altered Ca^{2+} influx. They produce higher levels of IL-13 and IL-4 in response to *Aspergillus fumigatus* infections, and lower levels of IL-10 compared with non-CF controls.[88] Defective tryptophan catabolism may also contribute to the abnormal T-cell phenotype in CF.[89] Pathogenic Th17 T-cells, with the production of high IL-17 levels,[90] have both an early and late contribution to CF lung pathophysiology. Although Th17 T-cells are critically important in host responses to infection, in CF they promote neutrophil recruitment into the lungs and induce expression of mucin-producing genes from the epithelium.[91] Treatments aimed at neutralization of IL-17 signaling reduced neutrophil recruitment into lungs of CF mice challenged with *P aeruginosa*, implicating IL-17 as a therapeutic target.[92] However, because IL-17 is central to controlling infections and stimulating $HCO3^-$ transport at the airway mucosa,[93] therapeutics aimed to decrease IL-17 may not be completely adequate in CF. Inflammation in CF may also be attributed to the defective activity of the regulatory T-cell.[94,95]

B Cells, Antibodies, and Autoantibodies in Cystic Fibrosis

The CF lung environment creates a unique milieu for B-cell development and maturation, as shown by changes in the transcriptional profile of CF B-cells.[96] Patients with CF have increased lung neogenesis of bronchial-associated lymphoid tissue and B-cell-activating factor of tumor necrosis factor family that regulates B-cell survival and maturation. CF patients infected with P aeruginosa present with high levels of circulating immunoglobulin G (IgG) (mostly IgG3 and IgG4), and increased levels of IgA.[97] Although high levels of antibodies against P aeruginosa are produced, the antibodies are not efficient, potentially due to inefficient bacterial opsonization and phagocytosis.[98]

Altered B-cell phenotype and elevated immune complexes can promote autoimmunity[99] contributing to CF lung damage, inefficient complement, and adaptive immune response.[100,101] Autoimmunity is present in 2% to 3% of CF patients including the presence of antineutrophil cytoplasmic autoantibodies that correlates with the efficiency in managing P aeruginosa infections and disease severity.[102,103] Autoantibodies against the bactericidal/permeability-increase (BPI) protein and the degraded form of SPLUNC1, important in the management of infections, are elevated in CF. BPI autoantibodies correlate with platelet numbers, impacting the inflammatory response to P aeruginosa, as well as efficient wound healing and clotting.[104,105]

In summary

- Inefficient anti-P aeruginosa neutralizing antibody isotypes highlight the defective adaptive immune response to lung infections in people with CF.
- CF pathophysiology may promote exposure to self-proteins, potentially contributing to autoimmunity and antibody-mediated platelet accumulation and activation.

POTENTIAL NEW PLAYERS MODIFYING THE IMMUNE RESPONSE IN PATIENTS WITH CYSTIC FIBROSIS
Innate Lymphoid Cells and Innate-like Lymphocytes

Innate lymphoid cells (ILCs) differentiate from lymphoid progenitors. In contrast to B- and T-cells that express antigen receptors and undergo clonal

selection and expansion when stimulated, ILCs mature into cells with specific phenotypes when exposed to microenvironmental cues, contributing to mucosal immune surveillance and activation of DCs. The CF lung microenvironment drives trans-differentiation of ILC precursors in specific types of ILCs (ie, ILC2) that secrete high IL-17A levels as well as contribute to mucin production and obstruction in CF airways.[106] Other innate-like lymphocytes such as mucosal-associated invariant T (MAIT) cells, γ δ T cells, and natural killer T (NKT) cells that share features with ILCs,[107] are also shown to be dysregulated in CF. MAITs are dramatically reduced in peripheral blood of patients with CF, and their reduction is positively correlated with P aeruginosa infection, pulmonary exacerbation, and increased severity of lung disease.[108,109] Patients with CF infected with P aeruginosa may have an increase in γ δ T cells[110] that contribute to IL-17A secretion in lung tissue, lymph nodes, and peripheral blood of patients with CF.[111] Finally, dysregulation of the invariant NKT population has been shown to be involved in attracting MΦ and neutrophils to the CF lungs.[112]

Platelets

Growing scientific evidence identifies platelets as critical players in immune processes, contributing to pulmonary inflammation and destruction in CF. Platelets isolated from patients with CF show an increased level of activation that correlates with the clinical and proinflammatory status of the patients.[113] CFTR modulator therapy can partially restore CF platelet dysfunction.[114] Hyperactivity of platelets can also enhance cardiovascular disease, as well as the incidence of neurologic events such as stroke in CF.[115,116]

Myeloid-Derived Suppressor Cells

Myeloid-derived suppressor cells (MDSCs) are a heterogeneous population of cells that derive from a pathologic state of activation of monocytes (M-MDSCs) and neutrophils (G-MDSCs) and have the key feature of inhibiting T-cell function. Studies using CF mice and samples from CF patients have shown that CF lungs have increased MDSC numbers—specifically G-MDSCs—that mediate T-cell suppression and have a detrimental impact on the adaptive immune response.[117,118]

Cell-to-Cell Communications via Extracellular Vesicles

Different types of cells in the lung communicate by the secretion and transfer of biological mediators (proteins, RNAs, lipids) through extracellular

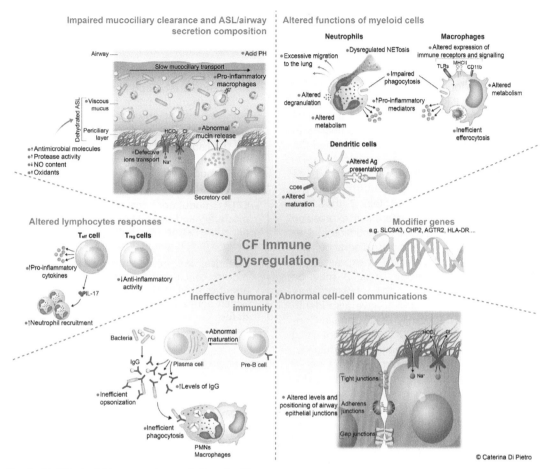

Fig. 2. Multifactorial immune dysregulations in CF.

vesicles (EVs) and exosomes. EVs can function by either promoting or inhibiting the immune responses defined by their contents. In CF, EVs promote lung inflammation and tissue damage.[119,120] Although less characterized, EVs are also abundantly secreted by neutrophils in CF lungs.[69] Bacterial-derived outer-membrane vesicles (OMVs) transport virulence factors, antibiotic-degrading enzymes, surface adherence factors, proteases, and enzymes that are important for nutrient acquisition and communication in the microbiome community. OMVs are also decoyed to prevent host immune cell attack by transferring information from the bacteria to host cells, disarming normal pathogen resolution strategies.[121] OMVs from *P aeruginosa* have been found to suppress MHC-related molecules in human lung MΦs as a strategy to evade the host immune response.[122]

Mesenchymal Stem Cells

MSCs have an immune-modulatory activity that may be beneficial in CF through their production of antimicrobial peptides, anti-inflammatory cytokines,[123,124] and EVs (MSC-EVs).[63] MSC and their products can be given as an allogeneic source, with no requirements for immunosuppression, but MSC donor selection is important for optimizing potency and potential efficacy.[125,126] The advantage of MSC therapeutics, over traditional anti-cytokine therapeutics, is the combined anti-microbial and anti-inflammatory function. Anti-cytokine therapy is counter-indicated in scenarios of infection, such as in CF.[127]

In summary

- Immune imbalance in CF is driven by many complementary mechanisms and diverse immune cell populations that requires further investigation.
- MSC and MSC-EVs hold promise as potential immune-modulatory therapeutics in CF.

IMMUNITY AND MODIFIER GENES IN CYSTIC FIBROSIS

Although mutations in the CFTR gene are the causative factor for the CF pathophysiology, genome-wide association studies have demonstrated that the severity of CF lung disease is influenced by gene variants located on other loci in the genome.[128] Several single nucleotide polymorphisms (SNPs) associated with the severity of CF lung disease are found at the human leukocyte antigen (HLA) class II locus.[128,129] Although the precise mechanisms by which SNPs in this locus modify the immune response in CF are unclear to date, the association between HLA-DR and CF lung disease severity is the most significant region in the genome. Among other modifier genes, there are the Na/H exchanger (*SLC9A3*)[130] and the Calcineurin Like EF-Hand Protein 2 that help controlling ASL pH. Their differential expression because of SNPs may change the antimicrobial responses[131] and the mucociliary clearance efficiency in CF airways. Variation in expression of the Angiotensin II Receptor Type 2 may be involved in controlling the inflammatory response.[132] Additional studies have also identified SNPs at the NLR Family Pyrin Domain Containing 3, NLR Family CARD Domain Containing 4, surfactant protein-D, and mannose-binding lectin. These genes are associated with increased *P aeruginosa* colonization and severity of lung disease in CF.[133,134] SNPs in genes that encode for immune mediators (eg, *IL-10*, *C3*, macrophage migration inhibitory factor, transforming growth factor beta, *IFN-γ*, and tumor necrosis factor α) have also been shown to correlate with CF lung pathology[135] (see also Anya T. Joynt and colleagues' article, "Genetics of Cystic Fibrosis: Clinical Implications," in this issue).

In summary

- Gene variants that modify the immune response contribute to the unique CF pathophysiology and the heterogeneity of disease severity in patients with the same CFTR mutations.

SUMMARY

Evidence suggests that CF patients have inherited and acquired factors that contribute to abnormal innate and adaptive immune regulation that support hyper-inflammation, defective bacterial clearance, and lung disease progression (**Fig. 2**). Effective, long-term therapies for CF will need to target and restore these inefficiencies of the immune response. More studies need to be pursued to understand the causes of dysregulated immunity in CF. Concurrent immune-supportive therapeutics with CFTR modulatory therapies, promise to provide CF patients with an improved quality of life.

CLINICS CARE POINTS

- CF patients have abnormal innate and adaptive immune regulation that support hyper-inflammation, defective bacterial clearance, and lung disease progression.

- More studies are needed to understand better the causes and consequences of dysregulated immunity in CF and to what extent CFTR modulator therapies correct the immune dysfunctions.

- CFTR modulator therapy has improved morbidity and mortality of the disease. Complications associated with long-term CF in older adults now need to be addressed.

- Effective, long-term therapies for CF may require concurrent immune-supportive therapeutics until there are curative treatments which permanently correct the CFTR genetic defect.

ACKNOWLEDGMENTS

The authors would like to thank Morgan Sutton BS (Graduate Student, St. Jude Graduate School of Biomedical Sciences, Memphis TN) for her edification and review of the article. This work was supported by The American Cystic Fibrosis Foundation (BONFIE20Y2-SCV to TLB; BRUS-CI20G0 to EMB), by The Marcus Foundation (CON211741 to TLB), and by the NIH (R01AI153422-01A1, R01HL157776-01A1 to EMB). The cartoon shown in Figure 2 is a creation by Caterina Di Pietro, Ph.D.

DISCLOSURE

The authors have nothing to disclose.

REFERENCES

1. Knowles MR, Boucher RC. Mucus clearance as a primary innate defense mechanism for mammalian airways. J Clin Invest 2002;109(5):571–7.
2. Esther CR Jr, Muhlebach MS, Ehre C, et al. Mucus accumulation in the lungs precedes structural changes and infection in children with cystic fibrosis. Sci Transl Med 2019;11(486).
3. Chen G, Sun L, Kato T, et al. IL-1beta dominates the promucin secretory cytokine profile in cystic fibrosis. J Clin Invest 2019;129(10):4433–50.
4. Montgomery ST, Mall MA, Kicic A, et al. Hypoxia and sterile inflammation in cystic fibrosis airways: mechanisms and potential therapies. Eur Respir J 2017;49(1).

5. Hoegger MJ, Fischer AJ, McMenimen, et al. Impaired mucus detachment disrupts mucociliary transport in a piglet model of cystic fibrosis. Science 2014;345(6198):818–22.

6. Tildy BE, Rogers DF. Therapeutic options for hydrating airway mucus in cystic fibrosis. Pharmacology 2015;95(3–4):117–32.

7. van Koningsbruggen-Rietschel S, Davies JC, Pressler T, et al. Inhaled dry powder alginate oligosaccharide in cystic fibrosis: a randomised, double-blind, placebo-controlled, crossover phase 2b study. ERJ Open Res 2020;6(4).

8. Martin SL, Saint-Criq V, Hwang TC, et al. Ion channels as targets to treat cystic fibrosis lung disease. J Cyst Fibros 2018;17(2S):S22–7.

9. Abou Alaiwa MH, Reznikov LR, Gansemer ND, et al. pH modulates the activity and synergism of the airway surface liquid antimicrobials beta-defensin-3 and LL-37. Proc Natl Acad Sci U S A 2014; 111(52):18703–8.

10. Rogan MP, Taggart CC, Greene CM, et al. Loss of microbicidal activity and increased formation of biofilm due to decreased lactoferrin activity in patients with cystic fibrosis. J Infect Dis 2004; 190(7):1245–53.

11. Ghio AJ, Roggli VL, Soukup JM, et al. Iron accumulates in the lavage and explanted lungs of cystic fibrosis patients. J Cyst Fibros 2013;12(4):390–8.

12. Moskwa P, Lorentzen D, Excoffon KJ, et al. A novel host defense system of airways is defective in cystic fibrosis. Am J Respir Crit Care Med 2007; 175(2):174–83.

13. Khanal S, Webster M, Niu N, et al. SPLUNC1: a novel marker of cystic fibrosis exacerbations. Eur Respir J 2021;58(5).

14. Berkebile AR, Bartlett JA, Abou Alaiwa M, et al. Airway Surface Liquid Has Innate Antiviral Activity That Is Reduced in Cystic Fibrosis. Am J Respir Cell Mol Biol 2020;62(1):104–11.

15. Tunney MM, Payne JE, McGrath SJ, et al. Activity of hypothiocyanite and lactoferrin (ALX-009) against respiratory cystic fibrosis pathogens in sputum. J Antimicrob Chemother 2018;73(12):3391–7.

16. Couroux P, Farias P, Rizvi L, et al. First clinical trials of novel ENaC targeting therapy, SPX-101, in healthy volunteers and adults with cystic fibrosis. Pulm Pharmacol Ther 2019;58:101819.

17. Goss CH, Kaneko Y, Khuu L, et al. Gallium disrupts bacterial iron metabolism and has therapeutic effects in mice and humans with lung infections. Sci Transl Med 2018;10(460):eaat7520.

18. Goldstein W, Doring G. Lysosomal-Enzymes from Polymorphonuclear Leukocytes and Proteinase-Inhibitors in Patients with Cystic-Fibrosis. Am Rev Respir Dis 1986;134(1):49–56.

19. Sagel SD, Wagner BD, Anthony MM, et al. Sputum biomarkers of inflammation and lung function decline in children with cystic fibrosis. Am J Respir Crit Care Med 2012;186(9):857–65.

20. Weldon S, McNally P, McAuley DF, et al. miR-31 dysregulation in cystic fibrosis airways contributes to increased pulmonary cathepsin S production. Am J Respir Crit Care Med 2014;190(2):165–74.

21. Witko-Sarsat V, Halbwachs-Mecarelli L, Schuster A, et al. Proteinase 3, a potent secretagogue in airways, is present in cystic fibrosis sputum. Am J Respir Cell Mol Biol 1999;20(4):729–36.

22. Garratt LW, Sutanto EN, Ling KM, et al. Australian Respiratory Early Surveillance Team for Cystic F. Matrix metalloproteinase activation by free neutrophil elastase contributes to bronchiectasis progression in early cystic fibrosis. Eur Respir J 2015;46(2):384–94.

23. Harris JK, Wagner BD, Zemanick ET, et al. Changes in Airway Microbiome and Inflammation with Ivacaftor Treatment in Patients with Cystic Fibrosis and the G551D Mutation. Ann Am Thorac Soc 2020;17(2):212–20.

24. Chalmers JD, Haworth CS, Metersky ML, et al. Investigators W. Phase 2 Trial of the DPP-1 Inhibitor Brensocatib in Bronchiectasis. N Engl J Med 2020;383(22):2127–37.

25. Shen XB, Chen X, Zhang ZY, et al. Cathepsin C inhibitors as anti-inflammatory drug discovery: Challenges and opportunities. Eur J Med Chem 2021; 225:113818.

26. Barth P, Bruijnzeel P, Wach A, et al. Single dose escalation studies with inhaled POL6014, a potent novel selective reversible inhibitor of human neutrophil elastase, in healthy volunteers and subjects with cystic fibrosis. J Cyst Fibros 2020;19(2):299–304.

27. Mejias JC, Forrest OA, Margaroli C, et al. Neutrophil-targeted, protease-activated pulmonary drug delivery blocks airway and systemic inflammation. JCI Insight 2019;4(23).

28. Bogdan C. Nitric oxide and the immune response. Nat Immunol 2001;2(10):907–16.

29. Grasemann H, Michler E, Wallot M, et al. Decreased concentration of exhaled nitric oxide (NO) in patients with cystic fibrosis. Pediatr Pulmonol 1997;24(3):173–7.

30. Kelley TJ, Drumm ML. Inducible nitric oxide synthase expression is reduced in cystic fibrosis murine and human airway epithelial cells. J Clin Invest 1998;102(6):1200–7.

31. Grasemann H, Schwiertz R, Matthiesen S, et al. Increased arginase activity in cystic fibrosis airways. Am J Respir Crit Care Med 2005;172(12): 1523–8.

32. Grasemann H, Gonska T, Avolio J, et al. Effect of ivacaftor therapy on exhaled nitric oxide in patients with cystic fibrosis. J Cyst Fibros 2015.

33. Bentur L, Gur M, Ashkenazi M, et al. Pilot study to test inhaled nitric oxide in cystic fibrosis patients

with refractory Mycobacterium abscessus lung infection. J Cyst Fibros 2020;19(2):225–31.

34. Galli F, Battistoni A, Gambari R, et al. Oxidative stress and antioxidant therapy in cystic fibrosis. Biochim Biophys Acta 2012;1822(5):690–713.

35. Veltman M, De Sanctis JB, Stolarczyk M, et al. CFTR Correctors and Antioxidants Partially Normalize Lipid Imbalance but not Abnormal Basal Inflammatory Cytokine Profile in CF Bronchial Epithelial Cells. Front Physiol 2021;12:619442.

36. Pohl C, Hermanns MI, Uboldi C, et al. Barrier functions and paracellular integrity in human cell culture models of the proximal respiratory unit. Eur J Pharm Biopharm 2009;72(2):339–49.

37. Huang S, Jornot L, Wiszniewski L, et al. Src signaling links mediators of inflammation to Cx43 gap junction channels in primary and transformed CFTR-expressing airway cells. Cell Commun Adhes 2003;10(4–6):279–85.

38. Molina SA, Stauffer B, Moriarty HK, et al. Junctional abnormalities in human airway epithelial cells expressing F508del CFTR. Am J Physiol Lung Cell Mol Physiol 2015;309(5):L475–87.

39. Weiser N, Molenda N, Urbanova K, et al. Paracellular permeability of bronchial epithelium is controlled by CFTR. Cell Physiol Biochem 2011; 28(2):289–96.

40. Asgrimsson V, Gudjonsson T, Gudmundsson GH, et al. Novel effects of azithromycin on tight junction proteins in human airway epithelia. Antimicrob Agents Chemother 2006;50(5):1805–12.

41. Akira S, Uematsu S, Takeuchi O. Pathogen recognition and innate immunity. Cell 2006;124(4): 783–801.

42. Bruscia EM, Bonfield TL. Cystic Fibrosis Lung Immunity: The Role of the Macrophage. J Innate Immun 2016;8(6):550–63.

43. Lara-Reyna S, Holbrook J, Jarosz-Griffiths HH, et al. Dysregulated signalling pathways in innate immune cells with cystic fibrosis mutations. Cell Mol Life Sci 2020;77(22):4485–503.

44. Riquelme SA, Prince A. Pseudomonas aeruginosa Consumption of Airway Metabolites Promotes Lung Infection. Pathogens 2021;10(8).

45. Zheng S, De BP, Choudhary S, et al. Impaired innate host defense causes susceptibility to respiratory virus infections in cystic fibrosis. Immunity 2003;18(5):619–30.

46. Stanton BA, Hampton TH, Ashare A. SARS-CoV-2 (COVID-19) and cystic fibrosis. Am J Physiol Lung Cell Mol Physiol 2020;319(3):L408–15.

47. Cigana C, Nicolis E, Pasetto M, et al. Anti-inflammatory effects of azithromycin in cystic fibrosis airway epithelial cells. Biochem Biophys Res Commun 2006;350(4):977–82.

48. Manti S, Parisi GF, Papale M, et al. Looking beyond pulmonary disease in COVID-19: A lesson from patients with cystic fibrosis. Med Hypotheses 2021;147:110481.

49. Iannitti RG, Napolioni V, Oikonomou V, et al. IL-1 receptor antagonist ameliorates inflammasome-dependent inflammation in murine and human cystic fibrosis. Nat Commun 2016;7:10791.

50. Deng J, Yu XQ, Wang PH. Inflammasome activation and Th17 responses. Mol Immunol 2019;107:142–64.

51. Flores-Vega V, Vargas-Roldán S, Lezana-Fernández J, et al. Bacterial Subversion of Autophagy in Cystic Fibrosis. Front Cell Infect Microbiol 2021;11:760922.

52. Freedman SD, Blanco PG, Zaman MM, et al. Association of cystic fibrosis with abnormalities in fatty acid metabolism. N Engl J Med 2004;350(6):560–9.

53. Recchiuti A, Mattoscio D, Isopi E. Roles, Actions, and Therapeutic Potential of Specialized Pro-resolving Lipid Mediators for the Treatment of Inflammation in Cystic Fibrosis. Front Pharmacol 2019;10:252.

54. Yang J, Eiserich JP, Cross CE, et al. Metabolomic profiling of regulatory lipid mediators in sputum from adult cystic fibrosis patients. Free Radic Biol Med 2012;53(1):160–71.

55. Ringholz FC, Buchanan PJ, Clarke DT, et al. Reduced 15-lipoxygenase 2 and lipoxin A4/leukotriene B4 ratio in children with cystic fibrosis. Eur Respir J 2014;44(2):394–404.

56. White NM, Jiang D, Burgess JD, et al. Altered cholesterol homeostasis in cultured and in vivo models of cystic fibrosis. Am J Physiol Lung Cell Mol Physiol 2007;292(2):L476–86.

57. Worgall TS. Lipid metabolism in cystic fibrosis. Curr Opin Clin Nutr Metab Care 2009;12(2):105–9.

58. Konstan MW, VanDevanter DR, Sawicki GS, et al. Association of High-Dose Ibuprofen Use, Lung Function Decline, and Long-Term Survival in Children with Cystic Fibrosis. Ann Am Thorac Soc 2018;15(4):485–93.

59. Youssef M, De Sanctis JB, Shah J, et al. Treatment of Allergic Asthma with Fenretinide Formulation (LAU-7b) Downregulates ORMDL Sphingolipid Biosynthesis Regulator 3 (Ormdl3) Expression and Normalizes Ceramide Imbalance. J Pharmacol Exp Ther 2020;373(3):476–87.

60. McElvaney OJ, Zaslona Z, Becker-Flegler K, et al. Specific Inhibition of the NLRP3 Inflammasome as an Antiinflammatory Strategy in Cystic Fibrosis. Am J Respir Crit Care Med 2019;200(11):1381–91.

61. Grasemann H, Grasemann C, Kurtz F, et al. Oral L-arginine supplementation in cystic fibrosis patients: a placebo-controlled study. Eur Respir J 2005; 25(1):62–8.

62. Nichols DP, Ziady AG, Shank SL, et al. The triterpenoid CDDO limits inflammation in preclinical models of cystic fibrosis lung disease. Am J Physiol Lung Cell Mol Physiol 2009;297(5):L828–36.

63. Sutton MT, Fletcher D, Ghosh SK, et al. Antimicrobial Properties of Mesenchymal Stem Cells: Therapeutic Potential for Cystic Fibrosis Infection, and Treatment. Stem Cells Int 2016;2016:5303048.

64. Munshi A, Mehic J, Creskey M, et al. A comprehensive proteomics profiling identifies NRP1 as a novel identity marker of human bone marrow mesenchymal stromal cell-derived small extracellular vesicles. Stem Cell Res Ther 2019;10(1):401.

65. Khan MA, Ali ZS, Sweezey N, et al. Progression of Cystic Fibrosis Lung Disease from Childhood to Adulthood: Neutrophils, Neutrophil Extracellular Trap (NET) Formation, and NET Degradation. Genes (Basel). 2019;10(3).

66. Jennings LK, Dreifus JE, Reichhardt C, et al. Pseudomonas aeruginosa aggregates in cystic fibrosis sputum produce exopolysaccharides that likely impede current therapies. Cell Rep 2021;34(8):108782.

67. Painter RG, Valentine VG, Lanson NA, et al. CFTR Expression in human neutrophils and the phagolysosomal chlorination defect in cystic fibrosis. Biochemistry 2006;45(34):10260–9.

68. Pohl K, Hayes E, Keenan J, et al. A neutrophil intrinsic impairment affecting Rab27a and degranulation in cystic fibrosis is corrected by CFTR potentiator therapy. Blood 2014;124(7):999–1009.

69. Giacalone VD, Margaroli C, Mall MA, et al. Neutrophil Adaptations upon Recruitment to the Lung: New Concepts and Implications for Homeostasis and Disease. Int J Mol Sci 2020;21(3).

70. Margaroli C, Moncada-Giraldo D, Gulick DA, et al. Transcriptional firing represses bactericidal activity in cystic fibrosis airway neutrophils. Cell Rep Med 2021;2(4):100239.

71. Konstan MW, Doring G, Heltshe SL, et al. A randomized double blind, placebo controlled phase 2 trial of BIIL 284 BS (an LTB4 receptor antagonist) for the treatment of lung disease in children and adults with cystic fibrosis. J Cyst Fibros 2014;13(2):148–55.

72. Elborn JS, Konstan MW, Taylor-Cousar JL, et al. Empire-CF study: A phase 2 clinical trial of leukotriene A4 hydrolase inhibitor acebilustat in adult subjects with cystic fibrosis. J Cyst Fibros 2021;20(6):1026–34.

73. Gillan JL, Davidson DJ, Gray RD. Targeting cystic fibrosis inflammation in the age of CFTR modulators: focus on macrophages. Eur Respir J 2021;57(6).

74. Morales-Nebreda L, Misharin AV, Perlman H, et al. The heterogeneity of lung macrophages in the susceptibility to disease. Eur Respir Rev 2015;24(137):505–9.

75. Hubeau C, Puchelle E, Gaillard D. Distinct pattern of immune cell population in the lung of human fetuses with cystic fibrosis. J Allergy Clin Immunol 2001;108(4):524–9.

76. Brennan S, Sly PD, Gangell CL, et al. Alveolar macrophages and CC chemokines are increased in children with cystic fibrosis. Eur Respir J 2009;34(3):655–61.

77. Schupp JC, Khanal S, Gomez JL, et al. Single Cell Transcriptional Archetypes of Airway Inflammation in Cystic Fibrosis. Am J Respir Crit Care Med 2020.

78. del Fresno C, Gomez-Pina V, Lores V, et al. Monocytes from cystic fibrosis patients are locked in an LPS tolerance state: down-regulation of TREM-1 as putative underlying mechanism. PLoS ONE 2008;3(7):e2667.

79. Avendano-Ortiz J, Llanos-Gonzalez E, Toledano V, et al. Pseudomonas aeruginosa colonization causes PD-L1 overexpression on monocytes, impairing the adaptive immune response in patients with cystic fibrosis. J Cyst Fibros 2019;18(5):630–5.

80. Sorio C, Montresor A, Bolomini-Vittori M, et al. Mutations of Cystic Fibrosis Transmembrane Conductance Regulator Gene Cause a Monocyte-Selective Adhesion Deficiency. Am J Respir Crit Care Med 2016;193(10):1123–33.

81. Hisert KB, Birkland TP, Schoenfelt KQ, et al. CFTR Modulator Therapy Enhances Peripheral Blood Monocyte Contributions to Immune Responses in People With Cystic Fibrosis. Front Pharmacol 2020;11:1219.

82. Jarosz-Griffiths HH, Scambler T, Wong CH, et al. Different CFTR modulator combinations downregulate inflammation differently in cystic fibrosis. Elife 2020;9.

83. Hisert KB, Birkland TP, Schoenfelt KQ, et al. Ivacaftor decreases monocyte sensitivity to interferon-gamma in people with cystic fibrosis. ERJ Open Res 2020;6(2).

84. Vandivier RW, Fadok VA, Hoffmann PR, et al. Elastase-mediated phosphatidylserine receptor cleavage impairs apoptotic cell clearance in cystic fibrosis and bronchiectasis. J Clin Invest 2002;109(5):661–70.

85. Ma J, Kummarapurugu AB, Hawkridge A, et al. Neutrophil elastase-regulated macrophage sheddome/secretome and phagocytic failure. Am J Physiol Lung Cell Mol Physiol 2021;321(3):L555–65.

86. Hofer TP, Frankenberger M, Heimbeck I, et al. Decreased expression of HLA-DQ and HLA-DR on cells of the monocytic lineage in cystic fibrosis. J Mol Med (Berl) 2014;92(12):1293–304.

87. Xu Y, Krause A, Limberis M, et al. Low sphingosine-1-phosphate impairs lung dendritic cells in cystic fibrosis. Am J Respir Cell Mol Biol 2013;48(2):250–7.

88. Roghanian A, Drost EM, MacNee W, et al. Inflammatory lung secretions inhibit dendritic cell

maturation and function via neutrophil elastase. Am J Respir Crit Care Med 2006;174(11):1189–98.

89. Mueller C, Braag SA, Keeler A, et al. Lack of cystic fibrosis transmembrane conductance regulator in CD3+ lymphocytes leads to aberrant cytokine secretion and hyperinflammatory adaptive immune responses. Am J Respir Cell Mol Biol 2011;44(6):922–9.

90. Iannitti RG, Carvalho A, Cunha C, et al. Th17/Treg imbalance in murine cystic fibrosis is linked to indoleamine 2,3-dioxygenase deficiency but corrected by kynurenines. Am J Respir Crit Care Med 2013;187(6):609–20.

91. Chan YR, Chen K, Duncan SR, et al. Patients with cystic fibrosis have inducible IL-17+IL-22+ memory cells in lung draining lymph nodes. J Allergy Clin Immunol 2013;131(4):1117–29, 1129.e1-5.

92. Iwanaga N, Kolls JK. Updates on T helper type 17 immunity in respiratory disease. Immunology 2019;156(1):3–8.

93. Hsu D, Taylor P, Fletcher D, et al. Interleukin-17 Pathophysiology and Therapeutic Intervention in Cystic Fibrosis Lung Infection and Inflammation. Infect Immun 2016;84(9):2410–21.

94. Rehman T, Karp PH, Tan P, et al. Inflammatory cytokines TNF-alpha and IL-17 enhance the efficacy of cystic fibrosis transmembrane conductance regulator modulators. J Clin Invest 2021;131(16).

95. Hector A, Schafer H, Poschel S, et al. Regulatory T-cell impairment in cystic fibrosis patients with chronic pseudomonas infection. Am J Respir Crit Care Med 2015;191(8):914–23.

96. McGuire JK. Regulatory T cells in cystic fibrosis lung disease. More answers, more questions. Am J Respir Crit Care Med 2015;191(8):866–8.

97. Ideozu JE, Rangaraj V, Abdala-Valencia H, et al. Transcriptional consequences of impaired immune cell responses induced by cystic fibrosis plasma characterized via dual RNA sequencing. BMC Med Genomics 2019;12(1):66.

98. Mauch RM, Rossi CL, Nolasco da Silva MT, et al. Secretory IgA-mediated immune response in saliva and early detection of Pseudomonas aeruginosa in the lower airways of pediatric cystic fibrosis patients. Med Microbiol Immunol 2019;208(2):205–13.

99. Mauch RM, Rossi CL, Ribeiro JD, et al. Assessment of IgG antibodies to Pseudomonas aeruginosa in patients with cystic fibrosis by an enzyme-linked immunosorbent assay (ELISA). Diagn Pathol 2014;9:158.

100. Kristiansen TA, Vanhee S, Yuan J. The influence of developmental timing on B cell diversity. Curr Opin Immunol 2018;51:7–13.

101. Moss RB. Mucosal humoral immunity in cystic fibrosis - a tangled web of failed proteostasis, infection and adaptive immunity. EBioMedicine 2020;60:103035.

102. Theprungsirikul J, Skopelja-Gardner S, Meagher RE, et al. Dissociation of systemic and mucosal autoimmunity in cystic fibrosis. J Cyst Fibros 2020;19(2):196–202.

103. Sposito F, McNamara PS, Hedrich CM. Vasculitis in Cystic Fibrosis. Front Pediatr 2020;8:585275.

104. Skopelja S, Hamilton BJ, Jones JD, et al. The role for neutrophil extracellular traps in cystic fibrosis autoimmunity. JCI Insight 2016;1(17):e88912.

105. Hovold G, Lindberg U, Ljungberg JK, et al. BPI-ANCA is expressed in the airways of cystic fibrosis patients and correlates to platelet numbers and Pseudomonas aeruginosa colonization. Respir Med 2020;170:105994.

106. Webster MJ, Reidel B, Tan CD, et al. SPLUNC1 degradation by the cystic fibrosis mucosal environment drives airway surface liquid dehydration. Eur Respir J 2018;52(4).

107. Lewis BW, Choudhary I, Paudel K, et al. The Innate Lymphoid System Is a Critical Player in the Manifestation of Mucoinflammatory Airway Disease in Mice. J Immunol 2020;205(6):1695–708.

108. Fan X, Rudensky AY. Hallmarks of Tissue-Resident Lymphocytes. Cell 2016;164(6):1198–211.

109. Smith DJ, Hill GR, Bell SC, et al. Reduced mucosal associated invariant T-cells are associated with increased disease severity and Pseudomonas aeruginosa infection in cystic fibrosis. PLoS One 2014;9(10):e109891.

110. Pincikova T, Paquin-Proulx D, Moll M, et al. Severely Impaired Control of Bacterial Infections in a Patient With Cystic Fibrosis Defective in Mucosal-Associated Invariant T Cells. Chest 2018;153(5):e93–6.

111. Raga S, Julia MR, Crespi C, et al. Gammadelta T lymphocytes from cystic fibrosis patients and healthy donors are high TNF-alpha and IFN-gamma-producers in response to Pseudomonas aeruginosa. Respir Res 2003;4:9.

112. Hagner M, Albrecht M, Guerra M, et al. IL-17A from innate and adaptive lymphocytes contributes to inflammation and damage in cystic fibrosis lung disease. Eur Respir J 2021;57(6).

113. Siegmann N, Worbs D, Effinger, et al. Invariant natural killer T (iNKT) cells prevent autoimmunity, but induce pulmonary inflammation in cystic fibrosis. Cell Physiol Biochem 2014;34(1):56–70.

114. Lindberg U, Svensson L, Hellmark T, et al. Increased platelet activation occurs in cystic fibrosis patients and correlates to clinical status. Thromb Res 2018;162:32–7.

115. Ortiz-Munoz G, Yu MA, Lefrancais E, et al. Cystic fibrosis transmembrane conductance regulator dysfunction in platelets drives lung hyperinflammation. J Clin Invest 2020;130(4):2041–53.

116. Hoffman M, Gerding JP, Zuckerman JB. Stroke and myocardial infarction following bronchial artery embolization in a cystic fibrosis patient. J Cyst Fibros 2017;16(1):161–2.

117. Ellis S, Rang C, Kotsimbos T, et al. CNS imaging studies in cystic fibrosis patients presenting with sudden neurological events. BMJ Open Respir Res 2019;6(1):e000456.

118. Oz HH, Zhou B, Voss P, et al. Pseudomonas aeruginosa Airway Infection Recruits and Modulates Neutrophilic Myeloid-Derived Suppressor Cells. Front Cell Infect Microbiol 2016;6:167.

119. Tucker SL, Sarr D, Rada B. Granulocytic Myeloid-Derived Suppressor Cells in Cystic Fibrosis. Front Immunol 2021;12:745326.

120. Koeppen K, Nymon A, Barnaby R, et al. CF monocyte-derived macrophages have an attenuated response to extracellular vesicles secreted by airway epithelial cells. Am J Physiol Lung Cell Mol Physiol 2021;320(4):L530–44.

121. Szul T, Bratcher PE, Fraser KB, et al. Toll-Like Receptor 4 Engagement Mediates Prolyl Endopeptidase Release from Airway Epithelia via Exosomes. Am J Respir Cell Mol Biol 2016;54(3):359–69.

122. Schwechheimer C, Kuehn MJ. Outer-membrane vesicles from Gram-negative bacteria: biogenesis and functions. Nat Rev Microbiol 2015;13(10):605–19.

123. Armstrong DA, Lee MK, Hazlett HF, et al. Extracellular Vesicles from Pseudomonas aeruginosa Suppress MHC-Related Molecules in Human Lung Macrophages. Immunohorizons 2020;4(8):508–19.

124. Sutton MT, Fletcher D, Episalla N, et al. Mesenchymal Stem Cell Soluble Mediators and Cystic Fibrosis. J Stem Cell Res Ther 2017;7(9).

125. Zulueta A, Colombo M, Peli V, et al. Lung mesenchymal stem cells-derived extracellular vesicles attenuate the inflammatory profile of Cystic Fibrosis epithelial cells. Cell Signal 2018;51:110–8.

126. van Heeckeren AM, Sutton MT, Fletcher DR, et al. Enhancing Cystic Fibrosis Immune Regulation. Front Pharmacol 2021;12:573065.

127. Bonfield TL, Sutton MT, Fletcher DR, et al. Donor-defined mesenchymal stem cell antimicrobial potency against nontuberculous mycobacterium. Stem Cells Transl Med 2021;10(8):1202–16.

128. Drutskaya MS, Efimov GA, Kruglov AA, et al. Can we design a better anti-cytokine therapy? J Leukoc Biol 2017;102(3):783–90.

129. Corvol H, Blackman SM, Boelle PY, et al. Genome-wide association meta-analysis identifies five modifier loci of lung disease severity in cystic fibrosis. Nat Commun 2015;6:8382.

130. Wright FA, Strug LJ, Doshi VK, et al. Genome-wide association and linkage identify modifier loci of lung disease severity in cystic fibrosis at 11p13 and 20q13.2. Nat Genet 2011;43(6):539–46.

131. Dorfman R, Taylor C, Lin F, et al. Members of Canadian Consortium for CFGS. Modulatory effect of the SLC9A3 gene on susceptibility to infections and pulmonary function in children with cystic fibrosis. Pediatr Pulmonol 2011;46(4):385–92.

132. Namkoong H, Omae Y, Asakura T, et al. Genome-wide association study in patients with pulmonary Mycobacterium avium complex disease. Eur Respir J 2021;58(2).

133. Darrah RJ, Jacono FJ, Joshi N, et al. AGTR2 absence or antagonism prevents cystic fibrosis pulmonary manifestations. J Cyst Fibros 2019;18(1):127–34.

134. Graustein AD, Berrington WR, Buckingham KJ, et al. Inflammasome Genetic Variants, Macrophage Function, and Clinical Outcomes in Cystic Fibrosis. Am J Respir Cell Mol Biol 2021;65(2):157–66.

135. Nourkami-Tutdibi N, Freitag K, Zemlin M, et al. Genetic Association With Pseudomonas aeruginosa Acquisition in Cystic Fibrosis: Influence of Surfactant Protein D and Mannose-Binding Lectin. Front Immunol 2021;12:587313.

136. Weiler CA, Drumm ML. Genetic influences on cystic fibrosis lung disease severity. Front Pharmacol 2013;4:40.

Novel Applications of Biomarkers and Personalized Medicine in Cystic Fibrosis

Jennifer S. Guimbellot, MD, PhD[a], David P. Nichols, MD[b], John J. Brewington, MD, MS[c,d,*]

KEYWORDS

• Personalized medicine • Cystic fibrosis • CFTR • CFTR modulator

KEY POINTS

- In order to further personalize care of people with cystic fibrosis (CF), several research approaches are being translated into patient care.
- Patient-derived model systems, including those from gastrointestinal, respiratory, and induced pluripotent stem cells can be used to select the optimal cystic fibrosis transmembrane conductance regulator modulator therapies across a diverse group of patients.
- Application of pharmacokinetic, pharmacodynamic, and pharmacogenetic approaches may help titrate dosing of CF-relevant therapies.
- Emerging sensitive disease markers will be better able to follow disease progression in an increasingly healthy population.
- Novel clinical trial design approaches are necessary to streamline care and identify new opportunities to further personalize treatment.

INTRODUCTION

Increasing therapeutic options for people with cystic fibrosis (PwCF) have increased the importance of personalized care decisions. Examples of this include: variable pancreatic enzyme replacement needs, targeted antimicrobial therapies, inhaled drug delivery devices, and now cystic fibrosis transmembrane conductance regulator (CFTR) modulator therapies prescribed based on particular *CFTR* genotypes. Modulators directly target an individual's abnormal CFTR protein(s)

to significantly affect disease morbidity when combined with traditional, symptom-based therapies.[1–6] Highly effective modulator therapies (HEMT) are now Food and Drug Administration (FDA) approved for approximately 90% of PwCF based on genotype, presenting new opportunities to personalize treatment decisions in an effort to maximize overall health.

To start, genotype-directed therapy with HEMT remains unavailable to a significant minority of PwCF. Among this cohort is a subset of patients harboring *CFTR* mutations that may benefit from

[a] Department of Pediatrics, Division of Pulmonary and Sleep Medicine, Gregory Fleming James Cystic Fibrosis Research Center, University of Alabama at Birmingham; 1600 7th Avenue South, ACC 620, Birmingham, AL 35233, USA; [b] Department of Pediatrics, Division of Pulmonary Medicine, Seattle Children's Hospital, University of Washington School of Medicine, Building Cure, 1920 Terry Avenue, Office 4-209, Seattle, WA 98109, USA; [c] Department of Pediatrics, University of Cincinnati College of Medicine, 3230 Eden Avenue, Cincinnati, OH 45267, USA; [d] Division of Pulmonary Medicine, Cincinnati Children's Hospital Medical Center, 3333 Burnet Avenue, MLC 2021, Cincinnati, OH 45229, USA
* Corresponding author. Division of Pulmonary Medicine, Cincinnati Children's Hospital Medical Center, 3333 Burnet Avenue, MLC 2021, Cincinnati, OH 45229.
E-mail address: john.brewington@cchmc.org

Clin Chest Med 43 (2022) 617–630
https://doi.org/10.1016/j.ccm.2022.06.005
0272-5231/22/© 2022 Elsevier Inc. All rights reserved.

existing drugs but currently has no pathway to therapy. Due to the population-specific prevalence of certain alleles (namely F508del), some racial or ethnic minority populations with CF are less likely to be eligible for HEMT.[7] Identifying less common mutations responsive to HEMT will improve care outcomes and may assist efforts to close existing inequities in health outcomes for minority populations, who have lower average lung function and increased symptoms compared with Caucasians with CF.[8,9] Second, the real-world pharmacology of HEMT and how individualized differences in drug absorption and distribution may affect clinical outcomes is poorly understood.[10] Ongoing research may help to inform patient drug titration.[11,12] Finally, the current standard-of-care is to continue previous symptom-based therapies (eg, airway clearance therapies, inhaled antibiotics), which will assuredly benefit some but not all individuals. Eliminating unnecessary therapies reduces risk, cost, and burden of care but must be approached cautiously.

Several research efforts will help to provide more personalized care recommendations: assays to identify the most effective modulator therapies, better understanding of how to personalize drug dosing, sensitive biomarkers relevant to an increasingly healthy population, and, finally, proven outcomes to evaluate response to changes or addition of new therapies. Herein, we will describe tools that are currently available or emerging to address these needs and advance personalized care in CF, which are summarized in **Fig. 1**. Most of the discussion will focus on CFTR modulator therapies, although attention will be paid to symptomatic therapies and the broader patient treatment composition. Much of the content will focus on emerging research studies with high translational potential because the current standard-of-care tools to personalize care are limited. We anticipate these approaches will become more commonplace in CF care during the coming years.

DISCUSSION
Therapeutic Selection

The emergence of a *CFTR* genotype-specific approach to modulator therapies has dramatically altered CF care but opportunities to improve overall outcomes and better personalize treatment decisions remain.[2–6] Individuals harboring certain rare *CFTR* variants may potentially benefit from CFTR modulators but have no straightforward pathway to access drug. In addition, population variance in therapeutic response remains wide, and single individuals may be eligible for more than one modulator drug. To optimize the

therapeutic benefit, tools are needed to identify the best available modulator treatment.

Many such tools exist and have aided in the development of the current care model, such as Fisher Rat Thyroid (FRT) cell lines that have been heavily used in CF research since the 1990s.[13] FRT cells facilitated preclinical development of HEMT, as well as FDA label expansion (the first such use of in vitro data). Although such heterologous and immortalized cell lines may improve therapeutic access for those with rare variants, they do not address individual variance in therapeutic response or ultrarare mutations present in single or very small numbers of individuals. To achieve this, patient-derived, personalized model systems are necessary.

Gastrointestinal organoids generated from rectal or intestinal biopsies have been used for this purpose.[14] Numerous studies have demonstrated the capacity of this model to quantify CFTR activity and pharmacologic rescue across both common and rare *CFTR* variant groups.[14–23] Organoid model data have been linked to historical cohort clinical data, supporting the relevance of this ex vivo model.[15,17,23] This model has been used at scale across several studies, primarily in Europe, and are used for individual drug selection through the human individualized treatment for cystic fibrosis (HIT-CF) study, which seeks to identify optimal therapies for individual subjects (https://www.hitcf.org/).[18] Although still research tools, these models are being actively translated into patient care where available.

Human bronchial epithelial cells are considered a gold standard in pulmonary research but procurement is invasive and rarely performed.[24] Alternatively, researchers have used human nasal epithelial (HNE) cells, which are easily obtained in even very young patients.[25–29] These cells are expanded and differentiated as either air–liquid interface (ALI) or organoid/spheroid cultures.[25,30–35] Both models quantify CFTR function and modulation, correlate internally, and have been used for common or rare *CFTR* genotype groups.[32,33,36,37] Numerous studies have tied model function to historical cohort data or patient-specific outcome measures, although often in small numbers.[33,36,38,39] More recent reports highlight the use of such data to inform off-label prescription of CFTR modulators supported by third-party payors to directly inform patient-specific care.[40]

Several gaps must continue to be addressed to further allow cell-based assays to inform clinical care. First, identifying the right model depends on the goal. As noted above, FRT cells have succeeded in generating regulatory change, whereas personalized models provide individual resolution.

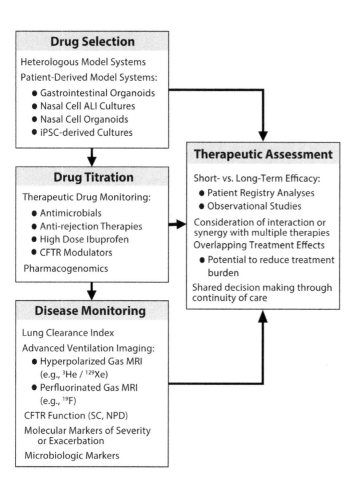

Drug Selection

Heterologous Model Systems

Patient-Derived Model Systems:
- Gastrointestinal Organoids
- Nasal Cell ALI Cultures
- Nasal Cell Organoids
- iPSC-derived Cultures

Drug Titration

Therapeutic Drug Monitoring:
- Antimicrobials
- Anti-rejection Therapies
- High Dose Ibuprofen
- CFTR Modulators

Pharmacogenomics

Disease Monitoring

Lung Clearance Index

Advanced Ventilation Imaging:
- Hyperpolarized Gas MRI
  (e.g., ³He / ¹²⁹Xe)
- Perfluorinated Gas MRI
  (e.g., ¹⁹F)

CFTR Function (SC, NPD)

Molecular Markers of Severity
  or Exacerbation

Microbiologic Markers

Therapeutic Assessment

Short- vs. Long-Term Efficacy:
- Patient Registry Analyses
- Observational Studies

Consideration of interaction or
synergy with multiple therapies
Overlapping Treatment Effects
- Potential to reduce treatment
  burden

Shared decision making through
continuity of care

Fig. 1. Overview of existing and emerging tools and approaches for personalized medicine in cystic fibrosis. ALI, air–liquid interface; CFTR, cystic fibrosis transmembrane conductance regulator; iPSC, induced pluripotent stem cell; NPD, nasal potential difference; SC, sweat chloride.

Additionally, the best tissue source remains unclear; all models carry strengths and weaknesses (summarized in **Table 1**), and selection is likely influenced by model availability. Next, although all models above approximate clinically relevant outcomes, understanding the accuracy of this approximation will be necessary in translating these measurements to compare therapeutic options. In order to fully translate such models into care, novel approaches for centralized testing, improved access, and drug approval/expansion will be needed. The success of the HIT-CF program may inform such work in HNE models.

Pharmacology and Pharmacogenomics— Approach to Personalized Therapies

Therapeutic drug monitoring (TDM) and pharmacogenomics (PGx) present a currently underutilized area for personalized CF care. Characterization of any novel medication includes pharmacokinetic (measures of drug exposure) and pharmacodynamic (relationship between drug exposure and response) (PK/PD) modeling in a

small group of patients. Once approved and expanded to the wider population, ongoing investigation can reveal additional areas for drug monitoring to manage side effect profiles and optimize therapy. In clinical practice, precision dosing of medications can have an important role in titrating dose to effect but requires specialized resources for rapid drug quantitation, relevant genotyping, and pharmacologic interpretation, which may not be universally available. TDM can improve personalized care by informing individual dosing strategies, even in the face of potential drug interactions.[41] In this section, the use of TDM and PGx for personalized medicine in clinical practice is discussed; these concepts are summarized in **Fig. 2**.

Variation in drug exposure among PwCF due to altered absorption, metabolism, distribution, and clearance of drugs is well recognized and known to have pronounced impact on drug efficacy.[42–45] For example, ciprofloxacin, metabolized by CYP3A4 and CYP1A2, has such a wide variation in plasma concentrations that some CF patients cannot reach therapeutic exposure with standard

Table 1
Comparison of commonly used patient-derived models for personalized cystic fibrosis transmembrane conductance regulator study

Model System	Sample Source	Expansion Capacity	Primary Measurement	Key Strengths	Limitations
Gastrointestinal organoids	Rectum, intestine	High	Fluid Efflux	Well characterized, high expansion and banking potential, generates large N for analysis	Limited adoption in North America
Bronchial cell ALI culture	Lower airway explants	Moderate	Chloride conductance/ Current	Extremely well characterized, relevant respiratory model	Invasive procurement, limited sample pool
Nasal cell ALI culture	Nasopharynx	Low	Chloride conductance/ current	Easy access to sample in all ages, recapitulates many bronchial cell culture characteristics	Small N with limited expansion
Nasal cell organoids	Nasopharynx	Low	Fluid efflux	Easy access to sample in all ages, recapitulates many bronchial cell culture characteristics	Small N with limited expansion
iPSC-derived models	Skin or blood fibroblasts	Very high	Chloride conductance/ current or fluid efflux	Very-high potential for expansion and banking, ease of sample access	Limited characterization in early development, time-intensive generation

dosing.[43] Similarly, tacrolimus, an immunosuppressant used in solid organ transplant, requires altered dosing in CF recipients versus non-CF to achieve therapeutic concentrations.[46] Currently, the most frequent indication for TDM in CF is the monitoring of antimicrobials.[45,47] PwCF tend to have higher clearance for many antimicrobials, necessitating increases in dosing requirements.[45]

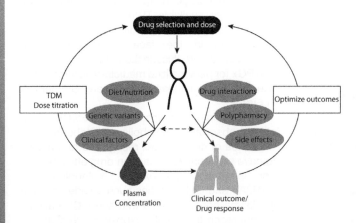

Fig. 2. Overview of concepts for drug titration. After dosing, plasma concentrations are influenced by many factors that overlap with those influencing drug response, including individual clinical characteristics (such as malabsorption, renal or liver disease, obesity, gender, and pregnancy), diet, pharmacogene variants, and concurrent medication use, among others. Clinical response depends, in part, on plasma concentration, which is one variable that can be monitored through TDM, allowing personalized dose adjustment, until optimized outcomes are reached.

TDM is most often used for antibiotics with a narrow therapeutic window, such as aminoglycosides and glycopeptides. Despite a high risk of dose-dependent toxicity, there remain unanswered questions for personalizing doses for these classes of antimicrobials in PwCF, such as frequency of blood sampling, methods for estimating individual drug exposure, and how to predict toxicity risks.[47–50] However, TDM can be very useful for monitoring other commonly used classes of antimicrobials because of the many differences PK/PD in PwCF, such as beta-lactams and oxazolidinones, to ensure therapeutic activity while reducing dose-dependent side effects.[45,47] To optimize personalized treatment and reduce adverse events, TDM could be used more frequently with antibiotics, not only those with narrow therapeutic indices.

For less frequently used antimicrobials, such as antifungals and antimycobacterials, TDM may also be used. Some antifungals require TDM to ensure the maintenance of therapeutic dosing or to avoid toxicity at higher concentrations.[51,52] For other antimicrobials, PwCF may need higher dosing to achieve therapeutic concentrations but due to high PK variability, TDM should be used to titrate dosing in pediatrics and adults.[51,53] Antimycobacterial drugs, typically used together in 3 to 4 drug regimens, are also of concern. Individuals with CF may have lower than expected concentrations of one or more antimycobacterial drugs, risking treatment failure.[54–56] Routine TDM can identify subtherapeutic concentrations on an ongoing basis to ensure treatment success. Moreover, achieving therapeutic concentrations quickly and efficiently with limited sampling approaches will require further study to improve precision approaches.

Outside of antimicrobials, drug titration in CF is typically completed based on empiric data—dose is increased until response is seen, or the maximum dosage is reached. One exception is for ibuprofen, which is used by a small fraction of eligible pwCF.[57,58] As a nonsteroidal anti-inflammatory drug, high-dose ibuprofen has been shown to reduce the rate of pulmonary decline and improve survival.[58,59] High-dose ibuprofen is primarily indicated for children aged younger than 18 years, at doses 3 to 4 times what is normally prescribed for other populations, and is accompanied by an increased risk of adverse effects that may be mitigated by gastrointestinal protection, TDM, appropriate patient selection, and temporary cessation when used concurrently with certain medications.[59] PK monitoring of peak blood levels to ensure target range (50–100 mg/mL) is required for use, which may be in part the reason for low uptake of this therapy in clinical practice. Another barrier to uptake includes the concurrent use of other medications, including CFTR modulators, which interact with ibuprofen, making TDM even more challenging.[41,60]

Titration of CFTR modulators has been proposed by a variety of investigators but is not currently used.[10,61–63] Lack of detailed PK data, the availability of assays for monitoring, and associations of concentrations with clinical response and adverse events all limit the progress of monitoring modulator concentrations for clinical care. There are, currently, no published studies on genetic variants that alter the concentration of any of the clinically available modulators, or clinical outcomes, despite detailed knowledge of the drug metabolism pathways involved and evidence of concentration–response relationships from both in vivo and in vitro studies.[1,12,64–67] The lack of PGx data can be mitigated by monitoring concentrations in plasma or tissue (such as from brushed nasal epithelia), an area for further study. Some studies suggest that epithelia may accumulate certain modulators at high concentrations, which may have detrimental impacts on CFTR rescue.[12,66,68,69] Therefore, a close relationship between the dose, plasma concentration, and CFTR rescue is likely to exist but is not yet understood. Some studies show that concentrations in clinical practice may exceed that required to reach maximum therapeutic response, but there have been no systematic studies to evaluate dose titration.[12,70] TDM of CFTR modulators would be useful to titrate dosing to balance beneficial clinical effect and undesirable side effects, such as liver injury.[71,72] Currently, empiric dose reductions are used for such adverse events, however, these reductions are not guided by TDM, and therefore may result in subtherapeutic concentrations of modulator compounds with detrimental long-term impacts.

With widespread use of HEMT, the CF community has experienced a shift in expectations for patient outcomes and long-term care. HEMT does not negate the need for other medications, and as PwCF age, they will still need therapies addressing manifestations of this disease. Personalizing therapy for each individual patient is complex without clear evidence to assist the clinician and patient in decision-making.[73] Transplant recipients with CF, in particular, require polypharmacy to manage immunosuppression, opportunistic infections, and CFTR dysfunction, making drug interactions a significant challenge. TDM is already used to manage antifungal and immunosuppressive drugs, and could aid in precision treatment with CFTR modulators in this group.[74–76] Because PwCF increasingly have successful pregnancies as a result of CFTR modulator therapy, TDM can also aid in maintaining therapeutic benefit for pregnant and nursing individuals with CF while balancing concerns regarding the exposure of the infant to these compounds.[77,78]

In addition, PGx represents a potential way to tailor precision approaches and is a currently underutilized resource in PwCF, with few CF-focused PGx guidelines outside of CFTR genotype determination for modulator eligibility.[79,80] This is despite the fact that several medications routinely used by PwCF have well-evidenced clinical guidelines for PGx implementation.[81] PwCF have repeated medication encounters over many years of use, increasing the opportunity for precision dosing using individual genetic information. As an example, the CYP3A superfamily including CYP3A4, CYP3A5, and CYP3A7 metabolize around 50% of available drugs but there is significant genetic variability in activity among individuals.[41] Although the relationship between genetic variation and clinical efficacy is not always consistent, there is substantial evidence these enzymes contribute to interindividual variation in dose requirements and drug response.[82–88] Implementation of PGx screening in PwCF could improve personalized approaches to therapy and dose selection, aid in the management of drug interactions, and potentially reduce adverse events.

Disease Monitoring Through Biomarkers

Several well-established disease markers are routinely used in the care of PwCF. Lung function, as measured by spirometry (primarily forced expiratory volume in 1 second, or FEV_1) has long served as a surrogate for disease severity. Indices of nutritional status, such as body mass index (BMI) or fat-soluble vitamin levels, are closely followed throughout life, and BMI is positively associated with FEV_1.[89] Bacterial growth from respiratory cultures is tracked, and the acquisition of key pathogens is a risk for rapid disease progression.[90–94] In the era of HEMT, however, the relevance and practicality of these disease markers may be shifting. Spirometry, for example, is expected to remain normal later into life with HEMT, highlighting the need for more sensitive measures in younger patients.[2,3,95–97] Similarly, as sputum production wanes, lower airway cultures may become more challenging. These changes highlight the need for novel biomarkers or surrogates of disease status and progression.

Multiple breath washout, or as it has evolved more recently, lung clearance index (LCI) is a technique that measures the time for a tracer gas to "wash out" the native gases, quantifying the degree of airways obstruction.[98,99] Numerous studies have found LCI to be more sensitive than spirometry for very mild disease and to change following therapies.[99,100] Moreover, as a passive maneuver, LCI is able to be performed in younger patients. There are shortcomings to LCI, however, including longer acquisition times, especially in advanced disease. Nonetheless, LCI is gaining traction, particularly in the detection of early disease.

Similarly, there have been significant advances in functional pulmonary imaging techniques. In particular, the use of hyperpolarized (typically ^{3}He or ^{129}Xe) or perfluorinated (^{19}F) gases as inhaled contrast agents have emerged to identify and quantify areas of gas trapping and ventilation inhomogeneity through MRI, avoiding ionizing radiation. These techniques, such as LCI, are more sensitive to early disease and to therapy-induced improvements.[101–103] Although hyperpolarized gas studies are currently limited to centers with research protocols to create the gases, ^{129}Xe is working toward FDA approval, which would increase availability for clinical use. Other functional imaging techniques, such as the capacity to quantify mucociliary clearance, are advancing in research and clinical trials.[104–107]

In vivo CFTR biomarkers such as sweat chloride (SC) and nasal potential difference (NPD) have not traditionally been used to monitor therapeutic benefit. With the emergence of HEMT, however, they are finding greater utility as measures of response to therapy.[2–6] Although the correlation between changes in SC or NPD and more physiologic disease markers, such as FEV_1, remains loose, these assays may still be useful in drug selection and monitoring for some.[108] Ongoing studies to understand the expected changes in SC on HEMT will provide relevance and seminormative data.[109]

Numerous additional biomarkers of CF disease severity have been evaluated over time but few are in routine clinical use. Such markers may be derived from blood, bronchoalveolar lavage fluid, exhaled breath condensate, or sputum, with several associating with disease severity or pulmonary exacerbation risk.[110–113] This is an area of focus in CF research, with a goal of identifying markers that will predict clinical change. This may include single assays or panels, potentially improving existing models of disease progression.[114] Predictive models will need to address the impact of HEMT, however, and modeling approaches created in the pre-HEMT era may not apply to patients on HEMT.

Respiratory cultures, most typically obtained from expectorated sputum, are a mainstay of CF care because the colonization of the airway with certain pathogens has been associated with increased decline in lung function.[91–94,115,116] The emergence of HEMT, however, has reduced the portion of the CF population capable of producing sputum reliably, and consensus on how best to replace these cultures is currently lacking. Induced sputum remains an option at centers with this capacity, whereas others have studied the use of exhaled breath analyses to identify particular pathogens of interest.[117,118] These approaches are presently limited to research studies at select institutions.

Personalized Care and Efficacy Evaluation

In CF, clinical care and prognosis have benefited from a well-organized, multidisciplinary delivery model partnered with thoughtful clinical care guidelines that seek to standardize outcomes across centers.[119–121] This systematic approach can work together with a personalized medicine paradigm to identify potentially effective therapies, determine the proper dose or regimen, and monitor for both safety and effectiveness in an individual. Optimizing CF care plans can be complex amid a wide range of therapeutic options. Three current challenges to personalizing care regimens are limited long-term, real-world efficacy data, sequential addition of new medications with little information on the impacts on existing therapies, and overlapping physiologic effects of highly effective CFTR modulator drugs with preexisting therapies targeting disease manifestations.

Those invested in the health care of PwCF have been remarkably successful in developing and applying new drugs and therapies for this population.[122] Strong commitment to research from individuals and families affected by CF, combined with robust clinical research networks and support from patient advocacy groups and foundations have enabled execution of well-designed controlled clinical trials despite the relatively small size of the disease population. This has also supported academic studies to address important questions that will not be prioritized in drug development but still impact care decisions and the lives of PwCF.[123–129] Nonetheless, the available and interested research study population is limited, particularly for disease manifestations found in a minority of patients (eg, CF-related diabetes, methicillin resistant *Staphylococcus aureus* (MRSA), nontuberculous mycobacteria, and so forth). Because of this, enrolling individuals into years-long prospective studies to assess the durability of effects seen in relatively short controlled clinical trials (eg, 6 months) is often impractical. It is recognized that the long-term benefits of many therapies may be smaller than those demonstrated in a short trial but rigorous assessment of the long-term impacts for most of our chronic treatments is often lacking. This gap is a key challenge when trying to individualize complex therapy regimens amid competing treatment options and burdensome daily care requirements.

High-quality CF patient registries exist in several countries to capture clinical care and health indices and are key resources when working to understand long-term effects of both common and uncommon therapies.[57] These registries can help to understand important questions not amenable to short-term controlled trials, such as rate of decline in lung function, survival, durability of clinical benefits over time, or interactions between sequentially added therapies.[130–135] Analyses of these databases are inherently observational and retrospective, limiting capacity to assign cause-and-effect but their contribution has been significant. Ultimately, key observations from registry analyses may require dedicated, prospective trials to more confidently assess the theories being tested. Withdrawal studies of longstanding therapies (discussed below) is an alternative approach to assessing whether such medications remain beneficial but should be based on strong scientific rationale.

A second challenge to personalizing care regimens in CF is the fact that new therapies are sequentially developed, approved, and endorsed in care guidelines with limited information on how they may affect common existing drugs. This is a natural and appropriate evolution of care for a progressive disease but it is important to consider whether new medications may be less effective when combined with existing drugs or may render existing therapies less effective. Beyond predictable drug–drug interactions (eg, overlapping hepatic metabolism), a current example of this is the widespread initiation of HEMT. Drugs such as elexacaftor/tezacaftor/ivacaftor (ETI) have proven to increase lung function, reduce pulmonary symptoms of CF, and reduce the risk of acute pulmonary exacerbations more than any other intervention to date.[2,3,95,136,137] These health outcomes mirror those of nearly all pulmonary-focused therapies used in CF, highlighting a third, related challenge: the opportunity to personalize care regimens by considering if overlapping effects of new and preexisting drugs can be understood well enough to decide if both remain beneficial and necessary.

Drugs such as inhaled dornase alfa and hypertonic saline support pulmonary health through targeted improvement in airway clearance of tenacious secretions but ETI has also been shown to improve mucociliary clearance and sputum properties (eg, viscosity), raising an important question of whether certain burdensome inhaled therapies are additionally benefiting airway clearance and lung function in PwCF taking ETI.[96,107,138] Modulators can also significantly reduce bacterial airway infections, which raises questions of the additional benefits of chronic suppressive inhaled antibiotics to microbiological or, more importantly, clinical status.[139,140] Similarly, the greatest impact of chronic azithromycin use shown in controlled trials is a reduction in the risk of acute pulmonary exacerbations, yet these events are increasingly uncommon for most people using ETI.[129,133,141,142] Finally, small studies of HEMT initiated at an early age show improved exocrine pancreatic function, which may allow some individuals to forego the need for pancreatic enzyme replacement therapy.[143,144] Modulators such as ETI have proven highly effective in populations with high use of many of these concomitant therapies, and care must be taken to minimize a risk of harm when testing withdrawal of preexisting drugs.

SUMMARY

The rapid pace of recent advancements in CF has led to significant improvements in patient outcomes and has created new opportunities to personalize care decisions. Numerous research tools have emerged to provide more personalized information and several are beginning to find use in the clinic. The capacity to identify and titrate optimal CF-specific therapies, coupled with the right disease markers and approach to follow clinical outcomes, is empowering refined care delivery that will ultimately improve patient experiences and outcomes. The tools highlighted here and others will continue to evolve, providing new ways to improve health outcomes over time.

Despite these exciting developments, some uncertainty often remains when making individual treatment decisions. This highlights the importance of continued regular care encounters and trusting relationships between patients, their families, and the care teams to discuss what is being learned from research and how it may apply to one's own treatment choices.[145] Often additional important factors must be considered, such as individual values affecting health-care participation and research, barriers to medication access or use, and comorbidities that affect overall prognosis. This ongoing engagement in joint decision-making remains a rewarding opportunity to tailor care, monitor health trajectory, and improve satisfaction for patients and providers alike. Tools to better personalize these discussions, as highlighted, should increasingly support this shared effort to maximize both health outcomes and quality of life.

CLINICS CARE POINTS

- Translation of research tools for therapeutic selection and titration may increase personalization of care in CF.
- Novel disease-relevant biomarkers, such as LCI and advanced MRI techniques, provide improved sensitivity to disease progression in an increasingly healthy population.
- Ongoing trials to streamline CF care and reduce treatment burden are required in the new era of HEMT.

DISCLOSURE

The authors have no conflicts of interest to disclose. The authors are supported by relevant grants from the Cystic Fibrosis Foundation (NAREN19R0, BREWIN20Y2-OUT, ROWE19R0, NICHOL20K0, SINGH19R0) and the National Institutes of Health (K23HL143167, K08HL144825, P30DK089507, P30DK072482, P30DK177467, R35HL135816).

REFERENCES

1. Accurso FJ, Rowe SM, Clancy JP, et al. Effect of VX-770 in persons with cystic fibrosis and the G551D-CFTR mutation. N Engl J Med 2010; 363(21):1991–2003.
2. Heijerman HGM, McKone EF, Downey DG, et al. Efficacy and safety of the elexacaftor plus tezacaftor plus ivacaftor combination regimen in people with cystic fibrosis homozygous for the F508del mutation: a double-blind, randomised, phase 3 trial. London, England): Lancet; 2019.
3. Middleton PG, Mall MA, Drevinek P, et al. Elexacaftor-Tezacaftor-Ivacaftor for Cystic Fibrosis with a Single Phe508del Allele. N Engl J Med 2019; 381(19):1809–19.
4. Ramsey BW, Davies J, McElvaney NG, et al. A CFTR potentiator in patients with cystic fibrosis and the G551D mutation. N Engl J Med 2011; 365(18):1663–72.

5. Rowe SM, Daines C, Ringshausen FC, et al. Teza-caftor-ivacaftor in residual-function heterozygotes with cystic fibrosis. N Engl J Med 2017;377(21): 2024–35.

6. Wainwright CE, Elborn JS, Ramsey BW, et al. Lu-macaftor-Ivacaftor in Patients with Cystic Fibrosis Homozygous for Phe508del CFTR. N Engl J Med 2015;373(3):220–31.

7. McGarry ME, McColley SA. Cystic fibrosis patients of minority race and ethnicity less likely eligible for CFTR modulators based on CFTR genotype. Pediatr Pulmonol 2021;56(6):1496–503.

8. DiMango E, Simpson K, Menten E, et al. Health Disparities among adults cared for at an urban cystic fibrosis program. Orphanet J rare Dis 2021;16(1): 332.

9. Quittner AL, Schechter MS, Rasouliyan L, et al. Impact of socioeconomic status, race, and ethnicity on quality of life in patients with cystic fibrosis in the United States. Chest 2010;137(3): 642–50.

10. Hanafin PO, Sermet-Gaudelus I, Griese M, et al. Insights into patient variability during ivacaftor-lumacaftor therapy in cystic fibrosis. Front Pharmacol 2021;12:577263.

11. van der Meer R, Wilms EB, Heijerman HGM. CFTR modulators: does one dose fit all? J Personalized Med 2021;11(6).

12. Guimbellot JS, Ryan KJ, Anderson JD, et al. Variable cellular ivacaftor concentrations in people with cystic fibrosis on modulator therapy. J Cystic Fibrosis 2020;19(5):742–5.

13. Sheppard DN, Carson MR, Ostedgaard LS, et al. Expression of cystic fibrosis transmembrane conductance regulator in a model epithelium. Am J Physiol 1994;266(4 Pt 1):L405–13.

14. Dekkers JF, Wiegerinck CL, de Jonge HR, et al. A functional CFTR assay using primary cystic fibrosis intestinal organoids. Nat Med 2013;19(7): 939–45.

15. Ramalho AS, Furstova E, Vonk AM, et al. Correction of CFTR function in intestinal organoids to guide treatment of Cystic Fibrosis. Eur Respir J 2020; 57(1):1902426.

16. Geurts MH, de Poel E, Amatngalim GD, et al. CRISPR-based adenine editors correct nonsense mutations in a cystic fibrosis organoid biobank. Cell stem cell 2020;26(4):503–10.

17. de Winter-de Groot KM, Janssens HM, van Uum RT, et al. Stratifying infants with cystic fibrosis for disease severity using intestinal organoid swelling as a biomarker of CFTR function. Eur Respir J 2018;52(3).

18. Noordhoek J, Gulmans V, van der Ent K, et al. Intestinal organoids and personalized medicine in cystic fibrosis: a successful patient-oriented research collaboration. Curr Opin Pulm Med 2016;22(6):610–6.

19. Beekman JM. Individualized medicine using intestinal responses to CFTR potentiators and correctors. Pediatr Pulmonol 2016;51(S44):S23–34.

20. Dekkers R, Vijftigschild LA, Vonk AM, et al. A bioassay using intestinal organoids to measure CFTR modulators in human plasma. J Cystic Fibrosis 2015;14(2):178–81.

21. de Poel E, Spelier S, Suen SWF, et al. Functional restoration of CFTR nonsense mutations in intestinal organoids. J Cyst Fibro 2021;21(2):246–53.

22. de Poel E, Spelier S, Korporaal R, et al. CFTR rescue in intestinal organoids with GLPG/ABBV-2737, ABBV/GLPG-2222 and ABBV/GLPG-2451 triple therapy. Front Mol Biosci 2021;8:698358.

23. Graeber SY, van Mourik P, Vonk AM, et al. Comparison of organoid swelling and in vivo biomarkers of CFTR function to determine effects of lumacaftor-ivacaftor in patients with cystic fibrosis homozygous for the F508del mutation. Am J Respir Crit Care Med 2020;202(11):1589–92.

24. Neuberger T, Burton B, Clark H, et al. Use of primary cultures of human bronchial epithelial cells isolated from cystic fibrosis patients for the preclinical testing of CFTR modulators. Methods Mol Biol (Clifton, NJ) 2011;741:39–54.

25. Brewington JJ, Filbrandt ET, LaRosa FJ 3rd, et al. Brushed nasal epithelial cells are a surrogate for bronchial epithelial CFTR studies. JCI Insight 2018;3(13).

26. Stokes AB, Kieninger E, Schogler A, et al. Comparison of three different brushing techniques to isolate and culture primary nasal epithelial cells from human subjects. Exp Lung Res 2014;40(7): 327–32.

27. Muller L, Brighton LE, Carson JL, et al. Culturing of human nasal epithelial cells at the air liquid interface. J Vis Exp 2013;80.

28. de Courcey F, Zholos AV, Atherton-Watson H, et al. Development of primary human nasal epithelial cell cultures for the study of cystic fibrosis pathophysiology. Am J Physiol Cell Physiol 2012;303(11):C1173–9.

29. Mosler K, Coraux C, Fragaki K, et al. Feasibility of nasal epithelial brushing for the study of airway epithelial functions in CF infants. J Cystic Fibros 2008;7(1):44–53.

30. Palechor-Ceron N, Suprynowicz FA, Upadhyay G, et al. Radiation induces diffusible feeder cell factor(s) that cooperate with ROCK inhibitor to conditionally reprogram and immortalize epithelial cells. Am J Pathol 2013;183(6):1862–70.

31. Liu X, Ory V, Chapman S, et al. ROCK inhibitor and feeder cells induce the conditional reprogramming of epithelial cells. Am J Pathol 2012;180(2): 599–607.

32. Brewington JJ, Filbrandt ET, LaRosa FJ 3rd, et al. Detection of CFTR function and modulation in primary human nasal cell spheroids. J Cyst Fibros 2017;17(1):26–33.

33. Anderson JD, Liu Z, Odom LV, et al. CFTR function and clinical response to modulators parallel nasal epithelial organoid swelling. Am J Physiol Lung Cell Mol Physiol 2021;321(1):L119–29.

34. Liu Z, Anderson JD, Deng L, et al. Human nasal epithelial organoids for therapeutic development in cystic fibrosis. Genes (Basel) 2020;11(6):603.

35. Guimbellot JS, Leach JM, Chaudhry IG, et al. Nasospheroids permit measurements of CFTR-dependent fluid transport. JCI insight 2017;2(22): e95734.

36. McGarry ME, Illek B, Ly NP, et al. In vivo and in vitro ivacaftor response in cystic fibrosis patients with residual CFTR function: N-of-1 studies. Pediatr Pulmonol 2017;52(4):472–9.

37. Ahmadi S, Bozoky Z, Di Paola M, et al. Phenotypic profiling of CFTR modulators in patient-derived respiratory epithelia. NPJ Genomic Med 2017;2:12.

38. Pranke I, Hatton A, Masson A, et al. Might brushed nasal cells Be a surrogate for CFTR modulator clinical response? Am J Respir Crit Care Med 2019; 199(1):123–6.

39. Pranke IM, Hatton A, Simonin J, et al. Correction of CFTR function in nasal epithelial cells from cystic fibrosis patients predicts improvement of respiratory function by CFTR modulators. Scientific Rep 2017;7(1):7375.

40. McCarthy C, Brewington JJ, Harkness B, et al. Personalised CFTR pharmacotherapeutic response testing and therapy of cystic fibrosis. Eur Respir J 2018;51(6):1702457.

41. Jordan CL, Noah TL, Henry MM. Therapeutic challenges posed by critical drug-drug interactions in cystic fibrosis. Pediatr Pulmonol 2016;51(S44): S61–70.

42. Dalboge CS, Nielsen XC, Dalhoff K, et al. Pharmacokinetic variability of clarithromycin and differences in CYP3A4 activity in patients with cystic fibrosis. J Cystic Fibros 2014;13(2):179–85.

43. Schultz AN, Hoiby N, Nielsen XC, et al. Individual pharmacokinetic variation leads to underdosing of ciprofloxacin in some cystic fibrosis patients. Pediatr Pulmonol 2017;52(3):319–23.

44. Rey E, Treluyer JM, Pons G. Drug disposition in cystic fibrosis. Clin Pharmacokinet 1998;35(4):313–29.

45. Castagnola E, Cangemi G, Mesini A, et al. Pharmacokinetics and pharmacodynamics of antibiotics in cystic fibrosis: a narrative review. Int J Antimicrob Agents 2021;58(3):106381.

46. Walker S, Habib S, Rose M, et al. Clinical use and bioavailability of tacrolimus in heart-lung and double lung transplant recipients with cystic fibrosis. Transplant Proc 1998;30(4):1519–20.

47. Huttner A, Harbarth S, Hope WW, et al. Therapeutic drug monitoring of the beta-lactam antibiotics: what is the evidence and which patients should we be using it for? J Antimicrob Chemother 2015; 70(12):3178–83.

48. Drennan PG, Thoma Y, Barry L, et al. Bayesian forecasting for intravenous tobramycin dosing in adults with cystic fibrosis using one versus two serum concentrations in a dosing interval. Ther Drug Monit 2021;43(4):505–11.

49. McDade EJ, Hewlett JL, Moonnumakal SP, et al. Evaluation of vancomycin dosing in pediatric cystic fibrosis patients. J Pediatr Pharmacol Ther 2016; 21(2):155–61.

50. Sherwin CM, Zobell JT, Stockmann C, et al. Pharmacokinetic and pharmacodynamic optimisation of intravenous tobramycin dosing among children with cystic fibrosis. J Pharmacokinet Pharmacodyn 2014;41(1):71–9.

51. Di Paolo M, Hewitt L, Nwanko E, et al. A retrospective 'real-world' cohort study of azole therapeutic drug monitoring and evolution of antifungal resistance in cystic fibrosis. JAC Antimicrob Resist 2021;3(1):dlab026.

52. Gothe F, Schmautz A, Hausler K, et al. Treating allergic bronchopulmonary aspergillosis with short-term prednisone and itraconazole in cystic fibrosis. J Allergy Clin Immunol Pract 2020;8(8): 2608–2614 e2603.

53. Bentley S, Davies JC, Gastine S, et al. Clinical pharmacokinetics and dose recommendations for posaconazole gastroresistant tablets in children with cystic fibrosis. J Antimicrob Chemother 2021; 76(12):3247–54.

54. Martiniano SL, Wagner BD, Brennan L, et al. Pharmacokinetics of oral antimycobacterials and dosing guidance for Mycobacterium avium complex treatment in cystic fibrosis. J Cyst Fibros 2021;20(5):772–8.

55. Cameron LH, Peloquin CA, Hiatt P, et al. Administration and monitoring of clofazimine for NTM infections in children with and without cystic fibrosis. J Cyst Fibros 2021;21(2):348–52.

56. Guimbellot JS, Acosta EP, Rowe SM. Sensitivity of ivacaftor to drug-drug interactions with rifampin, a cytochrome P450 3A4 inducer. Pediatr Pulmonol 2018;53(5):E6–8.

57. Knapp EA, Fink AK, Goss CH, et al. The cystic fibrosis foundation patient registry. design and methods of a national observational disease registry. Ann Am Thorac Soc 2016;13(7):1173–9.

58. Konstan MW, VanDevanter DR, Sawicki GS, et al. Association of high-dose ibuprofen use, lung function decline, and long-term survival in children with cystic fibrosis. Ann Am Thorac Soc 2018;15(4):485–93.

59. Lands LC, Stanojevic S. Oral non-steroidal anti-inflammatory drug therapy for lung disease in cystic

fibrosis. Cochrane database Syst Rev 2019;9: CD001505.

60. Bruch BA, Singh SB, Ramsey LJ, et al. Impact of a cystic fibrosis transmembrane conductance regulator (CFTR) modulator on high-dose ibuprofen therapy in pediatric cystic fibrosis patients. Pediatr Pulmonol 2018;53(8):1035–9.

61. Habler K, Kalla AS, Rychlik M, et al. Isotope dilution LC-MS/MS quantification of the cystic fibrosis transmembrane conductance regulator (CFTR) modulators ivacaftor, lumacaftor, tezacaftor, elexacaftor, and their major metabolites in human serum. Clin Chem Lab Med 2021;60(1):82–91.

62. Schneider EK, Reyes-Ortega F, Wilson JW, et al. Development of HPLC and LC-MS/MS methods for the analysis of ivacaftor, its major metabolites and lumacaftor in plasma and sputum of cystic fibrosis patients treated with ORKAMBI or KALYDECO. J Chromatogr B Analyt Technol Biomed Life Sci 2016;1038:57–62.

63. Reyes-Ortega F, Qiu F, Schneider-Futschik EK. Multiple reaction monitoring mass spectrometry for the drug monitoring of ivacaftor, tezacaftor, and elexacaftor treatment response in cystic fibrosis: a high-throughput method. ACS Pharmacol Transl Sci 2020;3(5):987–96.

64. Administration FaD. Drug approval package: trikafta. Available at: https://www.accessdata.fda. gov/drugsatfda_docs/nda/2019/212273Orig1s000 MultidisciplineR.pdf. Accessed July 30, 2020.

65. Administration FaD. Drug approval package: kalydeco (ivacaftor). Available at: https://www. accessdata.fda.gov/drugsatfda_docs/nda/2012/ 203188s000TOC.cfm. Accessed February 12, 2019.

66. Guhr Lee TN, Cholon DM, Quinney NL, et al. Accumulation and persistence of ivacaftor in airway epithelia with prolonged treatment. J Cyst Fibros 2020;19(5):746–51.

67. Van Goor F, Hadida S, Grootenhuis PD, et al. Rescue of CF airway epithelial cell function in vitro by a CFTR potentiator, VX-770. Proc Natl Acad Sci U S A 2009;106(44):18825–30.

68. Cholon DM, Quinney NL, Fulcher ML, et al. Potentiator ivacaftor abrogates pharmacological correction of DeltaF508 CFTR in cystic fibrosis. Sci translational Med 2014;6(246). 246ra296.

69. Avramescu RG, Kai Y, Xu H, et al. Mutation-specific downregulation of CFTR2 variants by gating potentiators. Hum Mol Genet 2017;26(24):4873–85.

70. Jeyaratnam J, van der Meer R, Berkers G, et al. Breast development in a 7 year old girl with CF treated with ivacaftor: an indication for personalized dosing? J Cyst Fibros 2021;20(5):e63–6.

71. Stylemans D, Francois S, Vincken S, et al. A case of self-limited drug induced liver injury under treatment with elexacaftor/tezacaftor/ivacaftor: when it is worth taking the risk. J Cyst Fibros 2021;20(4): 712–4.

72. Lowry S, Mogayzel PJ, Oshima K, et al. Drug-induced liver injury from elexacaftor/ivacaftor/tezacaftor. J Cyst Fibros 2021;21(2):e99–101.

73. Phan H. Treatment complexity in cystic fibrosis (CF): an increasing multifaceted challenge. Pediatr Pulmonol 2018;53(9):1174–6.

74. Smith M, Ryan KJ, Gutierrez H, et al. Ivacaftor-elexacaftor-tezacaftor and tacrolimus combination in cystic fibrosis. J Cyst Fibros 2021;21(1):e8–10.

75. McKinzie CJ, Doligalski CT, Lobritto SJ, et al. Use of elexacaftor/tezacaftor/ivacaftor in liver transplant patients with cystic fibrosis. J Cyst Fibros 2021; 21(2):227–9.

76. Chouchane I, Stremler-Lebel N, Reix P. Lumacaftor/ ivacaftor initiation in two liver transplantation patients under tacrolimus and antifungal azoles. Clin Case Rep 2019;7(4):616–8.

77. Qiu F, Habgood MD, Huang Y, et al. Entry of cystic fibrosis transmembrane conductance potentiator ivacaftor into the developing brain and lung. J Cyst Fibros 2021;20(5):857–64.

78. Taylor-Cousar JL, Jain R. Maternal and fetal outcomes following elexacaftor-tezacaftor-ivacaftor use during pregnancy and lactation. J Cyst Fibros 2021;20(3):402–6.

79. Wilk MA, Braun AT, Farrell PM, et al. Applying whole-genome sequencing in relation to phenotype and outcomes in siblings with cystic fibrosis. Cold Spring Harb Mol Case Stud 2020;6(1).

80. Carter SC, McKone EF. Pharmacogenetics of cystic fibrosis treatment. Pharmacogenomics 2016;17(13):1453–63.

81. Relling MV, Klein TE, Gammal RS, et al. The clinical pharmacogenetics implementation consortium: 10 Years later. Clin Pharmacol Ther 2020;107(1):171–5.

82. Provenzani A, Santeusanio A, Mathis E, et al. Pharmacogenetic considerations for optimizing tacrolimus dosing in liver and kidney transplant patients. World J Gastroenterol 2013;19(48):9156–73.

83. Shuker N, Bouamar R, van Schaik RH, et al. A randomized controlled trial comparing the efficacy of cyp3a5 genotype-based with body-weight-based tacrolimus dosing after living donor kidney transplantation. Am J Transplant 2016; 16(7):2085–96.

84. Pallet N, Etienne I, Buchler M, et al. Long-term clinical impact of adaptation of initial tacrolimus dosing to CYP3A5 genotype. Am J Transplant 2016;16(9): 2670–5.

85. Aouam K, Kolsi A, Kerkeni E, et al. Influence of combined CYP3A4 and CYP3A5 single-nucleotide polymorphisms on tacrolimus exposure in kidney transplant recipients: a study according to the post-transplant phase. Pharmacogenomics 2015; 16(18):2045–54.

86. Elens L, Bouamar R, Hesselink DA, et al. A new functional CYP3A4 intron 6 polymorphism significantly affects tacrolimus pharmacokinetics in kidney transplant recipients. Clin Chem 2011;57(11):1574–83.

87. Elens L, Hesselink DA, van Schaik RH, et al. The CYP3A4*22 allele affects the predictive value of a pharmacogenetic algorithm predicting tacrolimus predose concentrations. Br J Clin Pharmacol 2013;75(6):1545–7.

88. Elens L, van Schaik RH, Panin N, et al. Effect of a new functional CYP3A4 polymorphism on calcineurin inhibitors' dose requirements and trough blood levels in stable renal transplant patients. Pharmacogenomics 2011;12(10):1383–96.

89. 2020 Annual data report. Bethesda, Maryland: Cystic Fibrosis Foundation; 2020.

90. Cogen J, Emerson J, Sanders DB, et al. Risk factors for lung function decline in a large cohort of young cystic fibrosis patients. Pediatr Pulmonol 2015;50(8):763–70.

91. Harun SN, Wainwright C, Klein K, et al. A systematic review of studies examining the rate of lung function decline in patients with cystic fibrosis. Paediatr Respir Rev 2016;20:55–66.

92. Hubert D, Reglier-Poupet H, Sermet-Gaudelus I, et al. Association between Staphylococcus aureus alone or combined with Pseudomonas aeruginosa and the clinical condition of patients with cystic fibrosis. J Cyst Fibros 2013;12(5):497–503.

93. Kerem E, Viviani L, Zolin A, et al. Factors associated with FEV1 decline in cystic fibrosis: analysis of the ECFS patient registry. Eur Respir J 2014;43(1):125–33.

94. Zemanick ET, Emerson J, Thompson V, et al. Clinical outcomes after initial pseudomonas acquisition in cystic fibrosis. Pediatr Pulmonol 2015;50(1):42–8.

95. Nichols DP, Paynter AC, Heltshe SL, et al. Clinical effectiveness of elexacaftor/tezacftor/ivacaftor in people with cystic fibrosis. Am J Respir Crit Care Med 2021;205(5):529–39.

96. Rowe SM, Heltshe SL, Gonska T, et al. Clinical mechanism of the cystic fibrosis transmembrane conductance regulator potentiator ivacaftor in G551D-mediated cystic fibrosis. Am J Respir Crit Care Med 2014;190(2):175–84.

97. Davies JC, Wainwright CE, Canny GJ, et al. Efficacy and safety of ivacaftor in patients aged 6 to 11 years with cystic fibrosis with a G551D mutation. Am J Respir Crit Care Med 2013;187(11):1219–25.

98. Horsley AR, Gustafsson PM, Macleod KA, et al. Lung clearance index is a sensitive, repeatable and practical measure of airways disease in adults with cystic fibrosis. Thorax 2008;63(2):135–40.

99. Aurora P, Bush A, Gustafsson P, et al. Multiple-breath washout as a marker of lung disease in preschool children with cystic fibrosis. Am J Respir Crit Care Med 2005;171(3):249–56.

100. Amin R, Subbarao P, Jabar A, et al. Hypertonic saline improves the LCI in paediatric patients with CF with normal lung function. Thorax 2010;65(5):379–83.

101. Thomen RP, Walkup LL, Roach DJ, et al. Hyperpolarized (129)Xe for investigation of mild cystic fibrosis lung disease in pediatric patients. J Cyst Fibros 2017;16(2):275–82.

102. Rayment JH, Couch MJ, McDonald N, et al. Hyperpolarised (129)Xe magnetic resonance imaging to monitor treatment response in children with cystic fibrosis. Eur Respir J 2019;53(5):1802188.

103. Goralski JL, Chung SH, Glass TM, et al. Dynamic perfluorinated gas MRI reveals abnormal ventilation despite normal FEV1 in cystic fibrosis. JCI insight 2020;5(2).

104. Donaldson SH, Laube BL, Mogayzel P, et al. Effect of lumacaftor-ivacaftor on mucociliary clearance and clinical outcomes in cystic fibrosis: results from the PROSPECT MCC sub-study. J Cyst Fibros 2021;21(1):143–5.

105. Leung HM, Birket SE, Hyun C, et al. Intranasal micro-optical coherence tomography imaging for cystic fibrosis studies. Sci translational Med 2019;11(504):eaav3505.

106. Shei RJ, Peabody JE, Rowe SM. Functional anatomic imaging of the airway surface. Ann Am Thorac Soc 2018;15(Suppl 3):S177–83.

107. Donaldson SH, Laube BL, Corcoran TE, et al. Effect of ivacaftor on mucociliary clearance and clinical outcomes in cystic fibrosis patients with G551D-CFTR. JCI Insight 2018;3(24).

108. Fidler MC, Beusmans J, Panorchan P, et al. Correlation of sweat chloride and percent predicted FEV(1) in cystic fibrosis patients treated with ivacaftor. J Cyst Fibros 2017;16(1):41–4.

109. Zemanick ET, Konstan MW, VanDevanter DR, et al. Measuring the impact of CFTR modulation on sweat chloride in cystic fibrosis: rationale and design of the CHEC-SC study. J Cyst Fibros 2021;20(6):965–71.

110. Ishak A, Stick SM, Turkovic L, et al. BAL inflammatory markers can predict pulmonary exacerbations in children with cystic fibrosis. Chest 2020;158(6):2314–22.

111. Sagel SD, Kapsner RK, Osberg I. Induced sputum matrix metalloproteinase-9 correlates with lung function and airway inflammation in children with cystic fibrosis. Pediatr Pulmonol 2005;39(3):224–32.

112. Horati H, Janssens HM, Margaroli C, et al. Airway profile of bioactive lipids predicts early progression of lung disease in cystic fibrosis. J Cyst Fibros 2020;19(6):902–9.

113. Khanal S, Webster M, Niu N, et al. SPLUNC1: a novel marker of cystic fibrosis exacerbations. Eur Respir J 2021;58(5).

114. Wolfe C, Pestian T, Gecili E, et al. Cystic fibrosis point of personalized detection (CFPOPD): an interactive web application. JMIR Med Inform 2020;8(12):e23530.

115. Cogen JD, Faino AV, Onchiri F, et al. Association between number of intravenous antipseudomonal antibiotics and clinical outcomes of pediatric cystic fibrosis pulmonary exacerbations. Clin Infect Dis 2021;73(9):1589–96.

116. Lechtzin N, John M, Irizarry R, et al. Outcomes of adults with cystic fibrosis infected with antibiotic-resistant Pseudomonas aeruginosa. Respiration 2006;73(1):27–33.

117. Kos R, Brinkman P, Neerincx AH, et al. Targeted exhaled breath analysis for detection of Pseudomonas aeruginosa in cystic fibrosis patients. J Cyst Fibros 2021;21(1):e28–34.

118. Gilchrist FJ, Belcher J, Jones AM, et al. Exhaled breath hydrogen cyanide as a marker of early Pseudomonas aeruginosa infection in children with cystic fibrosis. ERJ Open Res 2015;1(2): 00044–2015.

119. Kapnadak SG, Dimango E, Hadjiliadis D, et al. Cystic Fibrosis Foundation consensus guidelines for the care of individuals with advanced cystic fibrosis lung disease. J Cyst Fibros 2020;19(3): 344–54.

120. Ramos KJ, Smith PJ, McKone EF, et al. Lung transplant referral for individuals with cystic fibrosis: cystic Fibrosis Foundation consensus guidelines. J Cyst Fibros 2019;18(3):321–33.

121. Ren CL, Morgan RL, Oermann C, et al. Cystic fibrosis foundation pulmonary guidelines. use of cystic fibrosis transmembrane conductance regulator modulator therapy in patients with cystic fibrosis. Ann Am Thorac Soc 2018;15(3):271–80.

122. Bell SC, Mall MA, Gutierrez H, et al. The future of cystic fibrosis care: a global perspective. Lancet Respir Med 2020;8(1):65–124.

123. Nichols DP, Singh PK, Baines A, et al. Testing the effects of combining azithromycin with inhaled tobramycin for P. aeruginosa in cystic fibrosis: a randomised, controlled clinical trial. Thorax; 2021.

124. Goss CH, Heltshe SL, West NE, et al. A randomized trial of antimicrobial duration for cystic fibrosis pulmonary exacerbation treatment. Am J Respir Crit Care Med 2021;204(11):1295–305.

125. Konstan MW, Byard PJ, Hoppel CL, et al. Effect of high-dose ibuprofen in patients with cystic fibrosis. N Engl J Med 1995;332:848–54.

126. Elkins MR, Robinson M, Rose BR, et al. A controlled trial of long-term inhaled hypertonic saline in patients with cystic fibrosis. N Engl J Med 2006;354(3):229–40.

127. Mayer-Hamblett N, Nichols DP, Odem-Davis K, et al. Evaluating the impact of stopping chronic therapies after modulator drug therapy in cystic fibrosis: the simplify clinical trial study design. Ann Am Thorac Soc 2021;18(8):1397–405.

128. Ratjen F, Davis SD, Stanojevic S, et al. Inhaled hypertonic saline in preschool children with cystic fibrosis (SHIP): a multicentre, randomised, double-blind, placebo-controlled trial. Lancet Respir Med 2019;7(9):802–9.

129. Saiman L, Marshall BC, Mayer-Hamblett N, et al. Azithromycin in patients with cystic fibrosis chronically infected with Pseudomonas aeruginosa: a randomized controlled trial. JAMA 2003;290: 1749–56.

130. Volkova N, Moy K, Evans J, et al. Disease progression in patients with cystic fibrosis treated with ivacaftor: data from national US and UK registries. J Cyst Fibros 2020;19(1):68–79.

131. Sawicki GS, Signorovitch JE, Zhang J, et al. Reduced mortality in cystic fibrosis patients treated with tobramycin inhalation solution. Pediatr Pulmonol 2012;47(1):44–52.

132. Denis A, Touzet S, Diabate L, et al. Quantifying long-term changes in lung function and exacerbations after initiation of azithromycin in cystic fibrosis. Ann Am Thorac Soc 2020;17(2): 195–201.

133. Nichols DP, Odem-Davis K, Cogen JD, et al. Pulmonary outcomes associated with long-term azithromycin therapy in cystic fibrosis. Am J Respir Crit Care Med 2020;201(4):430–7.

134. VanDyke RD, McPhail GL, Huang B, et al. Inhaled tobramycin effectively reduces FEV1 decline in cystic fibrosis. An instrumental variables analysis. Ann Am Thorac Soc 2013;10(3):205–12.

135. Schluchter MD, Konstan MW, Xue L, et al. Relationship between high-dose ibuprofen use and rate of decline in FEV1 among young patients with mild lung disease in the CFF Registry. Pediatr Pulmonol 2004;27:A385, 322.

136. Burgel PR, Durieu I, Chiron R, et al. Rapid improvement after starting elexacaftor-tezacaftor-ivacaftor in patients with cystic fibrosis and advanced pulmonary disease. Am J Respir Crit Care Med 2021;204(1):64–73.

137. O'Shea KM, O'Carroll OM, Carroll C, et al. Efficacy of elexacaftor/tezacaftor/ivacaftor in patients with cystic fibrosis and advanced lung disease. Eur Respir J 2021;57(2).

138. Donaldson SH, Bennett WD, Zeman KL, et al. Mucus clearance and lung function in cystic fibrosis with hypertonic saline. N Engl J Med 2006;354(3):241–50.

139. Hisert KB, Heltshe SL, Pope C, et al. Restoring cystic fibrosis transmembrane conductance regulator function reduces airway bacteria and inflammation in people with cystic fibrosis and chronic lung infections. Am J Respir Crit Care Med 2017; 195(12):1617–28.

140. Heltshe SL, Mayer-Hamblett N, Burns JL, et al. Pseudomonas aeruginosa in cystic fibrosis patients with G551D-CFTR treated with ivacaftor. Clin Infect Dis : official Publ Infect Dis Soc America 2015;60(5):703–12.

141. Mayer-Hamblett N, Retsch-Bogart G, Kloster M, et al. Azithromycin for early pseudomonas infection in cystic fibrosis. The OPTIMIZE Randomized Trial. Am J Respir Crit Care Med 2018;198(9):1177–87.

142. Saiman L, Anstead M, Mayer-Hamblett N, et al. Effect of azithromycin on pulmonary function in patients with cystic fibrosis uninfected with Pseudomonas aeruginosa: a randomized controlled trial. JAMA 2010;303:1707–15.

143. Rosenfeld M, Cunningham S, Harris WT, et al. An open-label extension study of ivacaftor in children with CF and a CFTR gating mutation initiating treatment at age 2-5years (KLIMB). J Cyst Fibros 2019; 18(6):838–43.

144. Rosenfeld M, Wainwright CE, Higgins M, et al. Ivacaftor treatment of cystic fibrosis in children aged 12 to <24 months and with a CFTR gating mutation (ARRIVAL): a phase 3 single-arm study. Lancet Respir Med 2018;6(7):545–53.

145. Breuer O, Shoseyov D, Koretz S, et al. Ethical dilemma: elexacaftor-tezacaftor-ivacaftor or lung transplantation in cystic fibrosis and end-stage lung disease? Chest 2021;161(3):773–80.

Emerging Approaches to Monitor and Modify Care in the Era of Cystic Fibrosis Transmembrane Conductance Regulators

Clemente J. Britto, MD[a],*, Felix Ratjen, MD, PhD, FRCP(C), FERS[b], John P. Clancy, MD[c]

KEYWORDS

- Cystic fibrosis • Disease monitoring • De-escalation of care • Lung clearance index
- Computed tomography • Patient-reported outcomes • Biomarkers

KEY POINTS

- Highly effective modulator therapy (HEMT) markedly improved clinical outcomes in cystic fibrosis, creating new challenges for long-term disease monitoring.
- Emerging approaches to monitor HEMT response include lung clearance index, developments in pulmonary imaging, patient-reported outcomes, and novel molecular biomarkers.
- Studies are underway to understand the value of these novel outcome measures in disease monitoring and treatment modification when indicated.

INTRODUCTION

Cystic fibrosis (CF) is a multisystem hereditary disease caused by mutations in the cystic fibrosis transmembrane conductance regulator (CFTR) gene, affecting more than 70,000 individuals worldwide.[1,2] CFTR modulators are small molecules that target mutant CFTR proteins to improve chloride channel processing and function. The recent, widespread adoption of triple modulator therapy with elexacaftor–tezacaftor–ivacaftor (ETI, an example of highly effective modulator therapy [HEMT]) had a profound impact on clinical outcomes, including improvements in lung function, exacerbation frequency, body weight, and quality of life.[3–5] (Please refer to Alex H. Gifford and colleagues' article, "Update on Clinical Outcomes of Highly Effective Modulator Therapy," in this issue.)

While this paradigm shift in our approach to CF care can be life-altering for many people with CF, it also uncovers the need to develop new methods to monitor the health of individuals receiving HEMT from a physiologic perspective. It also highlights the need to generate evidence that determines when de-escalation of symptomatic therapies is appropriate, as well as identifying patients with a limited or no response to HEMT who continue to benefit from symptomatic treatments or additional interventions.

In this article, we review emerging challenges in this new therapeutic era and discuss potential approaches to assess patients' responses to therapy and monitor long-term health by utilizing physiologic, imaging, and biomarker tools. We also discuss ongoing efforts to study the modification of respiratory therapies after the initiation of HEMT.

[a] Yale Adult Cystic Fibrosis Program, Division of Pulmonary, Critical Care, and Sleep Medicine, Department of Internal Medicine, Yale University School of Medicine; [b] Division of Respiratory Medicine, Translational Medicine, University of Toronto Hospital for Sick Children, 555 University Avenue, Toronto Ontario M5G 1X8, Canada; [c] Cystic Fibrosis Foundation, Bethesda, MD, USA
* Corresponding author.
E-mail address: clemente.britto@yale.edu

Clin Chest Med 43 (2022) 631–646
https://doi.org/10.1016/j.ccm.2022.06.006
0272-5231/22/© 2022 Elsevier Inc. All rights reserved.

MONITORING CLINICAL STATUS IN THE HIGHLY EFFECTIVE MODULATOR THERAPY-TREATED PATIENT

In recently reported pivotal phase 3 trials, ETI provided robust improvements in the forced expiratory volume in the first second (FEV_1), exacerbation frequency, respiratory symptoms, body mass index (BMI), and sweat chloride concentrations in subjects with at least one Phe508del CFTR mutation.[3,4,6–10] These observations raise questions about how health care providers should monitor physiologic parameters that assess the degree of modulator response and the extent to which established symptomatic treatments continue to provide benefit beyond the window of clinical trials. Indeed, recent results from the PROMISE study highlight the challenge of using established physiologic tests (eg, spirometry) in patients who initiate HEMT, with normalization of mean FEV_1 percent predicted values in a large portion of individuals within 1 month of starting treatment.[11] Disease monitoring may also have important implications for adjusting the use of established therapies, including decisions to de-escalate or continue therapies in a given patient. As with other therapies, the improvement observed in outcome measures was not uniform across all treated individuals. The CF research community is just beginning to examine the drivers of modulator response variability. A recent consideration is sex-based differential responses to modulators reported in modulator trials. Historically, females with CF tend to experience accelerated lung function decline, earlier *Pseudomonas aeruginosa* colonization, more frequent pulmonary exacerbations, and higher rates of CF complications and mortality than males.[12–18] Yet, some data suggest that females experience more robust responses than men to CFTR modulators, including exacerbation frequency and changes in sweat chloride.[19–21] Data for sex-based differences in ETI response are not yet conclusive and highlight the need to better understand the role of sex and other contributors in CFTR modulator response.[3–5,22,23] For further details on pharmacology and pharmacogenomics studies to understand these differences, see Jennifer S. Guimbellot and colleagues' article, "Novel Applications of Biomarkers and Personalized Medicine in Cystic Fibrosis," of this issue of The Clinics, covering novel applications of biomarkers and personalized medicine in CF.

There are no well-defined clinical monitoring guidelines to assess the degree of response to CFTR modulators over time or when to use or not use traditional symptomatic therapies to improve mucus clearance or to combat infection and inflammation, factors that may be mitigated by HEMT use. Indeed, all of the approved or commonly used therapies in CF were developed and demonstrated efficacy in the absence of HEMT, and all HEMT were evaluated in the setting of chronic symptomatic therapy use. Thus, it is unclear what the relative benefit of continuing symptomatic therapies is for a given CF patient in the context of HEMT treatment. Most CF patients in the United States and Europe are seen in quarterly clinics, where symptoms, lung function, nutritional status, microbiology, and assessment by multidisciplinary care team members are routinely reviewed.[24,25] Whether this monitoring frequency and intensity is warranted in all HEMT-treated patients is unknown, but the rapid pivot to virtual visits driven by the COVID-19 pandemic has raised questions about what aspects of disease monitoring require quarterly, face-to-face visits (and in which CF patients).[26–29] Although acute increases in FEV_1 are the primary outcome measure traditionally used to measure HEMT response in older children and adults, little is known regarding its long-term prediction of outcome measures, such as airway infection or future pulmonary decline. Long-term follow-up of patients treated with ivacaftor (another HEMT available for a small subset of CF patients since 2012) suggests that mortality, need for lung transplantation, detection of *P aeruginosa*, lung function decline, and the incidence of CF-related diabetes were reduced relative to controls from the CFF and UK patient registries.[30–32] Importantly, abnormalities across all of these domains persisted out to 5 years post-HEMT initiation, highlighting the need to better understand what clinical factors are associated with future clinical decline at the individual patient level.[33]

In addition to established pulmonary measurements, such as FEV_1 and microbiology, inflammatory biomarkers could potentially be used to quantify HEMT responses, as suggested by the ability of inflammation markers to predict the onset of bronchiectasis and their association with lung function decline.[34,35] To date, the data demonstrating robust changes in inflammatory biomarkers in response to HEMT are limited. Hisert and colleagues[36] reported that several sputum inflammatory biomarkers steadily declined over mo/y of follow-up in a small cohort of ivacaftor-treated CF adults. In contrast, changes in sputum inflammatory biomarkers did not demonstrate clear changes over 6 months of HEMT treatment in subjects initiating ivacaftor.[37] In addition to pulmonary outcome measures, assessment of pancreatic function through measures of stool elastase has demonstrated improvement of exocrine pancreatic function in many pediatric patients receiving HEMT (both in clinical trials and in post-approval studies).[38,39] Although monitoring airway, stool, and other biomarkers [eg, nutritional, patient-reported outcome (PRO) measures] may provide additional objective measures of improvement, there remains a gap in determining how reversible the various aspects of established CF disease are for a given patient. Finally, although sweat chloride and nasal potential difference have been used to diagnose CF and monitor aggregate HEMT responses in clinical trials, translation of these biomarkers into decision tools that inform individual therapies is limited. Indeed, although changes in sweat chloride correlate with improvements in FEV_1 at the population level, this relationship is insufficient to determine whether an HEMT response is complete or to guide decisions regarding de-escalation or retention of symptomatic pulmonary therapies.[11]

Quantifying Therapeutic Responses in the Era of Highly Effective Modulator Therapy

Since the previous *Cystic Fibrosis* issue of *The Clinics in Chest Medicine* in 2016, there has been a broad expansion of scientific methodologies useful to characterize a patient's response to modulators. Among these have emerged measures of lung function and mucociliary clearance, biomarker measurements, the growing application of pulmonary imaging in CF, and the development of molecular tools that provide HEMT response insights at a single-cell level (**Fig. 1**). These tools are at variable stages of development and application in HEMT-treated CF. The results of ongoing clinical research will begin to inform how they will influence the care of our HEMT-treated CF patients.

Lung Clearance Index, an Emerging Measure of Pulmonary Physiology in Cystic Fibrosis

Because lung function is an established surrogate of survival in people with CF, it is one of the most closely monitored parameters to assess therapeutic response to treatments, including HEMT.[3–5,11] Aggregate increases in FEV_1 observed in controlled clinical trials of ivacaftor and ETI suggest that an FEV_1 improvement of 10% could be anticipated for those who initiate HEMT. Yet, FEV_1 may be limited to detecting clinical improvement in those with normal values at the start of treatment, minimal or early disease, those with severe and irreversible lung damage, and those transitioning from one HEMT (eg, ivacaftor) to another (eg, ETI).[40–42]

In recent years the multiple breath washout/lung clearance index (MBW/LCI) has demonstrated increased sensitivity relative to FEV_1 to detect therapeutic effects (including CFTR modulators) and to monitor early CF lung disease when FEV_1 is often within normal range.[43–47] LCI measures ventilation homogeneity derived from a MBW of inert tracer gas. As it reflects ventilation throughout the respiratory tract, including the small airways, it seems to be a more sensitive marker of early airflow obstruction when not detectable by FEV_1 that mainly captures obstruction in larger airways. This technique has also been applied to infants, young children, and adults with mild pulmonary disease.[48–52] Numerous studies have correlated LCI with $FEV_1/FEV_{0.5}$.[53–55] Imaging studies have also shown a correlation between LCI and high-resolution computed tomography (HRCT) findings of bronchial wall thickening, mucus plugging, and bronchiectasis.[42] LCI has also been correlated to age, onset and type of infection, signs of inflammation on bronchoalveolar lavage, exhaled nitric oxide, and symptom scores.[56–59] Some limitations of LCI include its limited use in patients with moderate or severe lung disease,[60] a requirement for trained personnel and specialized equipment, and a poor correlation with bronchodilator response despite its good sensitivity to detect changes in ventilation associated with the use of hypertonic saline (HTS), dornase alfa, and treatment of pulmonary exacerbations.[49,51,59,61] Importantly, LCI can predict future spirometry impairment,[62–64] exertional limitation in children with normal FEV_1,[65] *P aeruginosa* colonization,[66] and exacerbations.[67,68] LCI has demonstrated improvements in clinical trials of ivacaftor, lumacaftor-ivacaftor, tezacaftor-ivacaftor, and ETI.[69–72] Recent studies have also sought to define the minimal clinical important difference (MCID) of LCI.[73,74] Although the MCID for LCI has not been defined, evidence suggests it can be used to identify patients at risk of future lung function decline.[45]

Pulmonary Imaging as a Disease Monitoring Tool in Cystic Fibrosis

Chest computed tomography (CT) is currently the gold standard for imaging pulmonary structures in CF. CT is a sensitive tool for characterizing CF lung disease progression.[75–77] Similar to other pulmonary imaging modalities, CT can provide information regarding air trapping, mucus plugging and structural damage, regional progression, and perfusion differences, among others. Several studies have reported that CT is more sensitive to detecting disease progression than FEV_1.[78–81] Further, CT can readily identify early signs of bronchiectasis, airway wall thickening, and air trapping

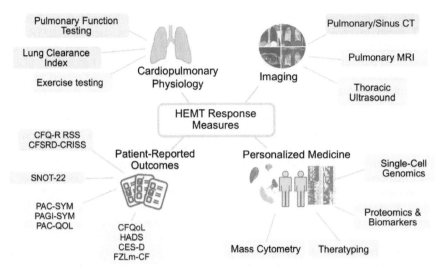

Fig. 1. Examples of established and emerging HEMT response measurements: overview of established and emerging strategies to monitor modulator response in four fields: cardiopulmonary physiology, pulmonary and paranasal sinus imaging, PROs, and personalized medicine. CES-D, Center for Epidemiologic Studies Depression Scale; FZLm-CF, Questions on Life Satisfaction for Children and Adults with CF; HADS, Hospital Anxiety Depression Scale; PAC-QOL, Patient Assessment of Constipation Quality of Life; PAC-SYM, Patient Assessment of Constipation Symptoms; PAGI-SYM, Patient Assessment of Gastrointestinal Symptoms; SNOT-22, Sinonasal Outcome Test-22.

that led to its incorporation into recent clinical trials and disease monitoring programs in children.[77,82,83] Baseline CT findings also predicted future bronchiectasis and relationship with airway inflammation and growth in a pediatric cohort. In addition, functional CT imaging has demonstrated improvements in air-trapping following initiation of lumacaftor/ivacaftor therapy.[84] A persistent hurdle in the development of broader CT monitoring strategies has been adopting a standardized scoring system to measure, grade, and follow CT findings over time in CF.[82,83,85–89] Furthermore, radiation exposure remains an important consideration for many practitioners before routine use to monitor the status and progression of lung disease after initiating HEMT.[90] Finally, although there is a sizable body of work investigating disease progression, there is minimal data regarding whether CT can detect improvement and/or the resolution of early pulmonary changes after initiation of HEMT.

The Perth-Rotterdam Annotated Grid Morphometric Analysis for CF (PRAGMA-CF) is a CT-based quantitative measure of lung disease used to evaluate the imaging progression of CF lung disease.[83] The Saline Hypertonic in Preschoolers + CT (SHIP-CT) trial is a phase 3, multicenter, randomized, double-blind, controlled trial assessing the impact of inhaled HTS on CF lung disease, as measured by chest CT imaging and LCI, using the PRAGMA-CF score.[91–93] The

application of PRAGMA-CF as a standardized approach to score lung disease progression highlights the importance of further developing scoring systems and centralizing the interpretation infrastructure to monitor disease progression and therapeutic response.

An emerging alternative to CT imaging that avoids radiation exposure is MRI.[43,77,94–97] In addition to being radiation-free, recent advancements, such as ultrashort echo time (UTE) provide comparable data to CT in terms of structural assessment.[98,99] MRI also offers the potential to assess additional pulmonary outcomes, such as lung perfusion, airway dynamics, and ventilation.[95,100,101] Although there is an ongoing need to standardize MRI platforms and scoring systems in CF and to link imaging findings to validated clinical outcomes, the pulmonary physiology insights gained through advanced MRI techniques may provide details with both the structural and functional resolution that when integrated with lung function measures may transform our ability to measure CF lung disease progression or response to therapy.[43,95,101]

Recent work shows that inhaled hyperpolarized noble gases (eg, 3He, ^{129}Xe) enable the visualization of regional ventilation differences to complement structural data. The Hyperpolarized Imaging for New Treatments (HyPOINT) trial is a prospective multicenter study in the United States and Canada that will evaluate the benefits of monitoring serial MRI structural and physiologic data to characterize lung disease progression in CF and how ETI modifies these findings. There are also ongoing efforts to improve the quality of MRI imaging to a resolution close to that of CT using UTE MRI in CF. UTE MRI revealed structural lung disease in patients as young as 23 months old.[94,95,102] These novel MRI approaches are highly sensitive to detect airway obstruction in CF, and in some studies, outperformed pulmonary function testing and LCI as measures of lung disease.[103–106]

Lung ultrasound is a relatively novel application in assessments of CF lung disease.[107–110] In one small study, lung ultrasound correlated incompletely with HRCT findings and lung function measurements,[110] and in another, a lung ultrasound score correlated strongly with LCI.[109] Although lung ultrasound could represent a valuable noninvasive imaging-resource with minimal adverse effects, it remains highly operator-dependent and will require further standardization prior to widespread use.

Developments in Cystic Fibrosis-Related Patient-Reported Outcomes

Improvements in PROs can help to facilitate the approval of new therapies as part of the The United States Food and Drug Administration mandate that therapy or intervention improves how a patient "feels, functions, or survives." They are also a crucial resource to understand the impact of modulators in clinical trials and in real-world settings. Numerous well-validated tools are available to assess PROs, including the Cystic Fibrosis Questionnaire-Revised (CFQ-R),[111–114] the Cystic Fibrosis Quality of Life (CFQoL) questionnaire,[115] and the Cystic Fibrosis Respiratory Symptom Diary - Chronic Respiratory Infection Symptom Score (CFRSD-CRISS).[116] In addition, tools, such as the Hospital Anxiety Depression Scale,[117] the Center for Epidemiologic Studies Depression Scale,[118] and the Questions on Life Satisfaction for Children and Adults with CF[117,119] provide insights into the quality of life and mental health parameters in CF. A recent survey revealed over 70 PRO collection instruments in use across 33 countries, of which CFQ-R was the most widely utilized.[120]

These tools provide insights into disease-specific symptoms, mental health, and quality-of-life parameters, giving an overview of an individual's perceived health and its trend compared with previous assessments. However, most of these instruments focus primarily on symptoms rather than objective data and were developed before

modulators were introduced into standard CF care. Modulators have brought challenges in the interpretation and optimization of these resources. For example, in the PROMISE trial[11] (an observational trial assessing the effectiveness of ETI), the CFQ-R Respiratory Domain (CFQ-R R domain) scores improved by 20.4 points (MCID = 5). However, this improvement may underestimate the impact of ETI on subjects who had a minimal disease or symptom scores at the start of treatment, and the effect that ETI would have had on individuals who were transitioning from a two-drug combination to ETI. This ceiling effect of PROs in the HEMT era becomes increasingly relevant as emerging data show that CFQ-R R domain scores and CFQoL may correlate poorly with lung function parameters in school-aged children.[121]

As modulators create new opportunities to re-evaluate and improve PROs in CF, there is renewed interest in organ-system-focused surveys that will enhance our ability to monitor symptoms in and outside of the lung over time. The CFQ-R Respiratory Symptom Scores, an example of this organ-system-specific focus, correlated well with CT findings of bronchiectasis and air trapping in a pediatric cohort over a 2-year follow-up period.[81] Similarly, the Sinonasal Outcome Test (SNOT-22) was developed to quantify the development and progression of upper airway symptoms in patients with CF and can predict the likelihood of symptom improvement after surgical intervention for chronic rhinosinusitis, and has been shown to improve following ETI administration.[10,122,123] Finally, a large multicenter prospective clinical trial investigating gastrointestinal (GI) symptoms in people with cystic fibrosis (GALAXY) has been recently completed. This study focused on assessing GI symptoms in patients with CF through multiple PRO questionnaires, including a Patient Assessment of Constipation Symptoms, Patient Assessment of Gastrointestinal Symptoms, Patient Assessment of Constipation Quality of Life, and a disease-specific questionnaire (Bristol Stool Scale and questions about fecal incontinence, and stool quality and frequency).[124,125]

Emerging Measures of Cardiopulmonary Physiology for Cystic Fibrosis Monitoring

Cardiopulmonary exercise testing (CPET)[47,126–128] provides a comprehensive assessment of cardiovascular, respiratory, and muscular physiology during exercise and may therefore be an informative tool to monitor functional status and respiratory improvements in HEMT-treated patients. Its detailed cardiac function, gas exchange, and anaerobic physiology data provide a wealth of information to monitor an individual's exertional progress over time.[129–132] CPET has been used in CF previously, primarily in the context of clinical trials and research, where impairment in peak oxygen uptake at maximal exercise was a prognostic indicator of survival.[133,134] More recently, CPET was used to identify high-risk clusters of patients with poor lung function, nutritional status, and exercise capacity,[126] and has been correlated with ventilation inhomogeneity in LCI.[135,136] Further, CPET has also been used to measure the impact of *P aeruginosa* colonization on exercise tolerance[137] and to predict mortality and progression to lung transplantation.[126,138–142] Finally, as with LCI, there is growing experience using CPET as a potential tool to follow modulator response.[126,143,144] Similar to other cardiopulmonary function tests, CPET can be limited by access to adequate infrastructure, staff to administer and interpret test findings, and its lack of sensitivity in younger CF patients, where CPET findings are largely within normal limits.[145] A less informative test than CPET, the six-minute walk (6MWT) test is a submaximal exercise stress test used to evaluate functional capacity and treatment effects.[146–149] This test measures the distance covered during ambulation for 6 min, taking into account exertional limitations and hypoxemic events. Although 6MWT may provide information in patients with moderate or severe exercise limitations, it is unlikely that they will be able to discern the presence of early disease, particularly in the case of children or individuals experiencing difficulties following instructions. In one study of 34 patients from 6 to 24 years of age, 6MWT Z-scores showed a significant but poor correlation with FEV1, BMI, CXR, and CT abnormalities.[150] Currently, limited data suggest that the 6MWT does not correlate with lung function measurements and may be challenging to perform in children.[151]

The Role of Real-World Studies in Monitoring Modulator Impact on Clinical Outcomes

Whereas novel tools to monitor infection, inflammation, and disease progression are increasingly available and more feasible, their clinical relevance, predictive ability, and performance characteristics must still be validated. Examining banked specimens from large study repositories linked to clinical data (eg, GOAL, PROMISE,[11] PROMISE pediatric cohorts, Study to Evaluate Biological & Clinical Effects of Significantly Corrected CFTR Function in Infants & Young Children [BEGIN, NCT04509050]) and studying long-term relationships between novel biomarkers, such as a change in sweat chloride concentration and clinical outcomes in patient registries (eg, CHEC-SC[152–154]) may identify markers of disease burden and potential patient phenotypes in the context of HEMT treatment. Ongoing real-world experience in large population studies of patients with CF receiving modulators will provide insights into disease marker development.[155,156] In addition to measuring established clinical outcomes noted earlier, the PROMISE trial generated an extensive resource of clinical data and biological samples that will enable future proteomic, genomic, and microbiologic analysis and the validation of these findings using clinical data after months of follow-up.[11] The study to evaluate the effects of CFTR modulators in infants and young children (BEGIN) and a pediatric cohort of the PROMISE will provide data specific to children and infants treated with modulators that may be crucial for the development and validation of markers of early disease, when established clinical outcome measures may be insensitive to detect mild disease.

An added benefit to measuring clinical outcomes and the collection of biospecimens from these cohorts will be the ability to understand disease development and response to modulators at a molecular level using personalized medicine. Our ability to profile individual CF patients based on genomic and biomarker data has recently expanded. Early studies of single-cell RNA sequencing in airway epithelial and immune cells provide data on the transcriptomic profiles of CF lung disease, dysfunctional host defense, and immunity programs within CF airways, and even enabled the discovery of novel airway epithelial cell types, such as the ionocytes.[157–159] In the HEMT era, these technologies may be applied to broadly characterize HEMT responses by epithelial and immune cells at an unprecedented single-cell and whole transcriptome resolution. Consistent with these studies, mass cytometry has been recently used to profile cell-specific marker expression and to immunophenotype CF immune cells and responses to inflammatory stimuli,[160] providing critical validation for genomic and computational findings. Finally, biomarkers of inflammation have been frequently used to understand responses to immunomodulatory therapies or modulators in CF.[161–163] Markers of CF airway inflammation, exacerbation, and disease progression measured from noninvasive clinical samples include electrolytes, inflammatory cytokines, host defense proteins, and tissue metalloproteinases.[35,97,164–168] Candidate sputum and systemic biomarkers of inflammation have generally not performed well in clinical trials, however, there is an emerging need to identify more sensitive predictors of clinical response using emerging technologies, such as multiplexed assays and proteomic screening.[169,170] Please refer to Jennifer S. Guimbellot and colleagues' article, "Novel Applications of Biomarkers and Personalized Medicine in Cystic Fibrosis," in this series for a comprehensive perspective on the application of these emerging strategies in CF.

Long-Term Health Monitoring and Personalization of Cystic Fibrosis Care

All available symptomatic therapies in CF were developed in the context of minimal or no CFTR activity, and thus, their relative benefit in the context of HEMT is unknown. As the modulator-treated CF population becomes healthier and lives longer, it is hoped that emerging markers of disease status can be combined with established outcome measures to understand the impact of modulators to monitor disease and guide changes in care.

Monitoring Disease Control

It is presumed that early use of HEMT (before the development of lung or other end-organ diseases) will delay the onset of CF pathology. Whereas this hypothesis has yet to be tested and will be informed by current and future trials of CFTR modulators, there is reason to believe that partial CFTR function in early life will delay or prevent CF disease. It is well known that patients with pancreatic-sufficient CF demonstrate numerous clinical features consistent with a milder clinical disease course than those with pancreatic-insufficient CF, including later age at diagnosis (in the absence of newborn screening), better lung function, later colonization with CF pathogens, improved growth, and longer survival.[171–173] Also, those with features of CF and diminished CFTR function but who fail to meet CF diagnostic criteria (eg, those with CFTR-related disorders) have a better overall prognosis than those diagnosed with CF.[174–176] It is also important to recognize that these patients are not disease-free and indeed can demonstrate both similar and unique features (eg, pancreatitis) to traditional CF, but often at an older age. Finally, the majority of adult CF patients receiving HEMT today and in the foreseeable future have established end-organ disease that is not reversible. Thus, the need for careful monitoring and intervention will be paramount as we learn to better care for this new HEMT-treated CF population. Many of the novel technologies described in this article may play an essential role in disease monitoring when established outcome measures, such as FEV$_1$, exacerbation frequency, growth, and microbiology may be stable or improved. There is early evidence to support this approach, as emerging pulmonary function tests (eg, MBW/LCI), imaging, and biomarker studies have shown increased sensitivity to detect early disease when compared with FEV$_1$.[35,82,166,177,178]

Defining the Level of Highly Effective Modulator Therapy Response

The approval of modulators for patients with rare CF-causing mutations (ie, patient subgroups with too few patients to conduct traditional clinical trials) has been driven by testing rare missense mutations in heterologous expression systems (eg, Fisher rat thyroid cells). This testing is an example of precision medicine in which those with uncommon mutations may be able to gain access to HEMT via standardized in vitro testing. In addition, there is emerging data that some patient-derived cell testing of modulators can predict clinical outcomes, such as changes in lung function and sweat chloride.[179,180] These measures are particularly relevant for personalized medicine and identifying CFTR modulator options for those with CFTR mutations that do not lend themselves well to testing in heterologous systems (eg, splice variants or other biosynthetic defects). Future studies should seek to quantify short-term benefits (to validate the preclinical systems), that these benefits are durable, and that results from personalized testing are readily reported to support access for those with similar rare mutations. Furthermore, normalizing the CFTR function of these rare mutations restored by modulators to wild-type CFTR function levels in vitro may help to understand those with substantial versus modest potential for modulator benefit.

Patients with more common mutations treated with HEMT based on clinical trial results (eg, F508del, G551D, and other gating mutations) may exhibit variable benefits from HEMT for a myriad of reasons, including baseline lung function or other markers of disease status, variable drug absorption, distribution, metabolism and/or excretion, drug–drug interactions or another defined cellular, molecular, and/or environmental contributors. Certainly, adherence is a critical factor to consider in those felt to have modest clinical benefit and has been described to be highly variable in a small cohort of ivacaftor-treated patients.[181] In the absence of routinely available serum drug level monitoring, health care providers will likely rely on established and emerging disease monitoring tools to assess modulator benefit. Defining these molecular biomarkers of modulator impact will be paramount in the next several years.

As an example, the relationship between sweat chloride changes and long-term clinical outcomes is the goal of the previously mentioned CHEC-SC study. Although clinical trials have not found sweat chloride changes to be clearly predictive of clinical outcomes such as lung function, standard and at-home sweat testing (eg, through wearable technologies[182]) could become part of a future panel of molecular and physiologic biomarkers. The identification of these future biomarkers may be informed by a review of data from large studies with established clinical outcome databases (eg, GOAL, PROMISE, RECOVER) and comparing/validating these with well-characterized samples from other CF-related studies (eg, PROSPECT study, Part A). Finally, the role of established and physiologic biomarkers, such as those discussed in this article, and their correlation with patient characteristics should be considered. Combinations of established clinical outcomes, surrogate clinical outcomes, and patient profiling data, including gene expression and cell-specific protein markers, can be used to identify subjects with varying degrees of modulator response. For example, patients may experience a limited FEV1 response on an initial assessment after initiation of HEMT but show gene expression changes in epithelial or immune cells consistent with a robust HEMT response. In this case, these patients could be monitored for a longer period in expectation of FEV1 improvements. In contrast, a similar subject with limited FEV1 response but no transcriptomic evidence of HEMT responsiveness would not be expected to improve, prompting the re-evaluation of current therapies and consideration of other treatments. Defining functional, imaging, genomics, and biomarkers response profiles could help personalize decisions to modify symptomatic treatments and target specific genes or markers in nonresponders. Notable examples of this application include "theratyping," the profiling of a patient's epithelial or immune cell response to modulators to predict clinical response to modulators,[161,183–185] and the development of wearable devices to measure epithelial chloride transport to monitor a patient's incremental response to modulators at home.[182,186–188] This topic is discussed in detail in article IV of this issue of *The Clinics*, titled *Novel applications of biomarkers and personalized medicine in cystic fibrosis.*

Guiding the Modification and Personalization of Symptomatic Therapies

Daily CF care often imposes a significant treatment burden, with several hours dedicated to airway clearance and respiratory therapies,[189–191] not to mention potentially numerous therapies to manage GI manifestations, CF-related diabetes, CF-related liver disease, and other disease manifestations. Following the approval of modulators and subsequent clinical improvements, many patients feel motivated to discontinue or de-escalate these therapies.[192,193] Symptomatic treatments were developed before modulator approval, limiting available data on their role in the HEMT era. Novel profiling and monitoring technologies, in addition to routinely used CF clinical outcomes, could accomplish this de-escalation in a stepwise, monitored approach. The SIMPLIFY trial will be the largest multicenter, randomized, controlled medication-withdrawal study in CF.[192,194] This study will evaluate the impact of discontinuing two standard-of-care respiratory therapies, dornase alpha[51,195,196] and HTS,[49,197,198] over 6 weeks in a planned population of approximately 800 individuals receiving ETI. Although this study focuses primarily on established clinical outcomes, including FEV_1 and exacerbation frequency, SIMPLIFY will also consider LCI changes after discontinuation of inhaled therapies. A similar, nonrandomized study of HTS and dornase alfa discontinuation with a more extended follow-up period is underway in the United Kingdom (CF STORM, EudraCT [European Union Drug Regulating Authorities Clinical Trials Database] number 2020 to 005864 to 77). This study will also focus on established measures of lung function, exacerbation frequency, and quality of life. Collecting imaging data and genomic/protein markers could inform the future design of similar trials, mainly focused on the de-escalation of respiratory therapies based on personalized HEMT response profiles. In addition to these studies, registry-based observational cohorts will inform our approach to clinical de-escalation. The Home-Reported Outcomes in People with Cystic Fibrosis Taking Highly Effective CFTR Modulator Therapy (HERO-2) study will monitor the impact of ETI on the daily use of chronic CF therapies using remote application-based PRO surveys and information from the CFF patient registry (NCT04798014), whereas the Qualitative Understanding of Experience with the SIMPLIFY Trial (QUEST) will monitor the experience of individuals with CF through qualitative patient interviews who discontinue standard-of-care respiratory therapies while on modulator therapy (NCT04320381). Although none of these studies will individually determine what features reliably identify candidates that should continue or can safely discontinue these inhaled therapies, it is hoped that this type of overlapping data and trial designs from controlled trials and real-world patient choices in their care will better define HEMT-treated patient phenotypes.

SUMMARY

Although the recent, widespread adoption of triple modulator therapy with ETI brought dramatic improvements in lung function, exacerbation frequency, nutrition, and quality of life, it also uncovered the need to develop new methods to monitor the health of individuals with CF when on HEMT. Most CF patients are frequently monitored through clinical symptoms, lung function, BMI, microbiology data, and a multidisciplinary care team assessment. FEV_1 has been the primary outcome measure used to quantify HEMT response in older children and adults. However, little is known regarding disease prognosis based on the assessment of an individual's clinical response.

The arrival of modulators coincided with a broad expansion of scientific methodologies that can help us better understand and characterize a patient's response to modulators. Among these have emerged measures of lung function, the growing application of pulmonary imaging in CF, and the adaptation of biomarker tools that could provide insights into HEMT responses at an unprecedented level of detail. Looking into the future, these emerging measures, along with new tools to measure PROs will offer a more comprehensive view of an individual's clinical trajectory when receiving HEMT.

Concurrent with clinical trials, data from real-world experience will continue to provide insights into the impact of modulators on CF disease progression and inform the development of early disease markers when established clinical outcome measures may be insensitive to early or mild disease. The combined application of these approaches has the potential to redefine HEMT-treated CF and has lasting effects in monitoring disease, profiling HEMT responses, and guiding the use of symptomatic therapies in a personalized fashion to ultimately enhance the quality of life and long-term outcomes of those with CF.

CLINICS CARE POINTS

- Highly effective modulator therapy (HEMT) markedly improved clinical outcomes in the majority of the cystic fibrosis population, creating new challenges for long-term disease monitoring.

- Emerging approaches to monitor HEMT response include lung clearance index, developments in pulmonary imaging, patient-reported outcomes, and novel molecular biomarkers.

- Imaging through pulmonary computed tomography, MRI, or ultrasound can provide insights into pulmonary anatomy and physiology.

- There are numerous studies underway to evaluate the impact of HEMT on these novel outcome measures and to determine an approach to de-escalate respiratory therapies on those receiving HEMT when indicated.

DISCLOSURE

C.J. Britto: Nothing to disclose relevant to this article, F. Ratjen: Nothing to disclose relevant to this article, J.P. Clancy: Nothing to disclose relevant to this article. To advance drug development and a search for a cure, the Cystic Fibrosis Foundation (CFF) has contracts with several companies to help fund the development of potential treatments and/or cures for CF. Pursuant to these contracts, CFF may receive milestone-based payments, equity interests, royalties on the net sales of therapies, and/or other forms of consideration. The resulting revenue received by the CFF is used in support of our mission.

REFERENCES

1. Shteinberg M, Haq IJ, Polineni D, et al. Cystic fibrosis. Lancet 2021;397:2195–211.
2. Cystic Fibrosis Foundation Patient Registry 2020 Annual Data Report Bethesda, Maryland ©2021 Cystic Fibrosis Foundation.
3. Middleton PG, et al. Elexacaftor–Tezacaftor–Ivacaftor for Cystic Fibrosis with a Single Phe508del Allele. N Engl J Med 2019;381:1809–19.
4. Heijerman HGM, et al. Efficacy and safety of the elexacaftor plus tezacaftor plus ivacaftor combination regimen in people with cystic fibrosis homozygous for the F508del mutation: a double-blind, randomised, phase 3 trial. Lancet 2019;394: 1940–8.
5. Burgel P-R, et al. Rapid improvement after starting elexacaftor-tezacaftor-ivacaftor in patients with cystic fibrosis and advanced pulmonary disease. Am J Respir Crit Care Med 2021. https://doi.org/10.1164/rccm.202011–204153OC.
6. Djavid AR, et al. Efficacy of elexacaftor/tezacaftor/ivacaftor in advanced cystic fibrosis lung disease. Ann Am Thorac Soc 2021. https://doi.org/10.1513/AnnalsATS.202102–202220RL.

7. Ridley K, Condren M. Elexacaftor-tezacaftor-ivacaftor: the first triple-combination cystic fibrosis transmembrane conductance regulator modulating therapy. J Pediatr Pharmacol Ther 2020;25:192–7.

8. Martin C, et al. Patient perspectives following initiation of elexacaftor-tezacaftor-ivacaftor in people with cystic fibrosis and advanced lung disease. Respir Med 2021;80:100829.

9. Egan ME. Cystic fibrosis transmembrane conductance receptor modulator therapy in cystic fibrosis, an update. Curr Opin Pediatr 2020;32:384–8.

10. DiMango E, et al. Effect of highly effective modulator treatment on sinonasal symptoms in cystic fibrosis. J Cyst Fibros 2021;20:460–3.

11. Nichols DP, et al. Clinical effectiveness of elexacaftor/Tezacftor/ivacaftor in people with cystic fibrosis. Am J Respir Crit Care Med 2021. https://doi.org/10.1164/rccm.202108–1986OC.

12. Rosenfeld M, Davis R, FitzSimmons S, et al. Gender gap in cystic fibrosis mortality. Am J Epidemiol 1997;145:794–803.

13. Holtrop M, et al. A prospective study of the effects of sex hormones on lung function and inflammation in women with cystic fibrosis. Ann Am Thorac Soc 2021. https://doi.org/10.1513/AnnalsATS.202008–1064OC.

14. Demko CA, Byard PJ, Davis PB. Gender differences in cystic fibrosis: Pseudomonas aeruginosa infection. J Clin Epidemiol 1995;48:1041–9.

15. Corey M, Farewell V. Determinants of mortality from cystic fibrosis in Canada, 1970–1989. Am J Epidemiol 1996;143:1007–17.

16. Chotirmall SH, et al. Effect of estrogen on pseudomonas mucoidy and exacerbations in cystic fibrosis. N Engl J Med 2012;366:1978–86.

17. Chotirmall SH, Greene CM, McElvaney NG. Immune, inflammatory and infectious consequences of estrogen in women with cystic fibrosis. Expert Rev Respir Med 2012;6:573–5.

18. Sutton S, Rosenbluth D, Raghavan D, et al. Effects of puberty on cystic fibrosis related pulmonary exacerbations in women versus men. Pediatr Pulmonol 2014;49:28–35.

19. Secunda KE, et al. Females with cystic fibrosis demonstrate a differential response profile to ivacaftor compared with males. Am J Respir Crit Care Med 2020;201:996–8.

20. Fidler MC, Beusmans J, Panorchan P, et al. Correlation of sweat chloride and percent predicted FEV1 in cystic fibrosis patients treated with ivacaftor. J Cyst Fibros 2017;16:41–4.

21. Aalbers BL, et al. Females with cystic fibrosis have a larger decrease in sweat chloride in response to lumacaftor/ivacaftor compared to males. J Cyst Fibros 2021;20:e7–11.

22. Huang Y, et al. Elexacaftor/tezacaftor/ivacaftor improved clinical outcomes in an N1303K-CFTR patient based on in vitro Experimental evidence. Am J Respir Crit Care Med 2021. https://doi.org/10.1164/rccm.202101–0090LE.

23. Barry PJ, et al. Triple therapy for cystic fibrosis Phe508del–gating and –residual function Genotypes. N Engl J Med 2021;385:815–25.

24. Agent P, Morison L, Prasad A. Standards for the clinical care of children and adults with cystic fibrosis in the UK–. Cystic Fibrosis Trust 2011;1:46.

25. Castellani C, et al. ECFS best practice guidelines: the 2018 revision. J Cyst Fibros 2018;17:153–78.

26. Hendra K, Neemuchwala F, Chan M, et al. Patient and provider experience with cystic fibrosis Telemedicine clinic. Front Pediatr 2021;9:784692.

27. Somerville LAL, et al. Real-world outcomes in cystic fibrosis Telemedicine clinical care in a time of a Global pandemic. Chest 2021. https://doi.org/10.1016/j.chest.2021.11.035.

28. Dixon E, et al. Telemedicine and cystic fibrosis: do we still need face-to-face clinics? Paediatr Respir Rev 2021. https://doi.org/10.1016/j.prrv.2021.05.002.

29. Compton M, et al. A Feasibility study of Urgent Implementation of cystic fibrosis multidisciplinary Telemedicine clinic in the face of COVID-19 pandemic: single-Center experience. Telemed. J E Health 2020;26:978–84.

30. Guimbellot J, et al. Effectiveness of ivacaftor in cystic fibrosis patients with non-G551D gating mutations. J Cyst Fibros 2019;18:102–9.

31. Volkova N, et al. Disease progression in patients with cystic fibrosis treated with ivacaftor: data from national US and UK registries. J Cyst Fibros 2020;19:68–79.

32. Hughes DA, et al. Clinical characteristics of Pseudomonas and Aspergillus co-infected cystic fibrosis patients: a UK registry study. J Cyst Fibros 2021. https://doi.org/10.1016/j.jcf.2021.04.007.

33. Burgel P-R, et al. Clinical response to lumacaftor-ivacaftor in patients with cystic fibrosis according to baseline lung function. J Cyst Fibros 2021;20:220–7.

34. Chalmers JD, et al. Neutrophil elastase activity is associated with exacerbations and lung function decline in bronchiectasis. Am J Respir Crit Care Med 2017;195:1384–93.

35. Mayer-Hamblett N, et al. Association between pulmonary function and sputum biomarkers in cystic fibrosis. Am J Respir Crit Care Med 2007;175:822–8.

36. Hisert KB, et al. Restoring cystic fibrosis transmembrane conductance regulator function reduces airway bacteria and inflammation in people with cystic fibrosis and chronic lung infections. Am J Respir Crit Care Med 2017;195:1617–28.

37. Rowe SM, et al. Clinical mechanism of the cystic fibrosis transmembrane conductance regulator

potentiator ivacaftor in G551D-mediated cystic fibrosis. Am J Respir Crit Care Med 2014;190: 175–84.

38. Davies JC, et al. Safety, pharmacokinetics, and pharmacodynamics of ivacaftor in patients aged 2–5 years with cystic fibrosis and a CFTR gating mutation (KIWI): an open-label, single-arm study. Lancet Respir Med 2016;4:107–15.

39. Rosenfeld M, et al. An open-label extension study of ivacaftor in children with CF and a CFTR gating mutation initiating treatment at age 2–5 years (KLIMB). J Cyst Fibros 2019;18:838–43.

40. Taylor-Robinson D, et al. Understanding the natural progression in %FEV1decline in patients with cystic fibrosis: a longitudinal study. Thorax 2012;67:860–6.

41. Breuer O, Caudri D, Stick S, et al. Predicting disease progression in cystic fibrosis. Expert Rev Respir Med 2018;12:905–17.

42. Ellemunter H, et al. Sensitivity of lung clearance index and chest computed tomography in early cf lung disease. Respir Med 2010;104:1834–42.

43. Stahl M, et al. Comparison of lung clearance index and magnetic resonance imaging for assessment of lung disease in children with cystic fibrosis. Am J Respir Crit Care Med 2017;195:349–59.

44. Kent L, et al. Lung clearance index: evidence for use in clinical trials in cystic fibrosis. J Cyst Fibros 2014;13:123–38.

45. Horsley AR, et al. Longitudinal assessment of lung clearance index to monitor disease progression in children and adults with cystic fibrosis. Thorax 2021. https://doi.org/10.1136/thoraxjnl-2021–216928.

46. Donaldson SH, et al. Effect of lumacaftor-ivacaftor on mucociliary clearance and clinical outcomes in cystic fibrosis: results from the PROSPECT MCC sub-study. J Cyst Fibros 2021. https://doi.org/10.1016/j.jcf.2021.05.004.

47. Hatziagorou E, et al. Toward the establishment of new clinical endpoints for cystic fibrosis: the role of lung clearance index and cardiopulmonary exercise testing. Front Pediatr 2021;9:635719.

48. Davies JC, et al. WS7. 6 Effect of ivacaftor on lung function in subjects with CF who have the G551D-CFTR mutation and mild lung disease: a comparison of lung clearance index (LCI) vs. spirometry. J Cyst Fibros 2012;S15.

49. Amin R, Subbarao P, Jabar A, Balkovec S, Jensen R, Kerrigan S, Gustafsson P, Ratjen F. Hypertonic saline improves the LCI in paediatric patients with CF with normal lung function. Thorax. 2010 May;65(5):379-83. doi:10.1136/thx.2009.125831. PMID: 20435858.

50. Voldby C, et al. Withdrawal of dornase alfa increases ventilation inhomogeneity in children with cystic fibrosis. J Cystic Fibrosis 2021. https://doi.org/10.1016/j.jcf.2021.02.004.

51. Amin R, et al. The effect of dornase alfa on ventilation inhomogeneity in patients with cystic fibrosis. Eur Respir J 2011;37:806–12.

52. Subbarao P, et al. Effect of hypertonic saline on lung clearance index in infants and preschool children with cf: a pilot study: 223. Pediatr Pulmonol 2012;47:301–2.

53. Horsley AR, et al. Lung clearance index is a sensitive, repeatable and practical measure of airways disease in adults with cystic fibrosis. Thorax 2008;63:135–40.

54. Aurora P, et al. Multiple-breath washout as a marker of lung disease in preschool children with cystic fibrosis. Am J Respir Crit Care Med 2005;171: 249–56.

55. Verbanck S, et al. Lung clearance index in adult cystic fibrosis patients: the role of convection-dependent lung units. Eur Respir J 2013;42: 380–8.

56. Cohen-Cymberknoh M, Kerem E, Ferkol T, et al. Airway inflammation in cystic fibrosis: molecular mechanisms and clinical implications. Thorax 2013;68:1157–62.

57. Ramsey KA, et al. Multiple-breath washout outcomes are sensitive to inflammation and infection in children with cystic fibrosis. Ann Am Thorac Soc 2017;14:1436–42.

58. Keen C, Gustafsson P, Lindblad A, et al. Low levels of exhaled nitric oxide are associated with impaired lung function in cystic fibrosis. Pediatr Pulmonol 2010;45:241–8.

59. Horsley AR, et al. Changes in physiological, functional and structural markers of cystic fibrosis lung disease with treatment of a pulmonary exacerbation. Thorax 2013;68:532–9.

60. Horsley A. Lung clearance index in the assessment of airways disease. Respir Med 2009;103:793–9.

61. Gustafsson PM. Peripheral airway involvement in CF and asthma compared by inert gas washout. Pediatr Pulmonol 2007;42:168–76.

62. Hardaker KM, et al. Abnormal preschool Lung Clearance Index (LCI) reflects clinical status and predicts lower spirometry later in childhood in cystic fibrosis. J Cyst Fibros 2019;18:721–7.

63. Aurora P, et al. Lung clearance index at 4 years predicts subsequent lung function in children with cystic fibrosis. Am J Respir Crit Care Med 2011; 183:752–8.

64. Davies G, et al. An observational study of the lung clearance index throughout childhood in cystic fibrosis: early years matter. Eur Respir J 2020; 56(4):2000006.

65. Chelabi R, Soumagne T, Guillien A, et al. In cystic fibrosis, lung clearance index is sensitive to detecting abnormalities appearing at exercise in children with normal spirometry. Respir Physiol Neurobiol 2018;247:9–11.

66. Hatziagorou E, et al. Can LCI predict new Pseudomonas aeruginosa colonization among CF patients? Eur Respir J 2017;50.

67. Hatziagorou E, Avramidou V, Kampouras A, et al. Clinical value of lung clearance index (LCI) among patients with cystic fibrosis. Eur Respir J 2014;44.

68. Perrem L, et al. Lung clearance index to Track acute respiratory Events in school-age children with cystic fibrosis. Am J Respir Crit Care Med 2021;203:977–86.

69. Davies J, et al. Assessment of clinical response to ivacaftor with lung clearance index in cystic fibrosis patients with a G551D- CFTR mutation and preserved spirometry: a randomised controlled trial. Lancet Respir Med 2013;1:630–8.

70. Davies JC, et al. A phase 3, double-blind, parallel-group study to evaluate the efficacy and safety of tezacaftor in combination with ivacaftor in participants 6 through 11 years of age with cystic fibrosis homozygous for F508del or heterozygous for the F508del-CFTR mutation and a residual function mutation. J Cystic Fibrosis 2021;20:68–77.

71. Shaw M, et al. Changes in LCI in F508del/F508del patients treated with lumacaftor/ivacaftor: results from the prospect study. J Cyst Fibros 2020;19: 931–3.

72. Group, V.-445-106 S. & Others. A phase 3 open-label study of elexacaftor/tezacaftor/ivacaftor in children 6 through 11 years of age with cystic fibrosis and at least one F508del allele. Am. J. Respir. Crit. Care Med 2021;203:1522–32.

73. Frauchiger BS, et al. Natural variability of clinically measured lung clearance index in children with cystic fibrosis. Eur Respir J 2021;58.

74. Svedberg M, Gustafsson PM, Robinson PD, et al. Variability of lung clearance index in clinically stable cystic fibrosis lung disease in school age children. J Cystic Fibrosis 2018;17:236–41.

75. Hall GL, et al. Air trapping on chest CT is associated with worse ventilation distribution in infants with cystic fibrosis diagnosed following newborn screening. PLoS One 2011;6:e23932.

76. Oikonomou A, et al. High resolution computed tomography of the chest in cystic fibrosis (CF): is simplification of scoring systems feasible? Eur Radiol 2008;18:538–47.

77. Szczesniak R, Turkovic L, Andrinopoulou E-R, et al. Chest imaging in cystic fibrosis studies: what counts, and can be counted? J Cyst Fibros 2017; 16:175–85.

78. de Jong PA, et al. Progressive damage on high resolution computed tomography despite stable lung function in cystic fibrosis. Eur Respir J 2004;23: 93–7.

79. Brody AS, et al. Computed tomography in the evaluation of cystic fibrosis lung disease. Am J Respir Crit Care Med 2005;172:1246–52.

80. Owens CM, et al. Lung Clearance Index and HRCT are complementary markers of lung abnormalities in young children with CF. Thorax 2011;66:481–8.

81. Tepper LA, et al. Tracking CF disease progression with CT and respiratory symptoms in a cohort of children aged 6-19 years. Pediatr Pulmonol 2014; 49:1182–9.

82. Ramsey KA, et al. Lung clearance index and structural lung disease on computed tomography in early cystic fibrosis. Am J Respir Crit Care Med 2016;193:60–7.

83. Rosenow T, et al. PRAGMA-CF. A quantitative structural lung disease computed tomography outcome in young children with cystic fibrosis. Am J Respir Crit Care Med 2015;191:1158–65.

84. Lauwers E, et al. The short-term effects of ORKAMBI (lumacaftor/ivacaftor) on regional and distal lung structures using functional respiratory imaging. Ther Adv Respir Dis 2021;15. 17534666211046774.

85. Brody AS, et al. High-resolution computed tomography of the chest in children with cystic fibrosis: support for use as an outcome surrogate. Pediatr Radiol 1999;29:731–5.

86. Brody AS, et al. High-resolution computed tomography in young patients with cystic fibrosis: distribution of abnormalities and correlation with pulmonary function tests. J Pediatr 2004;145:32–8.

87. Wainwright CE, et al. Effect of bronchoalveolar lavage–Directed therapy on Pseudomonas aeruginosa infection and structural lung Injury in children with cystic fibrosis: a randomized trial. JAMA 2011; 306:163–71.

88. Tepper LA, et al. Impact of bronchiectasis and trapped air on quality of life and exacerbations in cystic fibrosis. Eur Respir J 2013;42:371–9.

89. Kuo W, Perez-Rovira A, Andinopoulou ER, et al. WS08. 3 CF-CT and PRAGMA-CF scoring techniques compared using quantification with objective airway and artery dimensions of children with cystic fibrosis. J Cyst Fibros 2016;1:S13.

90. Pearce MS, et al. Radiation exposure from CT scans in childhood and subsequent risk of leukaemia and brain tumours: a retrospective cohort study. Lancet 2012;380:499–505.

91. Ratjen F, et al. Inhaled hypertonic saline in preschool children with cystic fibrosis (SHIP): a multicentre, randomised, double-blind, placebo-controlled trial. Lancet Respir Med 2019;7:802–9.

92. Tiddens H, et al. 539: effect of inhaled hypertonic saline on structural lung disease in preschool children with cystic fibrosis. The SHIP-CT study. J Cyst Fibros 2021;20:S255.

93. Tiddens HA, et al. P058 the effect of hypertonic saline treatment in pre-schoolers with cystic fibrosis on lung structure as measured by chest computed

tomography. SHIP-CT study. J Cyst Fibros 2021;20: S56.

94. Dournes G, et al. Lung morphology assessment of cystic fibrosis using MRI with ultra-short echo time at submillimeter spatial resolution. Eur Radiol 2016; 26:3811–20.

95. Woods JC, et al. Current state of the art MRI for the longitudinal assessment of cystic fibrosis. J Magn Reson Imaging 2020;52:1306–20.

96. Stahl M, et al. Magnetic resonance imaging detects progression of lung disease and impact of newborn screening in preschool children with cystic fibrosis. Am J Respir Crit Care Med 2021. https://doi.org/10.1164/rccm.202102–0278OC.

97. Chung, J. et al. Increased Inflammatory Markers Detected in Nasal Lavage Correlate with Paranasal Sinus Abnormalities at MRI in Adolescent Patients with Cystic Fibrosis. Antioxidants (Basel) 10, (2021).

98. Ciet P, et al. Comparison of chest-MRI to chest-ct to monitor cystic fibrosis lung disease. Pediatric Pulmonology Supplement 2010;33:362.

99. Failo R, et al. Lung morphology assessment using MRI: a robust ultra-short TR/TE 2D steady state free precession sequence used in cystic fibrosis patients. Magn Reson Med 2009;61:299–306.

100. Ciet P, et al. Spirometer-controlled cine magnetic resonance imaging used to diagnose tracheobronchomalacia in paediatric patients. Eur Respir J 2014;43:115–24.

101. Ley-Zaporozhan J, et al. Repeatability and reproducibility of quantitative whole-lung perfusion magnetic resonance imaging. J Thorac Imaging 2011; 26:230–9.

102. Thomen RP, et al. Regional structure-function in cystic fibrosis lung disease using hyperpolarized 129Xe and Ultrashort echo magnetic resonance imaging. Am J Respir Crit Care Med 2020;202: 290–2.

103. Smith LJ, et al. The assessment of short- and long-term changes in lung function in cystic fibrosis using 129Xe MRI. Eur Respir J 2020;56.

104. Koch MF, et al. Comparison of hyperpolarized 3He and 129Xe MR imaging in patients with cystic fibrosis. A108. Pathophysiology in DIFFUSE PARENCHYMAL. LUNG DISEASES 2019. https://doi.org/10.1164/ajrccm-conference.2019.199.1_meetingabstracts.a2567.

105. Bannier E, et al. Hyperpolarized 3He MR for sensitive imaging of ventilation function and treatment efficiency in young cystic fibrosis patients with normal lung function. Radiology 2010;255: 225–32.

106. Dournes G, et al. The clinical Use of lung MRI in cystic fibrosis: what, now, how? Chest 2021;159: 2205–17.

107. Strzelczuk-Judka L, Wojsyk-Banaszak I, Zakrzewska A, et al. Diagnostic value of chest ultrasound in children with cystic fibrosis - pilot study. PLoS One 2019;14:e0215786.

108. Ciuca I, Pop L, Marc M, et al. How useful is the lung ultrasound in cystic fibrosis? Eur Respir J 2016;48: 1261.

109. Ciuca IM, Dediu M, Pop LL. Lung clearance index and lung ultrasound in cystic fibrosis children. Eur Respir J 2018;52(62):OA4988.

110. Peixoto AO, et al. The Use of ultrasound as a tool to evaluate pulmonary disease in cystic fibrosis. Respir. Care 2020;65:293–303.

111. Quittner AL, Buu A, Messer MA, et al. Development and validation of the Cystic Fibrosis Questionnaire in the United States: a health-related quality-of-life measure for cystic fibrosis. Chest 2005;128: 2347–54.

112. Patrick DL, et al. Content validity—establishing and reporting the evidence in newly developed patient-reported outcomes (PRO) instruments for medical product evaluation: ISPOR PRO Good Research Practices Task Force report: part 2—assessing respondent understanding. Value Health 2011;14: 978–88.

113. Quittner AL, et al. Translation and linguistic validation of a disease-specific quality of life measure for cystic fibrosis. J Pediatr Psychol 2000;25:403–14.

114. Quittner AL, et al. Psychometric evaluation of the cystic fibrosis questionnaire-Revised in a national sample. Qual Life Res 2012;21:1267–78.

115. Gee L, Abbott J, Conway SP, et al. Development of a disease specific health related quality of life measure for adults and adolescents with cystic fibrosis. Thorax 2000;55:946–54.

116. Goss CH, Edwards TC, Ramsey BW, et al. Patient-reported respiratory symptoms in cystic fibrosis. J Cyst Fibros 2009;8:245–52.

117. Besier T, et al. Anxiety, depression, and life satisfaction in parents caring for children with cystic fibrosis. Pediatr Pulmonol 2011;46:672–82.

118. Smith BA, Modi AC, Quittner AL, et al. Depressive symptoms in children with cystic fibrosis and parents and its effects on adherence to airway clearance. Pediatr Pulmonol 2010;45:756–63.

119. Goldbeck L, Schmitz TG, Henrich G, et al. Questions on life satisfaction for adolescents and adults with cystic fibrosis: development of a disease-specific questionnaire. Chest 2003;123:42–8.

120. Coucke R, et al. 'Il faut continuer à poser des questions' patient reported outcome measures in cystic fibrosis: an anthropological perspective. J Cyst Fibros 2021;20:e108–13.

121. Pattie P, et al. Quality of life is poorly correlated to lung disease severity in school-aged children with cystic fibrosis. J Cyst Fibros 2021. https://doi.org/10.1016/j.jcf.2021.11.005.

122. Beswick DM, et al. Impact of CFTR therapy on chronic rhinosinusitis and health status: Deep learning CT analysis and patient reported outcomes. Ann Am Thorac Soc 2021. https://doi.org/10.1513/AnnalsATS.202101-203057OC.

123. Douglas JE, et al. Impact of novel CFTR modulator on sinonasal quality of life in adult patients with cystic fibrosis. Int Forum Allergy Rhinol 2021;11:201-3.

124. Freeman AJ, et al. Designing the GALAXY study: Partnering with the cystic fibrosis community to optimize assessment of gastrointestinal symptoms. J Cyst Fibros 2021;20:598-604.

125. Sathe M, et al. Utilization of electronic patient-reported outcome measures in cystic fibrosis research: application to the GALAXY study. J Cyst Fibros 2021;20:605-11.

126. Hebestreit H, et al. Cardiopulmonary exercise testing provides additional prognostic information in cystic fibrosis. Am J Respir Crit Care Med 2019;199:987-95.

127. Gruet M, Peyré-Tartaruga LA, Mely L, et al. The 1-minute Sit-to-Stand test in adults with cystic fibrosis: correlations with cardiopulmonary exercise test, 6-minute walk test, and Quadriceps Strength. Respir. Care 2016;61:1620-8.

128. Paolo MD, et al. Six-minute walk test vs cardiopulmonary exercise test in the assessment of exercise tolerance in adults with cystic fibrosis. Cystic Fibrosis 2017. https://doi.org/10.1183/1393003.congress-2017.pa1349.

129. Radtke T, et al. ERS statement on standardisation of cardiopulmonary exercise testing in chronic lung diseases. Eur Respir Rev 2019;28:180101.

130. Fletcher GF, et al. Exercise standards for testing and training: a scientific statement from the American Heart Association. Circulation 2013;128:873-934.

131. Orenstein DM. Assessment of exercise pulmonary function. Pediatr Lab Exerc Test 1993;141-63.

132. Orenstein DM, Nixon PA. Exercise performance and breathing patterns in cystic fibrosis: Male-female differences and influence of resting pulmonary function. Pediatr Pulmonol 1991;10:101-5.

133. Nixon PA, Orenstein DM, Kelsey SF, et al. The prognostic value of exercise testing in patients with cystic fibrosis. N. Engl. J Med 1992;327:1785-8.

134. Saynor ZL, Barker AR, Oades PJ, et al. Reproducibility of maximal cardiopulmonary exercise testing for young cystic fibrosis patients. J Cyst Fibros 2013;12:644-50.

135. Avramidou V, et al. Lung clearance index (LCI) as a predictor of exercise limitation among CF patients. Pediatr Pulmonol 2018;53:81-7.

136. Kampouras A, et al. Ventilation efficiency to exercise in patients with cystic fibrosis. Pediatr Pulmonol 2019;54:1584-90.

137. Kampouras A, et al. Does Pseudomonas aeruginosa colonization Affect exercise capacity in CF? Pulm Med 2019;2019:3786245.

138. Edgeworth D, et al. Improvement in exercise duration, lung function and well-being in G551D-cystic fibrosis patients: a double-blind, placebo-controlled, randomized, cross-over study with ivacaftor treatment. Clin Sci 2017;131:2037-45.

139. Urquhart DS, Saynor ZL. Exercise testing in cystic fibrosis: who and why? Paediatr Respir Rev 2018;27:28-32.

140. Radtke T, Faro A, Wong J, et al. Exercise testing in pediatric lung transplant candidates with cystic fibrosis. Pediatr Transpl 2011;15:294-9.

141. Vendrusculo FM, Heinzmann-Filho JP, da Silva, et al. Peak oxygen uptake and mortality in cystic fibrosis: systematic review and meta-analysis. Respir. Care 2019;64:91-8.

142. Pianosi P, Leblanc J, Almudevar A. Peak oxygen uptake and mortality in children with cystic fibrosis. Thorax 2005;60:50-4.

143. Ejiofor LCK, et al. Patients with cystic fibrosis and advanced lung disease benefit from lumacaftor/ivacaftor treatment. Pediatr Pulmonol 2020;55:3364-70.

144. Saynor ZL, Barker AR, Oades PJ, et al. The effect of ivacaftor in adolescents with cystic fibrosis (G551D mutation): an exercise physiology perspective. Pediatr Phys Ther 2014;26:454-61.

145. Lang RL, Stockton K, Wilson C, et al. Exercise testing for children with cystic fibrosis: a systematic review. Pediatr. Pulmonol 2020;55:1996-2010.

146. Brooks D, Solway S. ATS statement on six-minute walk test. Am J Respir Crit Care Med 2003;167:1287.

147. Barry SC, Gallagher CG. The repeatability of submaximal endurance exercise testing in cystic fibrosis. Pediatr Pulmonol 2007;42:75-82.

148. Enright PL, et al. The 6-min walk test: a quick measure of functional status in elderly adults. Chest 2003;123:387-98.

149. Cunha MT, Rozov T, de Oliveira, et al. Six-minute walk test in children and adolescents with cystic fibrosis. Pediatr Pulmonology 2006;41:618-22.

150. Stollar F, Rodrigues JC, Cunha MT, et al. Six minute walk test Z score: correlations with cystic fibrosis severity markers. J Cyst Fibros 2012;11:253-6.

151. Andrade Lima C, et al. Six-minute walk test as a determinant of the functional capacity of children and adolescents with cystic fibrosis: a systematic review. Respir. Med 2018;137:83-8.

152. Zemanick ET, et al. Measuring the impact of CFTR modulation on sweat chloride in cystic fibrosis: Rationale and design of the CHEC-SC study. J Cyst Fibros 2021;20:965-71.

153. Mayer-Hamblett N, et al. CFTR modulator-induced sweat chloride changes across the cystic fibrosis

population: first results from the CHEC-SC study. Pediatric Pulmonology 2019;54:S229. WILEY 111 RIVER ST, HOBOKEN 07030-5774, NJ USA.

154. Mayer-Hamblett N, et al. 555: clinical trial interest after establishment of modulator therapy: Interim CHEC-SC survey results. J Cyst Fibros 2021;20: S262.

155. Bessonova L, et al. Data from the US and UK cystic fibrosis registries support disease modification by CFTR modulation with ivacaftor. Thorax 2018;73: 731–40.

156. Higgins M, Volkova N, Moy K, et al. Real-world outcomes among patients with cystic fibrosis treated with ivacaftor: 2012–2016 experience. Pulm Ther 2020;6:141–9.

157. Schupp JC, et al. Single-cell transcriptional archetypes of airway inflammation in cystic fibrosis. Am J Respir Crit Care Med 2020;202:1419–29.

158. Plasschaert LW, et al. A single-cell atlas of the airway epithelium reveals the CFTR-rich pulmonary ionocyte. Nature 2018;560:377–81.

159. Okuda K, et al. Secretory cells dominate airway CFTR expression and function in human airway superficial epithelia. Am J Respir Crit Care Med 2021; 203:1275–89.

160. Yao Y, et al. Multiparameter single cell profiling of airway inflammatory cells. Cytometry B Clin Cytom 2017;92:12–20.

161. Hisert KB, et al. CFTR modulator therapy enhances peripheral blood monocyte contributions to immune responses in people with cystic fibrosis. Front. Pharmacol 2020;11:1219.

162. Westhölter D, et al. Pseudomonas aeruginosa infection, but not mono or dual-combination CFTR modulator therapy affects circulating regulatory T cells in an adult population with cystic fibrosis. J Cyst Fibros 2021. https://doi.org/10.1016/j.jcf. 2021.05.001.

163. Keown K, et al. Airway inflammation and host responses in the era of CFTR modulators. Int J Mol Sci 2020;21.

164. Levy H, et al. Inflammatory markers of lung disease in adult patients with cystic fibrosis. Pediatr Pulmonol 2007;42:256–62.

165. De Rose V. Mechanisms and markers of airway inflammation in cystic fibrosis. Eur Respir J 2002; 19:333–40.

166. Caudri D, et al. A screening tool to identify risk for bronchiectasis progression in children with cystic fibrosis. Pediatr Pulmonol 2021. https://doi.org/10. 1002/ppul.25712.

167. Jiang K, et al. RNA sequencing data from neutrophils of patients with cystic fibrosis reveals potential for developing biomarkers for pulmonary exacerbations. J Cystic Fibrosis 2019;18:194–202.

168. Short C, et al. A Short extension to multiple breath washout provides additional signal of distal airway disease in people with CF: a pilot study. J Cyst Fibros 2021. https://doi.org/10.1016/j.jcf.2021.06. 013.

169. Gharib SA, et al. Mapping the lung proteome in cystic fibrosis. J Proteome Res 2009;8:3020–8.

170. Khanal S, et al. SPLUNC1: a novel marker of cystic fibrosis exacerbations. Eur Respir J 2021. https:// doi.org/10.1183/13993003.00507–02020.

171. Muhlebach MS, et al. Anaerobic bacteria cultured from cystic fibrosis airways correlate to milder disease: a multisite study. Eur Respir J 2018;52.

172. Loubières Y, et al. Association between genetically determined pancreatic status and lung disease in adult cystic fibrosis patients. Chest 2002;121: 73–80.

173. Simanovsky N, et al. Differences in the pattern of structural abnormalities on CT scan in patients with cystic fibrosis and pancreatic sufficiency or insufficiency. Chest 2013;144:208–14.

174. Coffey MJ, Ooi CY. Pancreatitis in Cystic Fibrosis and CFTR-Related Disorder. In: Rodrigo, L., editor. Acute Pancreatitis [Internet]. London: IntechOpen; 2012 [cited 2022 Jul 11]. Available from: https:// www.intechopen.com/chapters/26187 doi: 10. 5772/27861.

175. Moskowitz SM, et al. Clinical practice and genetic counseling for cystic fibrosis and CFTR-related disorders. Genet Med 2008;10:851–68.

176. Paranjape SM, Zeitlin PL. Atypical cystic fibrosis and CFTR-related diseases. Clin Rev Allergy Immunol 2008;35:116–23.

177. Smith L, et al. Longitudinal monitoring of disease progression in children with mild CF using hyperpolarised gas MRI and LCI. Eur Respir J 2016;48.

178. Marshall H, et al. Detection of early subclinical lung disease in children with cystic fibrosis by lung ventilation imaging with hyperpolarised gas MRI. Thorax 2017;72:760–2.

179. Dekkers JF, et al. Characterizing responses to CFTR-modulating drugs using rectal organoids derived from subjects with cystic fibrosis. Sci Transl Med 2016;8:344ra84.

180. Pranke I, et al. Might brushed nasal cells be a surrogate for CFTR modulator clinical response? Am J Respir Crit Care Med 2019;199:123–6.

181. Siracusa CM, et al. Electronic monitoring reveals highly variable adherence patterns in patients prescribed ivacaftor. J Cyst Fibros 2015;14:621–6.

182. Ray TR, et al. Soft, skin-interfaced sweat stickers for cystic fibrosis diagnosis and management. Sci Transl Med 2021;13.

183. Pranke IM, et al. Correction of CFTR function in nasal epithelial cells from cystic fibrosis patients predicts improvement of respiratory function by CFTR modulators. Sci Rep 2017;7:7375.

184. Clancy JP, et al. CFTR modulator theratyping: current status, gaps and future directions. J Cyst Fibros 2019;18:22–34.

185. Sette G, et al. Theratyping cystic fibrosis in vitro in ALI-culture and organoid models generated from patient-derived nasal epithelial Conditionally Reprogrammed Stem Cells. Eur. Respir J 2021. https://doi.org/10.1183/13993003.00908–02021.

186. Choi D-H, Kitchen GB, Stewart KJ, et al. The dynamic response of sweat chloride to changes in exercise Load measured by a wearable sweat sensor. Scientific Rep 2020;10.

187. Vaquer A, Barón E, de la Rica R. Wearable Analytical platform with Enzyme-Modulated dynamic range for the Simultaneous Colorimetric detection of sweat Volume and sweat biomarkers. ACS Sens 2021;6:130–6.

188. Lechtzin N, et al. Rationale and design of a randomized trial of home electronic symptom and lung function monitoring to detect cystic fibrosis pulmonary exacerbations: the early intervention in cystic fibrosis exacerbation (eICE) trial. Contemp Clin Trials 2013;36:460–9.

189. Sawicki GS, Sellers DE, Robinson WM. High treatment burden in adults with cystic fibrosis: challenges to disease self-management. J Cyst Fibros 2009;8:91–6.

190. Sawicki GS, Goss CH. Tackling the increasing complexity of CF care. Pediatr Pulmonol 2015; 40(50 Suppl):S74–9.

191. Nichols DP, Kuk KN, Nick JA. Drug interactions and treatment burden as survival improves. Curr Opin Pulm Med 2015;21:617–25.

192. Mayer-Hamblett N, et al. Evaluating the impact of stopping chronic therapies after modulator drug therapy in cystic fibrosis: the SIMPLIFY clinical trial study design. Ann Am Thorac Soc 2021;18: 1397–405.

193. Narayanan S, Mainz JG, Gala S, et al. Adherence to therapies in cystic fibrosis: a targeted literature review. Expert Rev Respir Med 2017;11:129–45.

194. Davies G, et al. Characterising burden of treatment in cystic fibrosis to identify priority areas for clinical trials. J Cyst Fibros 2020;19:499–502.

195. Eisenberg JD, et al. Safety of repeated intermittent courses of aerosolized recombinant human deoxyribonuclease in patients with cystic fibrosis. J Pediatr 1997;131:118–24.

196. Fuchs HJ, et al. Effect of aerosolized recombinant human DNase on exacerbations of respiratory symptoms and on pulmonary function in patients with cystic fibrosis. N. Engl. J Med 1994;331: 637–42.

197. Donaldson SH, et al. Mucus clearance and lung function in cystic fibrosis with hypertonic saline. N. Engl. J Med 2006;354:241–50.

198. Elkins MR, et al. A controlled trial of long-term inhaled hypertonic saline in patients with cystic fibrosis. N. Engl. J Med 2006;354:229–40.

The Impact of Highly Effective Modulator Therapy on Cystic Fibrosis Microbiology and Inflammation

Lindsay J. Caverly, MD[a], Sebastián A. Riquelme, PhD[b],
Katherine B. Hisert, MD, PhD[c],*

KEYWORDS

- Inflammation • Infection • Cystic fibrosis transmembrane regulator • Modulator
- Highly effective cystic fibrosis transmembrane conductance regulator modulator therapy (HEMT)
- Cystic fibrosis

KEY POINTS

- Cystic fibrosis (CF) airway disease results from the complex interactions of 3 pathologic processes: (1) primary airway epithelial cell deficiency in CF transmembrane conductance regulator (CFTR) activity causing abnormal air surface liquid composition and impaired mucociliary clearance, (2) chronic airway infections, and (3) nonresolving inflammation.
- Highly effective CFTR modulator therapy (HEMT) acts to restore CFTR localization and function in the cell, enhancing mucociliary clearance and improving measures of pulmonary function; however, how HEMT changes airway infection and inflammation remains poorly understood.
- CF airway inflammation is a multifactorial process, and the impact of HEMT varies across the different contributors. Similarly, the impact of HEMT on inflammation and infection will differ across the different stages of CF lung disease.
- More research is needed to better understand how HEMT changes CF airway infection and inflammation to best predict how pulmonary disease will evolve in patients with CF receiving HEMT and to direct future treatment strategies.

INTRODUCTION: CYSTIC FIBROSIS AND CYSTIC FIBROSIS TRANSMEMBRANE CONDUCTANCE REGULATOR MODULATORS

Cystic fibrosis (CF), a multiorgan, life-limiting, autosomal-recessive genetic disease, develops when individuals possess disease-causing mutations in both copies of the gene encoding the CF transmembrane conductance regulator (CFTR).[1] CFTR functions as an anion channel,[2,3] and insufficient CFTR activity leads to decreased cellular transport of chloride and bicarbonate (and likely other anions), abnormal composition of secreted luminal fluids and other cellular impairments, and subsequent organ dysfunction.[4–6] Primary morbidity and mortality in CF result from a vicious cycle of impaired mucociliary clearance and chronic airway infection and inflammation, which causes progressive lung function decline and respiratory failure.[1] The prognosis for people

[a] Department of Pediatrics, University of Michigan Medical School, L2221 UH South, 1500 East Medical Center Drive, Ann Arbor, MI 48109-5212, USA; [b] Department of Pediatrics, College of Physicians and Surgeons, Columbia University, Columbia University Medical Center, 650West 168th Street, New York, NY 10032, USA; [c] Department of Medicine, National Jewish Health, Smith A550, 1400 Jackson Street, Denver, CO 80205, USA
* Corresponding author.
E-mail address: hisertk@njhealth.org

Clin Chest Med 43 (2022) 647–665
https://doi.org/10.1016/j.ccm.2022.06.007

with CF (PwCF) has changed markedly over the past several decades, largely because of developments in understanding of the molecular mechanisms that underlie CF.[7]

The biggest advance in the past decade was the identification of CFTR modulators, compounds that target the underlying molecular defect causing disease by increasing the abundance of functional CFTR protein in the cell.[6] The thousands of disease-causing mutations in the *CFTR* gene fall into 5 categories: (1) null mutations, (2) folding mutations, (3) gating mutations, (4) conductance mutations, and (5) insufficient protein production.[6,8] The first CFTR modulator, ivacaftor, was initially approved to treat G551D mutations, a class 3 mutation in which the CFTR channel folds and localizes correctly in the cell but does not open appropriately. Ivacaftor potentiates anion flux by increasing the open state of the CFTR channel.[9] In the approximately 5% of PwCF with G551D mutations, ivacaftor produces significant increases in lung function and weight gain and decreases in pulmonary exacerbation frequency.[10,11] Ivacaftor also markedly reduces sweat chloride,[10] the gold standard diagnostic test for CF, and the most direct measurement of CFTR anion transport activity.[12] Ivacaftor-induced changes thus became the benchmark for which subsequent modulators would be judged as highly effective CFTR modulator therapy (HEMT).[6]

Development then focused on discovery of modulators for the most common *CFTR* mutation, delta F508 (F508del). The F508del mutation is present in at least 1 copy in approximately 90% of PwCF, and approximately 50% are homozygous for this mutation.[13] Identifying molecules to correct the F508del mutation proved more challenging, as this mutation causes misfolding of the CFTR protein in the endoplasmic reticulum (ER), with subsequent destruction of most of the protein before it can reach the target location in the cell.[14] Initial combinations of modulators (ie, lumacaftor/ivacaftor and tezacaftor/ivacaftor) demonstrated efficacy in restoring CFTR activity in vitro[15–17] but induced only modest clinical and symptomatic changes in most PwCF[18–20] (and thus did not qualify as HEMT). The combination of 3 compounds, elexacaftor/tezacaftor/ivacaftor (ETI), was a breakthrough for enhancing CFTR channel activity in vivo in people with either 1 or 2 F508del mutations,[21,22] and ETI is now also considered HEMT.[6]

HEMT has been life changing for many PwCF, leading to significant decreases in respiratory symptoms and pulmonary exacerbations, and improvements in lung function and quality of life.[10,21,23–26] Although the dramatic changes in respiratory symptoms suggest that HEMT is altering the CF lung environment, the exact mechanisms by which CFTR modulators alter the CF airway are less clear. HEMT has been shown to increase mucociliary clearance.[27] Decreases in sweat chloride caused by HEMT correlate with increases in airway surface liquid (ASL) pH.[28] These findings are consistent with HEMT restoring chloride and bicarbonate secretion by epithelial cells in the airway, thus removing one major contributor to progressive airway damage in PwCF (**Fig. 1**A).

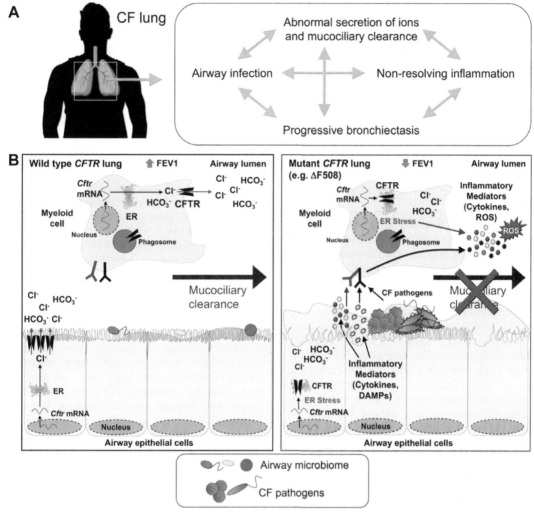

Fig. 1. Pulmonary damage in CF is associated with abnormal anion secretion, inflammation, and infection. *(A)* In contrast with healthy individuals, the CF lung exhibits many physiologic dysregulations, including abnormal secretion of ions and impaired mucociliary clearance, nonresolving inflammation, airway infection, and progressive bronchiectasis. These processes amplify each other and contribute to the long-term respiratory morbidity. *(B)* Impact of CFTR dysfunction (eg, F508del) on the many networks that promote airway injury. Lack of CFTR function in epithelial cells compromises airway anion balance favoring accumulation of an abnormal mucus layer that traps inhaled or aspirated bacteria. Certain CF pathogens with specific genetic and metabolic properties outcompete other members of the airway microbiome in the CF lung, which is detrimental for lung homeostasis. CFTR function deficiency in both epithelial and myeloid cells stimulates release of inflammatory mediators, which contribute to airway damage, release of damage-associated molecular patterns (DAMPs), and infection. These processes culminate in progressive pulmonary function decline and clinical deterioration.

However, the influence of HEMT on the complex interactions between ASL composition, mucus obstruction, infection, and inflammation is only beginning to be elucidated.

This article reviews the data regarding how HEMT impacts CF airway infection and inflammation, and describes the evolving understanding of the molecular and cellular mechanism by which HEMT induces these changes.

PULMONARY DAMAGE IN CF IS DUE TO INTERACTIONS BETWEEN AIRWAY INFLAMMATION, INFECTION, ABNORMAL ANION SECRETION, AND IMPAIRED MUCOCILIARY CLEARANCE

At baseline health, PwCF experience nonresolving low-grade inflammation in their airways, a process that is initiated by impaired anion secretion and impaired mucociliary clearance and then stoked by chronic airway infections (**Fig. 1**B). The intricate relationship between these processes becomes more complex as patients age and lung damage accumulates.

Before addressing how HEMT changes CF airway pathophysiology, one must first delineate the intersections of infection, inflammation, impaired ion transport, and impaired mucociliary clearance in the CF lung.

Cystic Fibrosis Transmembrane Conductance Regulator Dysfunction and Impaired Mucociliary Clearance Induces Inflammation Independent of Infection

Initial models of CF airway inflammation postulated that impaired mucociliary clearance led to bacterial airway infection, which stimulated the inflammatory response. Recent studies in human infants and newer animal models have suggested that lack of CFTR activity produces abnormal inflammation even in the absence of airway infection.[29] In young children with CF, levels of bronchoalveolar lavage (BAL) fluid inflammatory markers (eg, neutrophils, interleukin [IL]-8, extracellular DNA) correlate highly with the concentration of BAL mucins. These findings were observed in children without culture or molecular evidence of infection, and without radiologic (ie, computed tomography [CT] scan) evidence of airway damage, suggesting that mucous abnormalities and inflammation precede and may incite airway structural damage and infection.[30] Animal models also indicate that CF airway inflammation arises independent of infection.[31] When CF ferrets and pigs are administered sufficient antibiotics from birth to prevent airway infection, these animals still develop airway structural damage, mucus impaction, and neutrophilic airway inflammation.[32,33] These studies suggest that lack of CFTR activity on lung cells and resulting abnormalities in airway mucus and electrolytes promote inflammatory responses in the absence of infection.

Several mechanisms could account for these observations. Mucus obstruction in the airway and the associated hypoxia cause cellular stress, necrosis, and release of damage-associated molecular patterns (DAMPs), which trigger airway epithelial cell inflammatory responses[34,35] (see **Fig. 1**B). Abnormal composition of ASL has also been linked to aberrant immune cell responses. *Scnn1b-Tg* mice, which overexpress the epithelial sodium channel ENaC and develop dehydrated ASL, develop increased numbers of IL-17 secreting T cells, similar to cells seen in airways of PwCF; however, there is no increase in numbers of these cells in *Cftr*[−/−] mice, which do not develop spontaneous lung disease.[36]

Additionally, the structural cells of the airway and lung vasculature may promote inflammation when they lack sufficient CFTR activity. Endothelial cells lacking functional CFTR express IL-8 constitutively,[37] and epithelial cells lacking functional CFTR demonstrate enhanced and prolonged production of inflammatory cytokines IL-6 and IL-8 at baseline and after stimulation.[38–40] CF has thus been described as a disease of mucosal immune dysregulation.[41]

Chronic Infections Induce an Inflammatory Response

Bacterial airway infection occurs as early as infancy in CF, and CF airway microbiota measured by culture-independent analyses of BAL samples diverge from those of children with other airway diseases within the first few years of life.[42,43] Patterns in age-related pathogen prevalence in CF are well known and include predominance of *Staphylococcus aureus* and *Haemophilus influenzae* in early childhood, followed by increasing prevalence rates of CF pathogens (eg, *Pseudomonas aeruginosa*, methicillin-resistant *S aureus*, nontuberculous mycobacteria, *Achromobacter*, and *Burkholderia*) through adolescence and early adulthood.[13] Chronic airway infection with CF pathogens is associated with adverse clinical outcomes, including increased pulmonary exacerbations and accelerated lung function decline.[44–46] The relationship between airway infection and inflammation in CF begins in the first years of life, with obligate and facultative anaerobes detectable in BAL fluid and associated with increases in total bacterial load and inflammation. Subsequent infection with CF pathogens in early childhood is associated with further increases in inflammation.[47] The relative abundance of CF pathogens then increases throughout adolescence and adulthood in parallel with decreases in bacterial community diversity, progressive bronchiectasis, declining lung function, and increasing inflammation.[48–50] In this context, inflammation is largely a response to airway damage and chronic infections. In addition, studies that evaluate inflammatory cells and mediators before and following antibiotic regimens highlight how airway bacterial burden and composition strongly influence inflammatory responses in the CF airway.[51–55]

Immune Dysfunction as a Primary Consequence of Impaired Cystic Fibrosis Transmembrane Conductance Regulator Dysfunction on Immune Cells Exaggerates Inflammation

Although CFTR expression by epithelial cells accounts for much of the pathology manifest in

PwCF, CFTR is also expressed in immune cells.[56] Immune abnormalities observed in cells recovered from PwCF (compared with healthy donor cells) may be caused by lack of CFTR function on the immune cells or secondary effects of immune cells maturing within the unique airway and circulatory milieu generated by CF.[57–61] Studies in the past 2 decades, largely using animal models and *in vitro* cell systems that are free of the confounding presence of secondary effects of CF disease, have revealed how lack of functional CFTR alters responses of immune cells,[56,62] including neutrophils,[63,64] macrophages,[65] T cells,[36,66] B cells,[67,68] dendritic cells,[69] and platelets.[70] In CF animal models of airway infection or acute lung injury, inflammation is generally exaggerated compared with wild type animals; thus, restoration of CFTR activity by HEMT could potentially eliminate at least 1 contributor to deleterious inflammation.[32,71–73]

Multiple mechanisms have been proposed for how CFTR molecules participate in intracellular processes that regulate immune functions, including the contribution of CFTR ion transport to the phagolysosomal milieu,[74,75] CFTR's role as a scaffold to promote interactions of other proteins at the membrane,[76–78] and the requirement of CFTR for normal cellular responses to production of potentially toxic reactive oxygen species (ROS).[79] A more recent body of work demonstrates that CFTR dysfunction induces proinflammatory cellular metabolism.[80–82] These bioenergetic alterations are key for tissue homeostasis, as the same pathways that regulate ATP synthesis control the release of inflammatory mediators.[83,84] These abnormalities in cellular metabolism may be most critical in myeloid cells, as more than 95% of cells in the lumen of the CF airway are neutrophils and macrophages.[85,86] Resting myeloid cells, such as lung-resident macrophages, generate energy through oxidative phosphorylation (OXPHOS), a process that occurs in mitochondria (**Fig. 2**A). However, upon sensing of inflammatory stimuli such as bacterial ligands, OXPHOS is impaired, and, instead of generating energy, mitochondria become major sources of ROS.[87] If not adequately regulated, excess ROS can damage the airway mucosa. Recent studies have shown that CF macrophages exhibit mitochondrial dysfunction and excessive ROS production, even before infection.[88,89] This detrimental ROS accumulates in the CF lung and promotes protein aggregation and airway damage, contributing to long-term respiratory disease. In CF cells harboring class 2 *CFTR* mutations (protein processing mutations), ROS release is facilitated by reduced levels of phosphatase and tensin

homolog deleted on chromosome 10 (PTEN), which is a major metabolic checkpoint that requires CFTR to limit mitochondrial oxidative metabolism[90] (**Fig. 2**B). CFTR and PTEN form a metabolo-regulatory complex at the cell membrane, which is compromised in CF myeloid cells. The excessive ROS release by CF cells is worsened by infection, as *P aeruginosa*, a major CF pathogen, further reduces the function of PTEN in the cell.[41,88,90,91] Thus, pro-oxidant metabolic dysfunction in CF myeloid cells contributes to pulmonary injury.

Aerobic glycolysis (the Warburg effect) becomes the major mode of energy production in macrophages stimulated by bacteria, in which OXPHOS is impaired.[84] This metabolic pathway also contributes to inflammation.[83,92] Glycolysis promotes the synthesis of many inflammatory cytokines, including IL-1β and IL-6. These cytokines activate phagocytes to fight infection and can aggravate tissue damage if not adequately regulated.[41] Both CF macrophages and neutrophils exhibit a distinctive glycolytic signature that predisposes them to oversecrete inflammatory cytokines. In myeloid cells harboring class II *CFTR* mutations, this enhanced carbohydrate breakdown is facilitated by reduced function of the CFTR-PTEN complex. In response to different CF pathogens like *P aeruginosa*, *Burkholderia cenocepacia,* and *S aureus*, phagocytes harboring CFTR alterations that compromise PTEN function produce exaggerated levels of IL-1β, IL-6, and many oxidants that jeopardize pulmonary tissue integrity.[65,90,93,94]

Enhanced glycolysis is not exclusively associated to class 2 *CFTR* mutations, as cells exhibiting class 3 *CFTR* mutations (gating mutations) also trigger inflammatory pathways that require glucose catabolism to function. In cells harboring class 3 *CFTR* mutations, lack of chloride secretion promotes extracellular potassium (K^+) accumulation.[95] This K^+ activates the inflammasome, which is a major proinflammatory cytoplasmic complex that synthetizes IL-1β in response to glycolysis[6,9,83,96] (**Fig. 2**C). Additionally, the presence of class 2 *CFTR* mutations (whether 1 or 2 copies) can stimulate cellular oxidative metabolism independent of PTEN and extracellular K^+ accumulation (as illustrated in **Fig. 2**B for class 2 *CFTR* mutations). Accumulation of dysfunctional CFTR in the ER, as seen in cells harboring either F508del/F508del or G551D/F508del mutations, activates cell stress and the unfolded protein response (UPR).[96,97] In CF phagocytes, UPR triggers ROS generation, augmented glycolysis, and also synthesis of inflammatory cytokines that can damage the local mucosa, like IL-6 and tumor

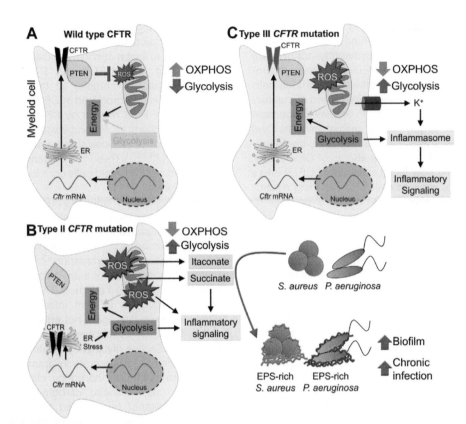

Fig. 2. CF myeloid cells exhibit proinflammatory metabolic dysregulation. (*A*) In healthy myeloid cells, WT CFTR interacts with many proteins at the cell membrane, including PTEN. PTEN not only restricts ROS generation, but also promotes OXPHOS and energy synthesis by mitochondria. Glycolysis is low, limiting the production of inflammatory mediators that rely on carbohydrate breakdown. (*B*) Myeloid cells harboring type II *CFTR* mutations accumulate CFTR in the endoplasmic reticulum (ER). This produces ER stress, promoting glycolysis and inflammatory signaling. Lack of surface-attached CFTR also compromises the ability of CF cells to regulate OXPHOS, prompting ROS release. One factor contributing to this OXPHOS dysregulation is reduced interaction of CFTR with PTEN. CFTR-PTEN complex dysfunction favors secretion of succinate and itaconate, which stimulate synthesis of extracellular polysaccharides (EPSs) and biofilm by *S aureus* and. *P aeruginosa*. (*C*) Myeloid cells harboring type III *CFTR* mutations secrete potassium, which activates inflammatory pathways that rely on glycolysis, such as the inflammasome. As a consequence of increased glycolysis, mitochondrial OXPHOS is jeopardized, contributing to ROS release and inflammatory damage.

necrosis factor alpha (TNFα).[96,98] Thus, glycolytic signaling enhanced by CFTR dysfunction also worsens CF lung inflammatory disease.

Immune Dysfunction Secondary to Cystic Fibrosis Chronic Disease Influences Inflammation

Many immune cells involved in CF airway disease are cells recruited from the circulation.[86,99–102] In the blood stream, and while migrating into lung tissue, these cells are exposed to circulating products of chronic infection and inflammation and other sequelae of CF (eg, protein calorie malnutrition, abnormal glucose control, or medications). These factors influence immune cell responses and may counteract the abnormalities caused by primary lack of CFTR function on these cells. For example, whereas macrophages lacking CFTR activity (either from mice, or matured in vitro from human blood monocytes) exhibit exaggerated lipopolysaccharide (LPS) responses,[73,103] monocytes studied ex vivo from PwCF exhibit an LPS-tolerant phenotype with decreased LPS responses.[104,105] Transcriptional profiling of peripheral blood mononuclear cells (PBMCs) from PwCF compared with healthy controls show a general downregulation of inflammatory genes, and this phenotype could be conferred on healthy donor cells by exposing them to CF plasma.[106] Functionally, immune cells from whole blood of healthy controls mount stronger Toll-like receptor (TLR)-mediated innate immune inflammatory responses (TMIIR) than cells from PwCF, and the

PwCF that demonstrated the most robust TMIIR also demonstrated better lung function.[58]

One hypothesis for why circulating immune cells may have blunted inflammatory responses in PwCF is that chronic infection in the airways results in a low-level leak of inflammatory mediators and bacterial products, including LPS, into the circulation.[107] Continuous exposure to low levels of inflammatory stimuli can cause immune cells to develop a tolerant phenotype.[108] Thus, PBMCs from PwCF with milder lung disease (ie, people who presumably are not leaking tolerogenic amounts of LPS and other inflammatory stimuli into the blood) produce more robust inflammatory responses to subsequent stimulation with bacterial ligands.[58] Complicating this hypothesis is the finding that levels of circulating markers of endothelial function in CF plasma are skewed to suggest more intact endothelial barrier function in PwCF compared with healthy controls.[109] However, this skewed response might also be associated with elevated endothelial damage, probably by an unbalanced inflammatory response, forcing the cells to oversynthetize these markers to stimulate tissue repair. Further studies are needed to understand the mechanisms of secondary effects of CFTR deficiency on immune cells.

CHANGES IN INFLAMMATION AND INFECTION AFTER INITIATION OF HIGHLY EFFECTIVE CYSTIC FIBROSIS TRANSMEMBRANE CONDUCTANCE REGULATOR MODULATOR THERAPY

Three types of studies have shaped understanding of how HEMT alters cellular responses, inflammation, and composition of airway microbiome in PwCF: in vitro studies of cells treated with HEMT, CF animal models, and human studies of response to HEMT (**Table 1**).

Highly Effective Cystic Fibrosis Transmembrane Conductance Regulator Modulator Therapy and In Vitro Cell Culture

Culturing cells in vitro in the presence of CFTR modulators reverses some CF immune cell defects. Defects in adhesion and trafficking observed in monocytes from PwCF and the genotype F508del homozygous could be reversed by addition of the CFTR corrector lumacaftor.[110] Similarly, impaired phagocytosis and killing of *P aeruginosa* by F508del homozygous human monocyte-derived macrophages were restored to levels seen in healthy control macrophages following culture with lumacaftor.[111] These studies confirm that deficient CFTR channel activity at the level of the immune cell is responsible for abnormal responses,

and restoration of CFTR activity by CFTR modulators is sufficient to remedy the impairments.

Some aberrant inflammatory responses observed in CF epithelial cells are also corrected by modulators. Treatment of in vitro cultured CF epithelial cells with various inflammatory stimuli results in marked increases in activation of the transcription factor nuclear factor kappa-B (NFKB) and secretion of the neutrophil chemoattractant IL-8, as compared to cells with functional CFTR.[39,112] Exposure of CFTR F508del homozygous epithelial cells in vitro to lumacaftor/ivacaftor markedly dampens the intracellular signaling cascade in response to inflammatory stimuli and transcription of IL-8.[113] Furthermore, if a CF epithelial cell monolayer is injured in vitro, treatment of the monolayer with lumacaftor/ivacaftor enhances repair.[114] Thus, HEMT directly dampens aberrant inflammation and helps restore homeostasis in CF both epithelial and immune cells. Interestingly, 2 studies recently demonstrated that exposure of epithelial cells to inflammatory mediators enhances their responsiveness to HEMT in vitro, manifested by improved CFTR function.[115,116] This result underscores the complex interactions between CFTR function and inflammation, and highlights the importance of assessing the chronic effects of HEMT on inflammation using animal models, and in human subjects.

Highly Effective Cystic Fibrosis Transmembrane Conductance Regulator Modulator Therapy and Animal Models of Cystic Fibrosis

Although in vitro studies provide direct evidence that HEMT alters cellular inflammatory responses, in vivo studies are required to understand how these HEMT-induced changes impact CF systemic and airway inflammation. Animal models permit manipulation of different contributors to systemic and airways disease with clearer interpretation of endpoints than in human studies, which can be confounded by genetic variability, behavioral differences, and environmental factors. However, studying chronic CF airway infection and inflammation has been challenging, because disrupting CFTR in smaller mammals has not recapitulated human CF lung disease.[31,117] CF rats develop abnormal airway mucus, impaired mucociliary clearance, and exaggerated airway inflammation,[71,118] but do not become spontaneously infected. Only the CF pig and ferret develop airway pathology similar to CF in people, including spontaneous bacterial airway infections.[31,117] Pigs, rats, and ferrets have been generated that express G551D CFTR, which

Table 1
Effects of highly effective cystic fibrosis transmembrane conductance regulator modulator therapy on infection, inflammation, and lung function in cystic fibrosis

Clinical Endpoints Known to Improve with HEMT	Pathways with Evidence of HEMT Modulation or Improvement	Active Areas of HEMT Impact Investigation
Infection		
Drug: ivacaftor (HEMT) Clinical observations: either decreased prevalence rates or delayed incidence of certain CF pathogens, such as *P aeruginosa, S aureus, S maltophilia*, and *Aspergillus*	Drug: ivacaftor (HEMT) or lumacaftor In vitro: Increased phenotypic polarization, phagocytosis, and bacterial killing by CF, both monocytes and macrophages	Impact of short and long-term HEMT on pathogen load, survival, and lifestyle (eg, biofilm, planktonic) in the CF airway Effect of HEMT on lung microbiome diversity and its influence on CF lung function Effect of antibiotic treatment and its interaction with HEMT Evaluation of confounding parameters (eg, lung function, comorbidities) on the long-term impact of HEMT on CF pathobiology
Inflammation		
Drug: ivacaftor (HEMT) Clinical observation: improved lung function and reduced airway accumulation of inflammation markers (eg, neutrophil elastase [NE], IL-8, IL-6, IL-1β)	Drug: ivacaftor (HEMT) In vivo: reduced airway damage and abundance of inflammation markers in CF ferrets and rats Drug: ivacaftor (HEMT), elexacaftor/tezacaftor/ ivacaftor (ETI) (HEMT), tezacaftor/ivacaftor (HEMT) Ex vivo: increased ability of different CF myeloid cells to regulate inflammation: (eg, more neutrophil apoptosis, augmented monocyte adhesion and trafficking, and reduced monocytes/ PBMCs inflammasome activation) Variable expression of cell activation markers, including IFNγ and TLR signalling	Influence of HEMT on myeloid and epithelial cell pathways that promote CF lung inflammatory damage: (eg, NFkB, inflammasome, extracellular potassium accumulation, hypoxia, recruitment of myeloid cells to the airway and regulation of their effector function) Impact of HEMT on adaptive immune cells that influence CF lung inflammation: subtypes of effector $CD4^+$ T cells (eg, T_H1, T_H2, T_H17), regulatory T cells (Tregs)
Metabolism		
	Drug: lumacaftor, lumacaftor/ ivacaftor *Ex vivo*: augmented PTEN levels in CF PBMCs	Effects of HEMT on oxidative metabolic pathways that contribute to CF lung damage (eg, ROS release, glycolysis, PTEN function, and synthesis of immunometabolites that fuel pathogen metabolism in the lung)

(continued on next page)

Table 1 (continued)		
Clinical Endpoints Known to Improve with HEMT	Pathways with Evidence of HEMT Modulation or Improvement	Active Areas of HEMT Impact Investigation
Lung function		
Drug: ivacaftor (HEMT), elexacaftor/tezacaftor/ivacaftor (ETI) (HEMT) Clinical observation: enhanced LCI, augmented FEV$_1$, increased mucociliary clearance, improvements in chest CT scan and MRI		How HEMT modulates lung function in hosts exhibiting chronic infection Utilization of CF animal models (eg, pig, ferrets, rats) Developing and testing new and more potent HEMT in these models

can be potentiated effectively by ivacaftor.[118–120] G551D-CFTR ferrets administered ivacaftor beginning in utero are spared airway pathology seen in CF ferrets not receiving modulators, but then develop airway inflammation when ivacaftor therapy is withdrawn.[119] G551D-CFTR rats raised for 6 months in the absence of ivacaftor demonstrate increased markers of airway inflammation in BAL fluid compared with wild-type rats. Levels of some markers interferon (IFNγ0, IL-1α, and IL-1β) normalized following 1 week of ivacaftor, whereas others did not (IL-6, TNFα),[71] indicating that restoration of CFTR activity in airways with established disease may not completely reverse inflammation, even in the absence of chronic infection. Experiments in these model systems in which chronic lung disease and associated infection are established followed by initiation of HEMT and characterization of how inflammation changes acutely and over time will provide important information to link cellular data generated in vitro with observations of PwCF on HEMT. In addition, pig and ferret models have the potential to better understand how chronic airway infections evolve in individuals with established lung disease and bronchiectasis who start treatment with HEMT.

EFFECTS OF HIGHLY EFFECTIVE CYSTIC FIBROSIS TRANSMEMBRANE CONDUCTANCE REGULATOR MODULATOR THERAPY ON INFLAMMATION AND INFECTION IN HUMAN SUBJECTS

Infection

Epidemiologic studies of culture-based data

The first study to prospectively evaluate PwCF starting HEMT was the GOAL (G551D ObservationAL) study, which followed individuals aged 6 and older with G551D *CFTR* mutations as they initiated treatment with ivacaftor.[27] Subjects in the

GOAL study had decreased prevalence rates of *P aeruginosa* and *Aspergillus* 1 year following ivacaftor initiation, with certain subjects (primarily those with better lung function and history of intermittent, as opposed to chronic, *P aeruginosa* infection) clearing their *P aeruginosa* infection.[121] Similarly, registry-based observational studies from the United States and United Kingdom of outcomes 3 years following ivacaftor approval identified decreased prevalence rates of most CF pathogens (*S aureus*, *P aeruginosa*, *Staphylococcus maltophilia*, *Aspergillus*), with NTM as the notable exception.[122] Although data on CFTR modulators other than ivacaftor are limited, a single-center analysis of patients on either ivacaftor or ivacaftor/lumacaftor showed delays in incident CF pathogen infection with *P aeruginosa* or *S aureus* in those on modulators compared with matched controls.[123] These studies demonstrate the likely significant impact that HEMT will have on reducing CF pathogen infection over time, with the greatest impact on those who start HEMT at younger ages with preserved lung function.[124] In addition to improving inflammation and mucociliary clearance, other potential mechanisms through which HEMT are likely to impact infection include direct antimicrobial activity of HEMT, HEMT synergy with antibiotics, and niche modification impacting pathogen virulence.[125–128]

Culture-independent studies

Culture-independent studies have been less consistent in showing impact of HEMT on CF airway infection, and overall have included variable changes in bacterial community diversity, bacterial load, and relative abundances of specific taxa (including CF pathogens and certain obligate and facultative anaerobes).[124,129–131] For example, although ivacaftor significantly increased mucociliary clearance in the GOAL study, no significant changes were noted in bacterial load, bacterial community diversity, or in inflammatory biomarkers in the first 6 months of treatment. These results contrast with a similar, prospective study of an Irish cohort of 12 adults with CF and G551D mutations starting ivacaftor.[132] This study observed a rapid (within the first week of therapy) and significant decrease in *P aeruginosa* burden across the first 6 months of treatment; however, *P aeruginosa* burden then increased by the end of the first year of treatment, and none of the subjects cleared their *P aeruginosa* infection, despite maintaining improvements in lung function, radiographic improvements, and sustained reduction in inflammatory markers. Subsequent studies have similarly shown no significant decreases in *P aeruginosa* burden or total bacterial load with ivacaftor treatment.[129] Several factors likely contribute to differences observed across studies, including differences in patient populations (eg, ages of subjects, *CFTR* mutations, severity of disease, types of airway infections, and use of CF therapies such as antibiotics) that may confound results or obscure signals. For example, ivacaftor-associated reductions in total bacterial load were observed in an Australian cohort, but only after controlling for changes in antibiotic exposure.[133] Future studies accounting for changes in antibiotic use and other potential confounders (eg, age, lung function, or comorbidities) across longer-term use of HEMT are needed to more fully understand the impact on HEMT on the many aspects of CF airway infection, including CF pathogens, bacterial load, anaerobes, and bacterial community structure.

Inflammation

Measurements of lung inflammation

Several modalities that assess overall lung health and function in patients with CF provide indirect measures of inflammation, including spirometry, lung clearance index (LCI), and radiologic imaging. HEMT improves airflow, as measured by forced expiratory volume in 1 second (FEV$_1$).[11,21,22] Multiple breath washout assesses ventilation heterogeneity in the lung, as reported by LCI,[134,135] and preliminary studies have demonstrated improvements in LCI with HEMT.[136,137] Likewise, radiology (eg, chest CT scan and MRI) can assess lung damage,[138–140] and studies of individuals before and after HEMT have demonstrated improvements in radiographic markers associated with inflammation.[130,132,141] However, these tests evaluate the complex endpoint of lung damage, with structural changes, mucus impaction, bronchoconstriction, and airway inflammation all potentially contributing.[142,143]

Direct measurements of airway inflammation (and infection) can be obtained by evaluating airway secretions (eg, BAL or induced or spontaneously expectorated sputum).[85,144] In CF, sputum biomarkers for quantitating airway inflammation, both for making clinical decisions and as endpoints in clinical trials, remain elusive.[145] However, higher concentrations of some airway inflammatory markers, such as neutrophil elastase (NE), correlate with severity of CF lung disease,[146–148] and also decrease in sputum following antibiotic treatment of CF pulmonary exacerbations.[51] In the GOAL study, no difference in sputum inflammatory cytokines and biomarkers was detected in specimens obtained 6 months after initiation of ivacaftor.[27,124] As with bacterial burden, this contrasted with the results of the Irish cohort study, in which initiation of ivacaftor was associated with a rapid and sustained (at >600 days) drop in sputum inflammatory biomarkers (NE, IL-8, and IL-1β).[132] These disparate results may reflect the fact that the GOAL study did not detect changes in bacterial burden in the airway following ivacaftor, whereas the Irish study did.

Because HEMT has led to decreased sputum production in many PwCF, alternate modalities for sampling airway inflammation are needed. A recent study reported on use of nasal lavage to obtain epithelial lining fluid (ENL),[149] and noted decreased levels of ENL IL-1β and IL-6 in subjects starting ivacaftor. Prior studies have shown that levels of inflammatory biomarkers in CF nasal lavage correlate with degree of sinus disease.[150] Whether nasal/upper airway inflammation mirrors bronchial/lower airway inflammation in CF, and whether HEMT alters upper airway and lower airway inflammation in a similar manner, remain to be determined. However, assays to evaluate CF airway inflammation that do not require lower airway specimens will be essential for characterizing CF lung inflammation in the era of HEMT.

Ex vivo studies of immune cell response

Investigations of how HEMT changes circulating immune cells can help elucidate how HEMT may influence lung inflammation, as circulating cells traffic to inflamed CF airways.[86,99,100] Some impairments described in CF immune cells are mitigated by initiation of HEMT. HEMT restored phenotypic polarization and phagocytosis in monocyte-derived macrophages (MDMs) generated from PwCF receiving ivacaftor to levels similar to those exhibited by healthy donor MDMs.[151] Delayed neutrophil apoptosis, thought to contribute to nonresolving CF airway inflammation, is corrected in individuals with CFTR-G551D mutations after initiation of ivacaftor.[152]

Dysregulated inflammasome activation is also thought to contribute to excessive inflammation in the CF airway.[91] Monocytes from individuals treated with ETI demonstrated decreased expression of the P2X7 receptor, which promotes ATP-induced inflammasome activation, and were more resistant to inflammasome activation than monocytes from the same individuals before receiving ETI.[153] Similar changes in inflammasome activation were seen in a study of PBMCs from PwCF homozygous for F508del mutations before and after initiation of tezacaftor/ivacaftor.[154] Inflammation resulting from abnormal cellular metabolism in CF cells is also likely to be dampened by CFTR modulators, which enhance CFTR channel stability and function, and are thus expected to restore interactions with key metabolic checkpoints at the cell membrane, such as PTEN. Administration of lumacaftor/ivacaftor to PwCF homozygous for F508del mutations increased PTEN levels in peripheral blood mononuclear cells.[90] Studies performed in vitro have demonstrated that ectopic PTEN expression in either F508del homozygous or control cells reduces mitochondrial ROS and glucose breakdown,[88] suggesting that HEMT will shift cellular metabolism in vivo to a less inflammatory state.

Other studies have characterized how HEMT alters circulating immune cell inflammatory phenotypes, using expression of different protein surface markers and cellular transcriptomes. Monocytes and neutrophils isolated from subjects at 1 and 6 months after initiation of ivacaftor exhibited decreases in expression of proteins associated with activation.[155] In a proteomic analysis, monocytes recovered 1 week after subjects started ivacaftor displayed changes in plasma membrane proteins, suggesting that cells had improved adhesion and trafficking and suppressed responses to the inflammatory cytokine IFNγ.[156] Follow-up studies of ex vivo monocytes from a separate cohort initiating ivacaftor demonstrated a marked reduction in monocyte responses to IFNγ.[157] In vitro functional studies of CF monocytes confirmed that impaired CFTR activity results in a monocyte adhesion deficiency, and this impairment is reversed by CFTR modulators.[110] Transcriptome analysis of PBMCs recovered from subjects in the GOAL cohort 1 month after starting ivacaftor revealed decreased transcription of genes involved in TLR signaling and other immune inflammatory pathways.[158] In contrast, transcriptomic analysis of monocytes isolated 1 week after initiation of ivacaftor identified an almost nonoverlapping set of differentially expressed genes (DEGs) compared with those identified in the GOAL cohort at 1 month after

initiation of ivacaftor, and these DEGs suggested that ivacaftor caused an overall more activated state of CF blood monocytes.[159] These disparate results may reflect the multiple ways in which CFTR dysfunction affects inflammation. For example, immune cells may acutely become more activated in the days after initiation of HEMT if there is a reduction in the immune tolerance previously described for CF monocytes[105] and leukocytes.[58] However, as HEMT leads to improvements in both pulmonary and systemic health over weeks to months, circulating immune cells may gradually be restored to a more quiescent and less activated state.

Some clinical complications seen in PwCF have been linked to sequelae of CFTR deficiency and immune impairments, including bronchiectasis and P aeruginosa airway infection, and may not be significantly improved by HEMT. For example, PwCF tend to have T cell responses skewed toward T_H2 and T_H17 lineages, phenotypes that cause exaggerated inflammation with poor infection-fighting potential.[36,160,161] In a study comparing T cells from PwCF with and without modulator treatment, no differences in T cell populations or concentrations of serum T cell-related cytokines were detected.[162] T cell populations from subjects with non-CF bronchiectasis were similar to those from subjects with CF, suggesting that bronchiectasis, and not CFTR dysfunction, drives skewing of T cell populations. These data highlight the multifactorial contributions to CF airway inflammation and indicate that some deleterious inflammation will likely persist despite HEMT in people with more advanced lung disease.

Cystic fibrosis macrophage oxidative metabolism contributes to bacterial adaptation to the cystic fibrosis transmembrane conductance regulator-mutant lung

Although recent studies have begun to shed light on the impact of HEMT on CF immune cell function, how these drugs influence the metabolism of CF phagocytes, and how changes in phagocyte metabolism will alter host-pathogen interaction in the CF lung, remain unknown. The pro-oxidative metabolic abnormalities of CF myeloid cells are associated with release of many metabolites, like succinate and itaconate, that participate in immune signaling but also trigger phenotypic changes in CF airway pathogens.[163] While succinate is a proinflammatory metabolite that supports synthesis of cytokines that can damage mucosal tissues, like IL-1β,[164] itaconate acts as a regulatory determinant rapidly synthetized in inflamed environments.[165] Itaconate not only limits the release of detrimental cytokines by effector phagocytes, but also maintains tissue homeostasis during inflammatory diseases. In contrast with healthy individuals, metabolomic analyses have shown that sputum and BAL fluid of PwCF accumulate succinate and itaconate.[166] Genetic and metabolic analyses of *P aeruginosa* isolates from chronic CF infections demonstrate metabolic adjustments consistent with exposure to abundant levels of succinate and itaconate.[166] In response to this metabolic pressure, *P aeruginosa* generates biofilms, which promote its ability to evade phagocytosis, antibiotics, complement and antibodies. CF host-adapted *P aeruginosa* strains upregulate specific genetic clusters that support the utilization of succinate and itaconate, indicating that CF airway immunometabolites nourish respiratory pathogens instead of promoting their eradication.[166] Similarly, *S aureus* also responds to CFTR-controlled immunometabolites. Longitudinal analysis of *S aureus* strains from PwCF demonstrates activation of specific genes in response to itaconate, including those involved in the generation of extracellular polysaccharides and biofilm.[167] These CF-adapted bacterial strains modify their own metabolism in response to itaconate, diverting their utilization of carbohydrates for the generation of biofilm in the lung.

These data strongly indicate that CF pathogens activate sophisticated mechanisms of pathogenesis in response to the oxidative metabolic environment set by CFTR-mutant lung cells and highlight the complex interactions between infection and inflammation in the CF airway.

Future studies in HEMT-treated PwCF should include characterization of immunometabolites in BAL and sputum, as well as how HEMT alters the presence and phenotypes of myeloid cells that participate in immunometabolite generation. It is likely that the metabolic effects of HEMT on the type of organisms recovered from CF airway will vary as a function of both the class of CFTR mutation studied and the metabolic preferences of the pathogen.

CONCLUDING REMARKS

HEMT promises to significantly improve lifespan and quality of life for most PwCF, largely because of HEMT's impact on almost all aspects of CF airway pathophysiology: mucus obstruction, ASL composition, infection, and inflammation. Although the improvements in CF airway infection and inflammation seen with HEMT are promising, these studies also emphasize the difficulty in determining which aspects of infection and inflammation will be resolved with HEMT and which may persist. CF airway inflammation (like inflammation in other chronic diseases) is not 1 process, but rather multiple immune processes initiated to eliminate infectious threats, repair damaged tissue, and attempt to restore homeostasis.[168] Although some contributors to CF inflammation are reversed directly by HEMT, others may be indirectly affected by HEMT, and others may not be affected at all. Similarly, HEMT's impact will likely differ across the CF population, with larger impact on infection and inflammation seen in individuals who start HEMT at a younger age, before the establishment of chronic infection and bronchiectasis. Finally, HEMT's impact on extrapulmonary manifestations of CF (eg, nutrition, intestinal inflammation, sinus disease) and on CF therapies (eg, reducing use of mucolytics and antibiotics) are likely indirect routes through which HEMT will continue to impact airway infection and inflammation.[169] Future studies are needed to continue to understand the mechanisms of the post-HEMT state, including further development of CF animal models to parse the intricate interactions between HEMT, metabolism, inflammation, and infection to continue to develop novel approaches for personalized care and optimal treatments for PwCF.

CLINICS CARE POINTS

- Highly effective modulator therapy (HEMT) improves lung function and quality of life for most people with cystic fibrosis (CF) and eligible CFTR mutations.

- There are multiple contributors to inflammation and infection in the lungs of people with CF.

- Lung inflammation and infection are not fully resolved by HEMT, especially in those people with CF with established or advanced lung disease.

DISCLOSURE

None of the authors has any commercial or financial conflicts of interest. L.J. Caverly receives funding from the National Institutes of Health (NIH) (K23HL136934) and the Cystic Fibrosis Foundation (CFF) (CAVERL20Y5). S.A. Riquelme receives funding from Vertex Research Innovation Award (PG010094), the CFF (RIQUEL21I0), and NIH (1R35HL135800). K.B. Hisert receives funding from the NIH (K08 HL136786) and the CFF (HISERT20A0 and HISERT19R3).

REFERENCES

1. Shteinberg M, Haq IJ, Polineni D, et al. Cystic fibrosis. Lancet 2021;397(10290):2195–211.
2. Csanady L, Vergani P, Gadsby DC. Structure, gating, and regulation of the CFTR anion channel. Physiol Rev 2019;99(1):707–38.
3. Infield DT, Strickland KM, Gaggar A, et al. The molecular evolution of function in the CFTR chloride channel. J Gen Physiol 2021;153(12):e202012625.
4. Stoltz DA, Meyerholz DK, Welsh MJ. Origins of cystic fibrosis lung disease. N Engl J Med 2015; 372(4):351–62.
5. Huang EN, Quach H, Lee JA, et al. A developmental role of the cystic fibrosis transmembrane conductance regulator in cystic fibrosis lung disease pathogenesis. Front Cell Dev Biol 2021;9:742891.
6. Mall MA, Mayer-Hamblett N, Rowe SM. Cystic fibrosis: emergence of highly effective targeted therapeutics and potential clinical implications. Am J Respir Crit Care Med 2020;201(10): 1193–208.
7. Elborn JS. Personalised medicine for cystic fibrosis: treating the basic defect. Eur Respir Rev 2013;22(127):3–5.
8. Brodlie M, Haq IJ, Roberts K, et al. Targeted therapies to improve CFTR function in cystic fibrosis. Genome Med 2015;7:101.
9. Van Goor F, Hadida S, Grootenhuis PD, et al. Rescue of CF airway epithelial cell function in vitro by a CFTR potentiator, VX-770. Proc Natl Acad Sci U S A 2009;106(44):18825–30.
10. Ramsey BW, Davies J, McElvaney NG, et al. A CFTR potentiator in patients with cystic fibrosis and the G551D mutation. N Engl J Med 2011; 365(18):1663–72.
11. Accurso FJ, Rowe SM, Clancy JP, et al. Effect of VX-770 in persons with cystic fibrosis and the G551D-CFTR mutation. N Engl J Med 2010; 363(21):1991–2003.
12. Cooke RE, Gochberg SH. Physiology of the sweat gland in cystic fibrosis of the pancreas. Pediatrics 1956;18(5):701–15.
13. Cystic fibrosis Foundation patient registry 2020 Annual data Report. Bethesda, MD: Cystic Fibrosis Foundation; 2021.
14. Ostedgaard LS, Meyerholz DK, Chen JH, et al. The DeltaF508 mutation causes CFTR misprocessing and cystic fibrosis-like disease in pigs. Sci Transl Med 2011;3(74). 74ra24.
15. Farinha CM, King-Underwood J, Sousa M, et al. Revertants, low temperature, and correctors reveal the mechanism of F508del-CFTR rescue by VX-809 and suggest multiple agents for full correction. Chem Biol 2013;20(7):943–55.
16. Van Goor F, Hadida S, Grootenhuis PD, et al. Correction of the F508del-CFTR protein processing defect in vitro by the investigational drug VX-809. Proc Natl Acad Sci U S A 2011; 108(46):18843–8.
17. Norman P. Novel picolinamide-based cystic fibrosis transmembrane regulator modulators: evaluation of WO2013038373, WO2013038376, WO2013038381, WO2013038386 and WO2013038390. Expert Opin Ther Pat 2014; 24(7):829–37.
18. Boyle MP, Bell SC, Konstan MW, et al. A CFTR corrector (lumacaftor) and a CFTR potentiator (ivacaftor) for treatment of patients with cystic fibrosis who have a phe508del CFTR mutation: a phase 2 randomised controlled trial. Lancet Respir Med 2014;2(7):527–38.
19. Wainwright CE, Elborn JS, Ramsey BW, et al. Lumacaftor-ivacaftor in patients with cystic fibrosis homozygous for Phe508del CFTR. N Engl J Med 2015;373(3):220–31.
20. Taylor-Cousar JL, Munck A, McKone EF, et al. Tezacaftor-ivacaftor in patients with cystic fibrosis homozygous for Phe508del. N Engl J Med 2017; 377(21):2013–23.
21. Heijerman HGM, McKone EF, Downey DG, et al. Efficacy and safety of the elexacaftor plus tezacaftor plus ivacaftor combination regimen in people with cystic fibrosis homozygous for the F508del mutation: a double-blind, randomised, phase 3 trial. Lancet 2019;394(10212):1940–8.
22. Middleton PG, Mall MA, Drevinek P, et al. Elexacaftor-tezacaftor-ivacaftor for cystic fibrosis with a single Phe508del allele. N Engl J Med 2019;381(19):1809–19.
23. Martin C, Burnet E, Ronayette-Preira A, et al. Patient perspectives following initiation of elexacaftor-tezacaftor-ivacaftor in people with cystic fibrosis and advanced lung disease. Respir Med Res 2021;80:100829.
24. Burgel PR, Durieu I, Chiron R, et al. Rapid improvement after starting elexacaftor-tezacaftor- ivacaftor in patients with cystic fibrosis and advanced pulmonary disease. Am J Respir Crit Care Med 2021;204(1):64–73.
25. DiMango E, Spielman DB, Overdevest J, et al. Effect of highly effective modulator therapy on quality of life in adults with cystic fibrosis. Int Forum Allergy Rhinol 2021;11(1):75–8.
26. Barry PJ, Taylor-Cousar JL. Triple combination cystic fibrosis transmembrane conductance regulator modulator therapy in the real world - opportunities and challenges. Curr Opin Pulm Med 2021; 27(6):554–66.
27. Rowe SM, Heltshe SL, Gonska T, et al. Clinical mechanism of the cystic fibrosis transmembrane conductance regulator potentiator ivacaftor in

G551D-mediated cystic fibrosis. Am J Respir Crit Care Med 2014;190(2):175–84.

28. Abou Alaiwa MH, Launspach JL, Grogan B, et al. Ivacaftor-induced sweat chloride reductions correlate with increases in airway surface liquid pH in cystic fibrosis. JCI insight 2018;3(15):e121468.

29. Balazs A, Mall MA. Mucus obstruction and inflammation in early cystic fibrosis lung disease: emerging role of the IL-1 signaling pathway. Pediatr Pulmonol 2019;54(Suppl 3):S5–12.

30. Esther CR Jr, Muhlebach MS, Ehre C, et al. Mucus accumulation in the lungs precedes structural changes and infection in children with cystic fibrosis. Sci Transl Med 2019;11(486).

31. Rosen BH, Chanson M, Gawenis LR, et al. Animal and model systems for studying cystic fibrosis. J Cyst Fibros 2018;17(2S):S28–34.

32. Rosen BH, Evans TIA, Moll SR, et al. Infection is not required for mucoinflammatory lung disease in CFTR-knockout ferrets. Am J Respir Crit Care Med 2018;197(10):1308–18.

33. Bouzek DC, Abou Alaiwa MH, Adam RJ, et al. Early lung disease exhibits bacteria-dependent and -independent abnormalities in cystic fibrosis pigs. Am J Respir Crit Care Med 2021;204(6):692–702.

34. Mall MA, Danahay H, Boucher RC. Emerging concepts and therapies for mucoobstructive lung disease. Ann Am Thorac Soc 2018;15(Suppl 3): S216–26.

35. Trojanek JB, Cobos-Correa A, Diemer S, et al. Airway mucus obstruction triggers macrophage activation and matrix metalloproteinase 12-dependent emphysema. Am J Respir Cell Mol Biol 2014;51(5):709–20.

36. Hector A, Schafer H, Poschel S, et al. Regulatory T-cell impairment in cystic fibrosis patients with chronic pseudomonas infection. Am J Respir Crit Care Med 2015;191(8):914–23.

37. Khalaf M, Scott-Ward T, Causer A, et al. Cystic fibrosis transmembrane conductance regulator (CFTR) in human lung microvascular endothelial cells controls oxidative stress, reactive oxygen-mediated cell signaling and inflammatory responses. Front Physiol 2020;11:879.

38. Bonfield TL, Konstan MW, Berger M. Altered respiratory epithelial cell cytokine production in cystic fibrosis. J Allergy Clin Immunol 1999;104(1):72–8.

39. Venkatakrishnan A, Stecenko AA, King G, et al. Exaggerated activation of nuclear factor-kappaB and altered IkappaB-beta processing in cystic fibrosis bronchial epithelial cells. Am J Respir Cell Mol Biol 2000;23(3):396–403.

40. Perez A, Issler AC, Cotton CU, et al. CFTR inhibition mimics the cystic fibrosis inflammatory profile. Am J Physiol Lung Cell Mol Physiol 2007;292(2): L383–95.

41. Cohen TS, Prince A. Cystic fibrosis: a mucosal immunodeficiency syndrome. Nat Med 2012;18(4): 509–19.

42. O'Connor JB, Mottlowitz MM, Wagner BD, et al. Divergence of bacterial communities in the lower airways of CF patients in early childhood. PloS One 2021;16(10):e0257838.

43. Frayman KB, Wylie KM, Armstrong DS, et al. Differences in the lower airway microbiota of infants with and without cystic fibrosis. J Cystic Fibrosis 2019; 18(5):646–52.

44. Gomez MI, Prince A. Opportunistic infections in lung disease: *Pseudomonas* infections in cystic fibrosis. Curr Opin Pharmacol 2007;7(3):244–51.

45. Hauser AR, Jain M, Bar-Meir M, et al. Clinical significance of microbial infection and adaptation in cystic fibrosis. Clin Microbiol Rev 2011;24(1):29–70.

46. Aaron SD, Ramotar K, Ferris W, et al. Adult cystic fibrosis exacerbations and new strains of *Pseudomonas aeruginosa*. Am J Respir Crit Care Med 2004;169(7):811–5.

47. Muhlebach MS, Zorn BT, Esther CR, et al. Initial acquisition and succession of the cystic fibrosis lung microbiome is associated with disease progression in infants and preschool children. PLoS Pathog 2018;14(1):e1006798.

48. Coburn B, Wang PW, Diaz Caballero J, et al. Lung microbiota across age and disease stage in cystic fibrosis. Sci Rep 2015;5:10241.

49. Zhao J, Schloss PD, Kalikin LM, et al. Decade-long bacterial community dynamics in cystic fibrosis airways. Proc Natl Acad Sci U S A 2012;109(15): 5809–14.

50. Frey DL, Boutin S, Dittrich SA, et al. Relationship between airway dysbiosis, inflammation and lung function in adults with cystic fibrosis. J Cystic Fibrosis 2021;20(5):754–60.

51. Horsley AR, Davies JC, Gray RD, et al. Changes in physiological, functional and structural markers of cystic fibrosis lung disease with treatment of a pulmonary exacerbation. Thorax 2013;68(6):532–9.

52. Liou TG, Adler FR, Keogh RH, et al. Sputum biomarkers and the prediction of clinical outcomes in patients with cystic fibrosis. PloS One 2012;7(8): e42748.

53. Downey DG, Brockbank S, Martin SL, et al. The effect of treatment of cystic fibrosis pulmonary exacerbations on airways and systemic inflammation. Pediatr Pulmonol 2007;42(8):729–35.

54. Ordonez CL, Henig NR, Mayer-Hamblett N, et al. Inflammatory and microbiologic markers in induced sputum after intravenous antibiotics in cystic fibrosis. Am J Respir Crit Care Med 2003; 168(12):1471–5.

55. Pittman JE, Wylie KM, Akers K, et al. Association of antibiotics, airway microbiome, and inflammation in

infants with cystic fibrosis. Ann Am Thorac Soc 2017;14(10):1548–55.

56. Bruscia EM, Bonfield TL. Innate and adaptive immunity in cystic fibrosis. Clin chest Med 2016; 37(1):17–29.

57. Moss RB, Hsu YP, Olds L. Cytokine dysregulation in activated cystic fibrosis (CF) peripheral lymphocytes. Clin Exp Immunol 2000;120(3):518–25.

58. Kosamo S, Hisert KB, Dmyterko V, et al. Strong toll-like receptor responses in cystic fibrosis patients are associated with higher lung function. J Cystic Fibrosis 2020;19(4):608–13.

59. Hartl D, Griese M, Kappler M, et al. Pulmonary T(H) 2 response in *Pseudomonas aeruginosa-* infected patients with cystic fibrosis. J Allergy Clin Immunol 2006;117(1):204–11.

60. Brennan S, Sly PD, Gangell CL, et al. Alveolar macrophages and CC chemokines are increased in children with cystic fibrosis. Eur Respir J 2009; 34(3):655–61.

61. Lindberg U, Svensson L, Hellmark T, et al. Increased platelet activation occurs in cystic fibrosis patients and correlates to clinical status. Thromb Res 2018;162:32–7.

62. Lara-Reyna S, Holbrook J, Jarosz-Griffiths HH, et al. Dysregulated signalling pathways in innate immune cells with cystic fibrosis mutations. Cell Mol Life Sci 2020;77(22):4485–503.

63. Ng HP, Zhou Y, Song K, et al. Neutrophil-mediated phagocytic host defense defect in myeloid Cftr-inactivated mice. PloS One 2014;9(9): e106813.

64. Su X, Looney MR, Su HE, et al. Role of CFTR expressed by neutrophils in modulating acute lung inflammation and injury in mice. Inflamm Res 2011;60(7):619–32.

65. Bruscia EM, Bonfield TL. Cystic fibrosis lung immunity: the role of the macrophage. J Innate Immun 2016;8(6):550–63.

66. Duan Y, Li G, Xu M, et al. CFTR is a negative regulator of gamma delta T cell IFN-gamma production and antitumor immunity. Cell Mol Immunol 2021; 18(8):1934–44.

67. Collin AM, Lecocq M, Noel S, et al. Lung immunoglobulin A immunity dysregulation in cystic fibrosis. EBioMedicine 2020;60:102974.

68. Polverino F, Lu B, Quintero JR, et al. CFTR regulates B cell activation and lymphoid follicle development. Respir Res 2019;20(1):133.

69. Xu Y, Tertilt C, Krause A, et al. Influence of the cystic fibrosis transmembrane conductance regulator on expression of lipid metabolism-related genes in dendritic cells. Respir Res 2009;10:26.

70. Ortiz-Munoz G, Yu MA, Lefrancais E, et al. Cystic fibrosis transmembrane conductance regulator dysfunction in platelets drives lung hyperinflammation. J Clin Invest 2020;130(4):2041–53.

71. Green M, Lindgren N, Henderson A, et al. Ivacaftor partially corrects airway inflammation in a humanized G551D rat. Am J Physiol Lung Cell Mol Physiol 2021;320(6):L1093–100.

72. Bonfield TL, Hodges CA, Cotton CU, et al. Absence of the cystic fibrosis transmembrane regulator (Cftr) from myeloid-derived cells slows resolution of inflammation and infection. J Leukoc Biol 2012;92(5):1111–22.

73. Bruscia EM, Zhang PX, Ferreira E, et al. Macrophages directly contribute to the exaggerated inflammatory response in cystic fibrosis transmembrane conductance regulator-/- mice. Am J Respir Cell Mol Biol 2009;40(3):295–304.

74. Lukasiak A, Zajac M. The distribution and role of the CFTR protein in the intracellular compartments. Membranes (Basel) 2021;11(11).

75. Zhou Y, Song K, Painter RG, et al. Cystic fibrosis transmembrane conductance regulator recruitment to phagosomes in neutrophils. J innate Immun 2013;5(3):219–30.

76. Guggino WB, Stanton BA. New insights into cystic fibrosis: molecular switches that regulate CFTR. Nat Rev Mol Cell Biol 2006;7(6):426–36.

77. Zhang PX, Murray TS, Villella VR, et al. Reduced caveolin-1 promotes hyperinflammation due to abnormal heme oxygenase-1 localization in lipopolysaccharide-challenged macrophages with dysfunctional cystic fibrosis transmembrane conductance regulator. J Immunol 2013;190(10):5196–206.

78. Kunzelmann K, Mehta A. CFTR: a hub for kinases and crosstalk of cAMP and Ca2+. FEBS J 2013; 280(18):4417–29.

79. Di Pietro C, Oz HH, Murray TS, et al. Targeting the heme oxygenase 1/carbon monoxide pathway to resolve lung hyper-inflammation and restore a regulated immune response in cystic fibrosis. Front Pharmacol 2020;11:1059.

80. DiBattista A, McIntosh N, Lamoureux M, et al. Metabolic signatures of cystic fibrosis identified in dried blood spots for newborn screening without carrier identification. J Proteome Res 2019;18(3): 841–54.

81. Bardon A. Cystic fibrosis. Carbohydrate metabolism in CF and in animal models for CF. Acta Paediatr Scand Suppl 1987;332:1–30.

82. Bardon A, Ceder O, Kollberg H. Increased activity of four glycolytic enzymes in cultured fibroblasts from cystic fibrosis patients. Res Commun Chem Pathol Pharmacol 1986;51(3):405–8.

83. Soto-Heredero G, Gomez de Las Heras MM, Gabande-Rodriguez E, et al. Glycolysis - a key player in the inflammatory response. FEBS J 2020; 287(16):3350–69.

84. Kelly B, O'Neill LA. Metabolic reprogramming in macrophages and dendritic cells in innate immunity. Cell Res 2015;25(7):771–84.

85. Henig NR, Tonelli MR, Pier MV, et al. Sputum induction as a research tool for sampling the airways of subjects with cystic fibrosis. Thorax 2001;56(4): 306–11.

86. Hisert KB, Liles WC, Manicone AM. A flow cytometric method for isolating cystic fibrosis airway macrophages from expectorated sputum. Am J Respir Cell Mol Biol 2019;61(1):42–50.

87. Mills EL, Kelly B, Logan A, et al. Succinate dehydrogenase supports metabolic repurposing of mitochondria to drive inflammatory macrophages. Cell 2016;167(2):457–70.e3.

88. Riquelme SA, Lozano C, Moustafa AM, et al. CFTR-PTEN-dependent mitochondrial metabolic dysfunction promotes *Pseudomonas aeruginosa* airway infection. Sci Transl Med 2019;11(499): eaav4634.

89. Luciani A, Villella VR, Esposito S, et al. Defective CFTR induces aggresome formation and lung inflammation in cystic fibrosis through ROS-mediated autophagy inhibition. Nat Cell Biol 2010;12(9):863–75.

90. Riquelme SA, Hopkins BD, Wolfe AL, et al. Cystic fibrosis transmembrane conductance regulator attaches tumor suppressor PTEN to the membrane and promotes anti Pseudomonas aeruginosa immunity. Immunity 2017;47(6): 1169–81.e7.

91. Iannitti RG, Napolioni V, Oikonomou V, et al. IL-1 receptor antagonist ameliorates inflammasome-dependent inflammation in murine and human cystic fibrosis. Nat Commun 2016;7:10791.

92. Buck MD, Sowell RT, Kaech SM, et al. Metabolic instruction of immunity. Cell 2017;169(4):570–86.

93. Kopp BT, Abdulrahman BA, Khweek AA, et al. Exaggerated inflammatory responses mediated by Burkholderia cenocepacia in human macrophages derived from Cystic fibrosis patients. Biochem Biophys Res Commun 2012;424(2): 221–7.

94. Meyer M, Huaux F, Gavilanes X, et al. Azithromycin reduces exaggerated cytokine production by M1 alveolar macrophages in cystic fibrosis. Am J Respir Cell Mol Biol 2009;41(5):590–602.

95. Scambler T, Jarosz-Griffiths HH, Lara-Reyna S, et al. ENaC-mediated sodium influx exacerbates NLRP3-dependent inflammation in cystic fibrosis. Elife 2019;8:e49248.

96. Lara-Reyna S, Scambler T, Holbrook J, et al. Metabolic reprograming of cystic fibrosis macrophages via the IRE1alpha arm of the unfolded protein response results in exacerbated inflammation. Front Immunol 2019;10:1789.

97. Ribeiro CM, Boucher RC. Role of endoplasmic reticulum stress in cystic fibrosis-related airway inflammatory responses. Proc Am Thorac Soc 2010;7(6):387–94.

98. Ribeiro CM, Lubamba BA. Role of IRE1alpha/XBP-1 in cystic fibrosis airway inflammation. Int J Mol Sci 2017;18(1):118.

99. Garratt LW, Wright AK, Ranganathan SC, et al. Small macrophages are present in early childhood respiratory disease. J Cyst Fibros 2012;11(3): 201–8.

100. Schupp JC, Khanal S, Gomez JL, et al. Single-cell transcriptional archetypes of airway inflammation in cystic fibrosis. Am J Respir Crit Care Med 2020; 202(10):1419–29.

101. Wright AK, Rao S, Range S, et al. Pivotal advance: expansion of small sputum macrophages in CF: failure to express MARCO and mannose receptors. J Leukoc Biol 2009;86(3):479–89. Pubmed Exact.

102. Regamey N, Tsartsali L, Hilliard TN, et al. Distinct patterns of inflammation in the airway lumen and bronchial mucosa of children with cystic fibrosis. Thorax 2012;67(2):164–70.

103. Bruscia EM, Zhang PX, Satoh A, et al. Abnormal trafficking and degradation of TLR4 underlie the elevated inflammatory response in cystic fibrosis. J Immunol 2011;186(12):6990–8.

104. del Fresno C, Garcia-Rio F, Gomez-Pina V, et al. Potent phagocytic activity with impaired antigen presentation identifying lipopolysaccharide-tolerant human monocytes: demonstration in isolated monocytes from cystic fibrosis patients. J Immunol 2009;182(10):6494–507.

105. del Fresno C, Gomez-Pina V, Lores V, et al. Monocytes from cystic fibrosis patients are locked in an LPS tolerance state: down-regulation of TREM-1 as putative underlying mechanism. PloS one 2008; 3(7):e2667.

106. Zhang X, Pan A, Jia S, et al. Cystic fibrosis plasma blunts the immune response to bacterial infection. Am J Respir Cell Mol Biol 2019;61(3):301–11.

107. del Campo R, Martinez E, del Fresno C, et al. Translocated LPS might cause endotoxin tolerance in circulating monocytes of cystic fibrosis patients. PloS One 2011;6(12):e29577.

108. Biswas SK, Lopez-Collazo E. Endotoxin tolerance: new mechanisms, molecules and clinical significance. Trends Immunol 2009;30(10):475–87.

109. Bhatraju PK, Hisert KB, Aitken ML, et al. Higher plasma endothelial markers in adults with cystic fibrosis compared with healthy age-matched control subjects. Ann Am Thorac Soc 2019;16(6): 768–71.

110. Sorio C, Montresor A, Bolomini-Vittori M, et al. Mutations of cystic fibrosis transmembrane conductance regulator (CFTR) gene cause a monocyte-selective adhesion deficiency. Am J Respir Crit Care Med 2016;193(10):1123–33.

111. Barnaby R, Koeppen K, Nymon A, et al. Lumacaftor (VX-809) restores the ability of CF macrophages

to phagocytose and kill Pseudomonas aeruginosa. Am J Physiol Lung Cell Mol Physiol 2018;314(3): L432–8.

112. Aldallal N, McNaughton EE, Manzel LJ, et al. Inflammatory response in airway epithelial cells isolated from patients with cystic fibrosis. Am J Respir Crit Care Med 2002;166(9):1248–56.

113. Ruffin M, Roussel L, Maille E, et al. Vx-809/Vx-770 treatment reduces inflammatory response to Pseudomonas aeruginosa in primary differentiated cystic fibrosis bronchial epithelial cells. Am J Physiol Lung Cell Mol Physiol 2018;314(4):L635–41.

114. Adam D, Bilodeau C, Sognigbe L, et al. CFTR rescue with VX-809 and VX-770 favors the repair of primary airway epithelial cell cultures from patients with class II mutations in the presence of Pseudomonas aeruginosa exoproducts. J Cyst Fibros 2018;17(6):705–14.

115. Gentzsch M, Cholon DM, Quinney NL, et al. Airway epithelial inflammation in vitro augments the rescue of mutant CFTR by current CFTR modulator therapies. Front Pharmacol 2021;12:628722.

116. Rehman T, Karp PH, Tan P, et al. Inflammatory cytokines TNF-alpha and IL-17 enhance the efficacy of cystic fibrosis transmembrane conductance regulator modulators. J Clin Invest 2021;131(16): e150398.

117. Xu J, Livraghi-Butrico A, Hou X, et al. Phenotypes of CF rabbits generated by CRISPR/Cas9- mediated disruption of the CFTR gene. JCI insight 2021;6(1):e139813.

118. Birket SE, Davis JM, Fernandez-Petty CM, et al. Ivacaftor reverses airway mucus abnormalities in a rat model harboring a humanized G551D-CFTR. Am J Respir Crit Care Med 2020;202(9): 1271–82.

119. Sun X, Yi Y, Yan Z, et al. In utero and postnatal VX-770 administration rescues multiorgan disease in a ferret model of cystic fibrosis. Sci Transl Med 2019; 11(485):eaau7531.

120. Ernst SE, Stoltz DA, Samuel M, et al. Poster Session, poster #447: development of a G551D porcine model of cystic fibrosis. Pediatr Pulmonol 2019;54(Suppl 2):S155–480.

121. Heltshe SL, Mayer-Hamblett N, Burns JL, et al. Pseudomonas aeruginosa in cystic fibrosis patients with G551D-CFTR treated with ivacaftor. Clin Infect Dis 2015;60(5):703–12.

122. Bessonova L, Volkova N, Higgins M, et al. Data from the US and UK cystic fibrosis registries support disease modification by CFTR modulation with ivacaftor. Thorax 2018;73(8):731–40.

123. Singh SB, McLearn-Montz AJ, Milavetz F, et al. Pathogen acquisition in patients with cystic fibrosis receiving ivacaftor or lumacaftor/ivacaftor. Pediatr Pulmonol 2019;54(8):1200–8.

124. Harris JK, Wagner BD, Zemanick ET, et al. Changes in airway microbiome and inflammation with ivacaftor treatment in patients with cystic fibrosis and the G551D mutation. Ann Am Thorac Soc 2020;17(2):212–20.

125. Cho DY, Lim DJ, Mackey C, et al. Ivacaftor, a cystic fibrosis transmembrane conductance regulator potentiator, enhances ciprofloxacin activity against Pseudomonas aeruginosa. Am J Rhinol Allergy 2019;33(2):129–36.

126. Reznikov LR, Abou Alaiwa MH, Dohrn CL, et al. Antibacterial properties of the CFTR potentiator ivacaftor. J Cyst Fibros 2014;13(5):515–9.

127. Rogers GB, Taylor SL, Hoffman LR, et al. The impact of CFTR modulator therapies on CF airway microbiology. J Cyst Fibros 2020;19(3): 359–64.

128. Payne JE, Dubois AV, Ingram RJ, et al. Activity of innate antimicrobial peptides and ivacaftor against clinical cystic fibrosis respiratory pathogens. Int J Antimicrob Agents 2017;50(3):427–35.

129. Einarsson GG, Ronan NJ, Mooney D, et al. Extended-culture and culture-independent molecular analysis of the airway microbiota in cystic fibrosis following CFTR modulation with ivacaftor. J Cyst Fibros 2021;20(5):747–53.

130. Ronan NJ, Einarsson GG, Twomey M, et al. CORK study in cystic fibrosis: sustained improvements in Ultra-low-dose chest CT scores after CFTR modulation with ivacaftor. Chest 2018;153(2):395–403.

131. Yi B, Dalpke AH, Boutin S. Changes in the cystic fibrosis airway microbiome in response to CFTR modulator therapy. Front Cell Infect Microbiol 2021;11:548613.

132. Hisert KB, Heltshe SL, Pope C, et al. Restoring CFTR function reduces airway bacteria and inflammation in people with cystic fibrosis and chronic lung infections. Am J Respir Crit Care Med 2017; 195(12):1617–28.

133. Peleg AY, Choo JM, Langan KM, et al. Antibiotic exposure and interpersonal variance mask the effect of ivacaftor on respiratory microbiota composition. J Cyst Fibros 2018;17(1):50–6.

134. Kent L, Reix P, Innes JA, et al. Lung clearance index: evidence for use in clinical trials in cystic fibrosis. J Cyst Fibros 2014;13(2):123–38.

135. Ramsey KA, Foong RE, Grdosic J, et al. Multiple breath washout outcomes are sensitive to inflammation and infection in children with cystic fibrosis. Ann Am Thorac Soc 2017;14(9):1436–42.

136. Davies J, Sheridan H, Bell N, et al. Assessment of clinical response to ivacaftor with lung clearance index in cystic fibrosis patients with a G551D-CFTR mutation and preserved spirometry: a randomised controlled trial. Lancet Respir Med 2013; 1(8):630–8.

137. Stylemans D, Darquenne C, Schuermans D, et al. Peripheral lung effect of elexacaftor/tezacaftor/ivacaftor in adult cystic fibrosis. J Cyst Fibros 2022; 21(1):160–3.

138. Brody AS, Sucharew H, Campbell JD, et al. Computed tomography correlates with pulmonary exacerbations in children with cystic fibrosis. Am J Respir Crit Care Med 2005;172(9):1128–32.

139. Sanders DB, Li Z, Brody AS. Chest computed tomography predicts the frequency of pulmonary exacerbations in children with cystic fibrosis. Ann Am Thorac Soc 2015;12(1):64–9.

140. McBennett K, MacAskill CJ, Keshock E, et al. Magnetic resonance imaging of cystic fibrosis: multi-organ imaging in the age of CFTR modulator therapies. J Cyst Fibros 2021;21(2):e148–57.

141. Chassagnon G, Hubert D, Fajac I, et al. Long-term computed tomographic changes in cystic fibrosis patients treated with ivacaftor. Eur Respir J 2016; 48(1):249–52.

142. O'Neal WK, Knowles MR. Cystic fibrosis disease modifiers: complex genetics defines the phenotypic diversity in a monogenic disease. Annu Rev Genomics Hum Genet 2018;19:201–22.

143. Sepahzad A, Morris-Rosendahl DJ, Davies JC. Cystic fibrosis lung disease modifiers and their relevance in the new era of precision medicine. Genes (Basel) 2021;12(4):562.

144. Giddings O, Esther CR Jr. Mapping targetable inflammation and outcomes with cystic fibrosis biomarkers. Pediatr Pulmonol 2017;52(S48): S21–8.

145. Perrem L, Ratjen F. Designing clinical trials for anti-inflammatory therapies in cystic fibrosis. Front Pharmacol 2020;11:576293.

146. Mayer-Hamblett N, Aitken ML, Accurso FJ, et al. Association between pulmonary function and sputum biomarkers in cystic fibrosis. Am J Respir Crit Care Med 2007;175(8):822–8.

147. Sagel SD, Wagner BD, Anthony MM, et al. Sputum biomarkers of inflammation and lung function decline in children with cystic fibrosis. Am J Respir Crit Care Med 2012;186(9):857–65.

148. Khanal S, Webster M, Niu N, et al. SPLUNC1: a novel marker of cystic fibrosis exacerbations. Eur Respir J 2021;58(5):2000507.

149. Mainz JG, Arnold C, Wittstock K, et al. Ivacaftor reduces inflammatory mediators in upper airway lining fluid from cystic fibrosis patients with a G551D mutation: serial non-invasive home-based collection of upper airway lining fluid. Front Immunol 2021;12:642180.

150. Chung J, Wunnemann F, Salomon J, et al. Increased inflammatory markers detected in nasal lavage correlate with paranasal sinus abnormalities at MRI in adolescent patients with cystic fibrosis. Antioxidants (Basel) 2021;10(9):1412.

151. Zhang S, Shrestha CL, Kopp BT. Cystic fibrosis transmembrane conductance regulator (CFTR) modulators have differential effects on cystic fibrosis macrophage function. Sci Rep 2018;8(1): 17066.

152. Gray RD, Hardisty G, Regan KH, et al. Delayed neutrophil apoptosis enhances NET formation in cystic fibrosis. Thorax 2018;73(2):134–44.

153. Gabillard-Lefort C, Casey M, Glasgow AMA, et al. Trikafta rescues CFTR and lowers monocyte P2X7R-induced inflammasome activation in cystic fibrosis. Am J Respir Crit Care Med 2022;205(7): 783–94.

154. Jarosz-Griffiths HH, Scambler T, Wong CH, et al. Different CFTR modulator combinations downregulate inflammation differently in cystic fibrosis. Elife 2020;9:e54556.

155. Bratcher PE, Rowe SM, Reeves G, et al. Alterations in blood leukocytes of G551D-bearing cystic fibrosis patients undergoing treatment with ivacaftor. J Cyst Fibros 2015;15(1):67–73.

156. Hisert KB, Schoenfelt KQ, Cooke G, et al. Ivacaftor-induced proteomic changes suggest monocyte defects may contribute to the pathogenesis of cystic fibrosis. Am J Respir Cell Mol Biol 2016; 54(4):594–7.

157. Hisert KB, Birkland TP, Schoenfelt KQ, et al. Ivacaftor decreases monocyte sensitivity to interferon-gamma in people with cystic fibrosis. ERJ Open Res 2020;6(2).

158. Sun T, Sun Z, Jiang Y, et al. Transcriptomic responses to ivacaftor and prediction of ivacaftor clinical responsiveness. Am J Respir Cell Mol Biol 2019;61(5):643–52.

159. Hisert KB, Birkland TP, Schoenfelt KQ, et al. CFTR modulator therapy enhances peripheral blood monocyte contributions to immune responses in people with cystic fibrosis. Front Pharmacol 2020; 11:1219.

160. Iwanaga N, Kolls JK. Updates on T helper type 17 immunity in respiratory disease. Immunology 2019; 156(1):3–8.

161. Mulcahy EM, Hudson JB, Beggs SA, et al. High peripheral blood th17 percent associated with poor lung function in cystic fibrosis. PloS One 2015; 10(3):e0120912.

162. Westholter D, Beckert H, Strassburg S, et al. Pseudomonas aeruginosa infection, but not mono or dual-combination CFTR modulator therapy affects circulating regulatory T cells in an adult population with cystic fibrosis. J Cyst Fibros 2021;20(6):1072–9.

163. Ryan DG, O'Neill LAJ. Krebs cycle reborn in macrophage immunometabolism. Annu Rev Immunol 2020;38:289–313.

164. Tannahill GM, Curtis AM, Adamik J, et al. Succinate is an inflammatory signal that induces IL-1beta through HIF-1alpha. Nature 2013;496(7444):238–42.

165. Lampropoulou V, Sergushichev A, Bambouskova M, et al. Itaconate links inhibition of succinate dehydrogenase with macrophage metabolic remodeling and regulation of inflammation. Cell Metab 2016;24(1): 158–66.

166. Riquelme SA, Liimatta K, Wong Fok Lung T, et al. Pseudomonas aeruginosa Utilizes host- derived itaconate to redirect its metabolism to promote biofilm formation. Cell Metab 2020;31(6): 1091–106.e6.

167. Tomlinson KL, Lung TWF, Dach F, et al. Staphylococcus aureus induces an itaconate-dominated immunometabolic response that drives biofilm formation. Nat Commun 2021;12(1):1399.

168. Medzhitov R. Origin and physiological roles of inflammation. Nature 2008;454(7203):428–35.

169. Sergeev V, Chou FY, Lam GY, et al. The extrapulmonary effects of cystic fibrosis transmembrane conductance regulator modulators in cystic fibrosis. Ann Am Thorac Soc 2020;17(2):147–54.

Novel Approaches to Multidrug-Resistant Infections in Cystic Fibrosis

Thomas S. Murray, MD, PhD[a],*, Gail Stanley, MD[b,c,d],*,
Jonathan L. Koff, MD[c,d,e],*

KEYWORDS

- Cystic fibrosis • Multidrug-resistant organisms • Bacteriophage • Gallium

KEY POINTS

- Despite the introduction of cystic fibrosis transmembrane conductance regulator (CFTR) modulator therapy, multidrug-resistant organism (MDRO) pulmonary infections remain a significant problem for patients with cystic fibrosis (CF), and new therapeutic strategies are needed.
- Standard antibiotic dosing regimens may produce subtherapeutic levels for patients with CF, as the pharmacokinetics/pharmacodynamics often differ from patients without CF.
- Novel therapies, such as gallium and bacteriophage(s), are emerging as exciting options to treat MDRO infections but additional studies are required to determine the optimal dosing, and patient populations, which will benefit the most.

INTRODUCTION

Chronic Multidrug-Resistant Organism Infections in Cystic Fibrosis

Patients with cystic fibrosis (CF) are colonized early in life with bacteria and treated with repeated cycles of antibiotics. This leads to the emergence of pathogenic chronic multidrug-resistant organism (MDROs), defined as microorganisms resistant to one or more different classes of antibiotics.[1] Organisms that are problematic include, but are not limited to, the gram-positive methicillin-resistant *Staphylococcus aureus* (MRSA), and a variety of gram-negative organisms that include *Pseudomonas aeruginosa, Burkholderia sp., Stenotrophomonas maltophilia, Achromobacter xylosoxidans,* and nontuberculous mycobacteria (NTM). In 2019, 16.9% of *P. aeruginosa* infections in patients with CF were multidrug-

resistant (MDR), while more than 50% of patients had a respiratory culture that grew MRSA.[2] As highly effective cystic fibrosis transmembrane conductance regulator (CFTR) modulator therapy is introduced at younger ages, there is optimism that this will reduce the incidence and/or severity of chronic infections and decrease the acquisition of new pathogens.[3,4] However, this is tempered by the observation that while the initiation of ivacaftor initially leads to decreases in *P. aeruginosa*, this effect is not maintained long term.[5] In addition, for some individuals with CF currently on CFTR modulator therapy, evidence suggests there is little change to the microbes in the airway.[6] Therefore, antibiotics remain integral to treatment regimens during pulmonary exacerbations,[4] and novel antimicrobial approaches or interventions are needed to treat these infections.

[a] Department of Pediatrics, Section Infectious Diseases and Global Health, Yale University School of Medicine, PO Box 208064, 333 Cedar Street, New Haven, CT 06520-8064, USA; [b] Department of Internal Medicine, Section Pulmonary, Critical Care and Sleep Medicine, Yale University School of Medicine, PO Box 208057, 300 Cedar Street TAC-441 South, New Haven, CT 06520-8057, USA; [c] Adult Cystic Fibrosis Program; [d] Yale University Center for Phage Biology & Therapy; [e] Department of Internal Medicine, Section Pulmonary, Critical Care and Sleep Medicine, Yale University School of Medicine, PO Box 208057, 300 Cedar Street TAC-455A South, New Haven, CT 06520-8057, USA
* Corresponding authors.
E-mail addresses: Thomas.s.murray@yale.edu (T.S.M.); gail.stanley@yale.edu (G.S.); jon.koff@yale.edu (J.L.K.)

Clin Chest Med 43 (2022) 667–676
https://doi.org/10.1016/j.ccm.2022.06.008

Several different therapeutic approaches have been tried in recent years to improve outcomes for patients with CF with chronic MDRO pulmonary infection (**Table 1**). One such approach is to improve the efficacy of existing antibiotics by optimizing the pharmacokinetics/pharmacodynamics (PK/PD), which may be achieved by altering the dosing regimen.[7] Another strategy to extend the benefits of a currently available drug (eg, vancomycin, ciprofloxacin, levofloxacin, and amikacin), is to develop an inhaled formulation that allows for higher concentrations in the lung while reducing systemic adverse effects.[8–10] Finally, existing beta-lactam drugs, such as ceftazidime and meropenem, have been combined with novel beta-lactamase inhibitors to create new drugs that target gram-negative MDROs that produce extended-spectrum beta-lactamases (ESBLs) and carbapenemases.[11]

While optimizing the delivery of existing drugs has been helpful, it is not surprising that resistant organisms continue to emerge. The above approaches also highlight the limitation of the existing antibiotic pipeline where few new drugs with novel mechanisms of action have been introduced in recent years. The result is innovative therapies currently being studied that either: (1) target the host to improve the immune response to infection [for example, granulocyte macrophage-colony stimulating factor (GM-CSF)] or (2) target the organism with a completely different class of molecule(s) that have antimicrobial activity (eg, gallium or bacteriophages).

DISCUSSION
Optimizing the Pharmacokinetics/Pharmacodynamics of Available Antibiotics

Based on pancreatic insufficiency and impaired gastrointestinal tract absorption, increased renal and hepatic drug clearance, and increased volume of distribution of hydrophilic drugs[12–14] standard antimicrobial dosing may not be appropriate for patients with CF as they require higher and/or more frequent drug administration to achieve therapeutic levels.[15–17] One review of anti-MRSA agents found that for both intravenous (IV) and oral administration, none of the currently

Table 1
Novel approaches to treat MDRO infections in patients with CF

Strategy	Examples	Advantages	Disadvantages
Extended antibiotic infusion/increased dosing	Meropenem	Optimizes existing drugs based on PK/PD studies in patients with CF	Daily activities hampered by long times with IV infusion, potential for adverse effects with higher dosing
Newer antimicrobial agents (eg, novel b-lactam/b-lactamase combinations)	Ceftazidime/avibactam Ceftolozane/tazobactam	Additional efficacy against organisms that produce B-lactamases.	Emergence of resistant organisms
Inhaled existing antimicrobials	Vancomycin	Avoid systemic adverse effects while achieving higher concentrations at the infection site	Limited efficacy data for most new formulations.
Novel inhaled antimicrobial Inhaled agents that enhance the immune response	Nitric oxide Granulocyte monocyte-colony stimulating factor	May provide benefit for difficult-to-treat organisms such as M. abscessus	Limited data from clinical studies. Optimal dosing not clear may require frequent dosing
Phage		No off-target effects on human cells, Has the potential to revert antibiotic resistance	Phage-resistant bacteria are well-described
Gallium		IV therapy is well-tolerated	Only IV administration has been studied to date

Abbreviations: IV, Intravenous; MDRO, multidrug-resistant organism; PK/PD, pharmacokinetics/pharmacodynamics.

recommended doses for any of the studied drugs achieved therapeutic levels for a sufficient time.[15] In each case either a higher dose or more frequent dosing was recommended to achieve the required minimum inhibitory concentrations (MICs) for the appropriate time. For certain beta-lactam antibiotics, such as meropenem, continuous infusions increase the time the drug concentration is above the MIC, which increases drug activity against isolates with higher MICs.[17,18] These data highlight the importance of studying the PK/PD of novel antimicrobials in CF children and adults as they come to market because suboptimal dosing will potentially select for resistant strains.[19]

CLINICS CARE POINTS

- When prescribing CF antimicrobial therapy, do not necessarily rely on "standard" dosing established for the general population;
- For a given drug, examine the literature for PK/PD data to determine the optimal therapeutic regimen and required drug monitoring in CF;
- Continuous infusions are an option for select beta-lactams.

Newer Systemic Antimicrobials for Multidrug-Resistant Organisms Therapy

Gram-negative organisms (eg, *P. aeruginosa, Burkholderia* sp)

Existing beta-lactam antibiotics combined with novel beta-lactamase inhibitors have produced a number of newer drugs with potent *in vitro* activity against select MDR isolates when a primary driver of antimicrobial resistance is the production of ESBLs or carbapenemases.[11] Two examples that have been used in CF to treat MDR organisms are ceftazidime-avibactam and ceftolozane-tazobactam.[19–25] A case series of 8 adults with advanced CF lung disease complicated by MDR *P. aeruginosa* and/or *Burkholderia* infection who received 15 courses of ceftazidime-avibactam showed a clinical response in 13/15 (86.7%) patients with no serious adverse events reported.[24] However, *in vitro P. aeruginosa* resistance to ceftazidime-avibactam is well described and should be considered before using this agent.[21,23,26]

Ceftolozane-tazobactam has prominent *P. aeruginosa* activity with higher rates of *in vitro* susceptibility compared with ceftazidime-avibactam.[11] A study of 21 patients with MDR *P. aeruginosa* treated with ceftolozane-tazobactam with or without additional anti-pseudomonal antibiotics included 6 patients with CF. Of these patients with CF, 5 (83%) demonstrated a successful

clinical response; the one patient who did not improve had ceftolozane-tazobactam-resistant isolates.[27] Additional individual case reports have suggested success with ceftolozane-avibactam for CF adults who have pulmonary exacerbations and respiratory cultures with MDR gram-negative bacteria.[28–30] While the existing data are generally in adults, ceftolozane-avibactam has also been proposed as an option for children with MDR *P. aeruginosa* refractory to standard therapies.[20]

Meropenem-vaborbactam is another new beta-lactam/beta-lactamase inhibitor combination. It differs from those previously discussed in that it does not provide additional activity against meropenem-resistant *P. aeruginosa*. However, it is efficacious against other MDR CF pathogens such as *Burkholderia* sp and *S. maltophilia*,[31] but there are little data on its clinical use for patients with CF. Additional combinations of beta-lactams and beta-lactamase inhibitors have been approved or are at various stages of clinical development.[11] An alternative novel approach is to use a beta-lactamase inhibitor from one of these new combinations to restore susceptibility of a different beta-lactam. For example, piperacillin susceptibility can be restored by the avibactam from ceftazidime-avibactam for MDR *Burkholderia* CF isolates resistant to piperacillin.[32] The relebactam from imipenem-relebactam can restore amoxicillin susceptibility to the resistant NTM, *Mycobacterium abscessus,* by inhibiting the mycobacterial beta-lactamases that degrade amoxicillin.[33]

Cefiderocol is a novel cephalosporin/siderophore that enters bacteria through the iron-uptake system and has activity against MDR gram negatives including *P. aeruginosa*.[34] It has been proposed as a potential salvage therapy for MDR gram negatives but very little data are available to support its use in CF.[35] One study of 8 patients with CF who received 12 courses of cefiderocol for MDR *A. xylosoxidans* noted a clinical response after 11/12 (91.7%) courses, but only one patient cleared the infection.[36] Additional studies are needed to determine if there is a role for cefiderocol when other agents have failed to generate a clinical response.

Although the correlation between *in vitro* antibiotic resistance and clinical outcomes is often absent in CF,[37,38] it is important to note that variable rates of *in vitro* resistance have been described for all of the above antibiotics.[11,25,27,39] Mechanisms of resistance to these agents include, but are not limited to, increased activity of efflux pumps, porin mutations, and overexpression of the AmpC beta-lactamase.[11,40] Additionally, none of the currently available new beta-lactam/beta-lactamase inhibitors bind class B metalloprotease b-lactamases, such that isolates with these enzymes will remain resistant.[11]

CLINICS CARE POINTS

- There are several new combinations of cephalosporins and beta-lactamase inhibitors for different MDR gram-negative pathogens.
- Based on the mechanism of action of specific drugs and the resistance mechanisms of some bacteria, antibiotic efficacy varies.
- While *in vitro* susceptibility testing does not correlate with clinical outcomes in CF, resistance to these new agents is described and worth monitoring.

Methicillin-Resistant S. aureus

Fewer new agents have been developed in recent years for MRSA treatment. Ceftaroline is a fifth-generation IV cephalosporin that targets the penicillin-binding protein 2A, which confers methicillin resistance to *S. aureus*. As with other antimicrobials, the PK/PD of ceftaroline in CF may require nonstandard dosing to achieve therapeutic levels.[15,41] There are little data for the use of ceftaroline to treat MRSA-associated pulmonary exacerbations.[42,43] One retrospective study of 90 patients with CF who received ceftaroline compared with 90 patients treated with vancomycin showed no difference in forced expiratory volume in 1 second (FEV1), which suggested equivalence between the 2 drugs.[42] Thus, ceftaroline may be an option for patients with renal dysfunction or those who are unable to tolerate vancomycin for other reasons. Importantly, carbapenem use in patients with CF has been linked to ceftaroline resistance, which makes susceptibility testing a consideration for patients who have previously received carbapenems for MDR gram-negative organisms.[44]

Novel Inhaled Therapies in Development

Inhaled delivery of existing antimicrobials. Concerns about the systemic toxicity of commonly used antimicrobials have led to the study of inhaled formulations that allow for high concentrations of drug delivery to the lungs with fewer systemic side effects.[9,10,45] A number of currently available antibiotics are being studied as inhalation therapy to address unmet needs for patients with CF. Phase 1 safety and PK studies of dry powder inhaled vancomycin in healthy adults and patients with CF elicited optimism. However, subsequent studies including a phase III randomized, multicenter, double-blinded, placebo-controlled study to evaluate the effectiveness of inhaled vancomycin in patients with CF ages 6 and older with MRSA (clinicaltrials.gov NCT03181932), did not meet the primary endpoints: improved lung function (FEV1% predicted) and decreased frequency of pulmonary exacerbations when compared with placebo.[46] In addition, a strategy to investigate the use of inhaled vancomycin for MRSA eradication was studied (clinicaltrials.gov NCT01594827). This trial enrolled 29 subjects; there were no differences in the rates of MRSA eradication, and inhaled vancomycin may be associated with increased rates of bronchospasm.[47] A recently completed phase I dose-escalation study examined inhaled teicoplanin, another anti-MRSA drug in patients with CF; the study results are pending at this time (clinicaltrials.gov NCT04176328).

For gram-negative organisms, an inhaled form of levofloxacin was evaluated in a phase III trial (clinicaltrials.gov NCT01180634). There was no difference between inhaled levofloxacin compared with placebo in the primary outcome of time to next pulmonary exacerbation. However, there was a statistically significant improvement in the treatment arm with respect to secondary outcomes of lung function and decreased microbial burden in the sputum.[48] Thus, inhaled levofloxacin has been approved in the European Union and Canada for adults.[49] Other antibiotics are also under development as inhaled therapy in areas with a significant clinical need. Oral clofazimine is a standard agent for the treatment of Mycobacterial infections that is being developed as an inhaled therapy, which has shown promise in a mouse model of NTM infection.[50]

Novel inhaled agents. In addition to new combinations and formulations of existing antibiotics, there are advances in developing inhaled administration of molecules integral to the host immune response to infection, especially for MDR *M. abscessus*.[51] These pathogens reside in host macrophages within the lung, thus there is a need to achieve high intracellular drug levels for treatment success. Two of the drugs furthest along in clinical development are inhaled nitric oxide (iNO) gas and GM-CSF.

NO as an antimicrobial. NO is a gas with both direct and indirect antimicrobial properties derived from L-arginine by iNO synthase, which is released by epithelial cells, macrophages, and other immune cells in response to infection.[52] NO production is reduced in CF, which is a potential mechanism for susceptibility to bacterial and viral infections.[53,54] Case reports describe the use of inhaled NO to decrease MDR-NTM numbers in the respiratory tract of patients that have failed traditional therapy, with an associated improvement in clinical symptoms.[55–57] A small phase 1 safety trial in patients with CF demonstrated that inhaled NO given five times daily (at 160 ppm) was safe when given over a 14-day period.[58] While there was an initial drop in the number of NTM recovered with improved lung function, sustained microbial clearance from the sputum was not achieved.[58] Another study looked at a higher inhaled NO dose in a single patient but was discontinued due to adverse effects.[55] While NTM clearance was not achieved, the patient had improved exercise tolerance and lung function.[55] A phase II clinical trial of inhaled NO in patients with CF (clinicaltrials.gov NCT02498535) was terminated due to COVID-19 thus, additional studies are required to determine appropriate dosing and confirm long-term benefits. Inhaled NO is also under investigation in patients with CF with *Pseudomonas*, *Staphylococcus*, or *Stenotrophomonas* (clinicaltrials.gov NCT02498535). A multi-center, randomized, placebo-controlled, phase II clinical trial has been completed and we await the reported results.[59]

GM-CSF as an antimicrobial. GM-CSF is released by alveolar macrophages in response to microbes, including NTM, and exogenous GM-CSF therapy is being studied as an antiinfective. Two patients with CF refractory to conventional therapy for *M abscessus* responded to inhaled GM-CSF, one in combination with antibiotics, and the other with GM-CSF alone.[60] A phase II clinical trial of inhaled GM-CSF for patients with CF with NTM (clinicaltrials.gov NCT03597347) was terminated early due to COVID-19 as well as changes in CF care that affected the primary outcome[61]. However, analysis of the primary outcome (sputum NTM culture conversion to negative after 48 weeks) showed that no significant sputum culture conversions occurred in the inhaled GM-CSF group. Based on these results, the use of inhaled GM-CSF in CF for NTM has been discontinued.

CLINICS CARE POINTS

- NO and GM-CSF are naturally produced by the immune system in response to infection.
- Inhaled NO and GM-CSF have been studied as adjuvant therapy for common CF bacterial infections, and highly resistant organisms such as NTM.
- Additional clinical studies are needed to establish the correct dosing and to determine whether there is a clinical benefit.

Novel Molecules with Antimicrobial Activity

Gallium is a metal that is used commercially in electronic circuits and semiconductors and is approved for clinical use in diagnostic procedures, and as a therapeutic in cancer and bone metabolism. Iron is an essential element for bacteria growth and metabolism. Bacteria use siderophores to scavenge iron from the environment. Gallium (Ga^{3+}) is similar enough in structure to ferric ion (Fe^{3+}), and will bind bacteria siderophores with high affinity.[62] However, Ga3+ cannot be reduced under physiologic conditions, rendering gallium-loaded enzymes inactive. Thus, gallium offers an opportunity to be used to disrupt bacterial iron metabolism,[63] which has been described as a "Trojan horse" strategy.[64] This potential use is particularly relevant in CF because gallium's antibacterial activity has been observed against *P. aeruginosa* and NTM,[63] and has an advantage for therapy because it is already FDA approved for clinical use for other conditions.

A phase II study (IGNITE; clinicaltrials.gov NCT02354859) investigated the safety and efficacy of IV gallium nitrate for 5 consecutive days in CF adults with chronic *P. aeruginosa*. While there was not a change in lung function (by 5% percent predicted), there was a significant decrease in *P. aeruginosa*, and gallium was well tolerated (CFF.org Clinical Trial Finder & clinicaltrials.gov NCT02354859), although we wait peer-reviewed published results. A limitation of this approach is the use of IV therapy in individuals with chronic *P. aeruginosa*, which would potentially require long-term IV access. However, in this patient population, IV therapies are already commonly used. Investigating the role of gallium during acute pulmonary exacerbations may be warranted. In addition, the potential for an inhaled formulation may be more appealing. Gallium was also found to be effective against NTM.[65] The ABATE trial (clinicaltrials.gov NCT04294043) is currently enrolling to study the safety and tolerability of inhaled gallium for NTM (*Mycobacterium avium* or *abscessus*) in an open-label multi-center trial.

Bacteriophages (phages) are viruses that infect and kill bacteria. Phage therapy is the application of lytic phages to treat bacterial infections.[66] Here, the strategy of using a natural competitor of bacteria, especially an MDRO or emerging pan-drug-resistant bacteria, could be described as "the enemy of my enemy is my friend."

The biosphere contains an estimated 10^{31} phages,[67] which means that natural exposure to phages occurs continuously throughout human life via contact with the environment (eg, food consumption and inhalation of particles suspended in the air). Phages are present on human skin[68] and in the gut,[69] and because humans have evolved with constant phage exposure, phages have generally been accepted as safe, provided they have been produced in a pharmaceutical-grade manner and are free of host bacteria endo-toxins.[70,71] As phages are the most numerous organisms on the planet, there are estimated to be 10:1 more phages than bacteria[67] which suggests an opportunity to find naturally occurring phages that infect bacterial pathogens of interest. In addition, phages can be genetically engineered to be used therapeutically.[72]

It is important to note that there are limited data on the safety and efficacy of phage therapy in traditionally defined clinical studies. However, the Eliava Institute in Georgia and the Ludwik Hirszfeld Institute in Poland have provided phage therapy to many patients.[73] There is an increasing experience in the United States with FDA-approved compassionate cases and clinical trials,[70] although early attempts to show phage therapy efficacy in randomized clinical trials have been largely unsuccessful. The lack of efficacy in clinical trials may be attributed to poor study design, challenges in phage stabilization, or administration of phage at concentrations too low to be therapeutically active. One hypothetical concern with phage therapy is a toxic response caused by target pathogen lysis that releases bacterial toxins (eg, lipopolysaccharides and other virulence factors) that could trigger an inflammatory response. It is important to highlight that this effect has not been observed in animal studies of phage therapy. Notably, studies have shown that exposure to clinically relevant beta-lactam antibiotics leads to a higher release of bacterial endotoxin compared with phages.[74]

Specific to CF, there are case reports of the addition of phage therapy to standard clinical care in compassionate cases.[75] These include pediatric and adult patients whereby phage therapy was delivered either via nebulization or IV to target bacteria such as P. aeruginosa, S. aureus, or A. xylosoxidans.[75] Since the publication of these reports, interest in phage therapy in the United States has increased with several phage therapy programs starting or expanding [Tailored Antibacterials & Innovative Laboratories for Phage Research (TAILφR) at Baylor University, Army & Navy Laboratories, Mayo Clinic, Center for Phage Technology (CPT) at Texas A&M University, Center for Innovative Phage Applications & Therapeutics (IPATH) at University of California, San Diego, University of Pittsburgh (expertise in NTM phage), Center for Phage Biology & Therapy at Yale University]. Current or planned clinical trials to investigate phage therapy to treat P. aeruginosa are independently investigating single phage (clinicaltrials.gov NCT04684641) or phage cocktails (multiple phages given at the same time; clinicaltrials.gov NCT04596319 & NCT05010577), and different routes of administration (eg, nebulized vs IV).

It will be important to study each of these approaches. For example, while phage cocktails may provide a broader range of coverage for a specific bacterium, there is evidence that cocktails may increase genetic mutations in P. aeruginosa that could result in increased virulence.[76] Such an effect will need to be investigated in clinical strains of P. aeruginosa and other bacteria. In addition, there is evidence that multiple phages may interfere with phage replication within the same bacteria, potentially reducing the effectiveness of phage therapy.[77] However, single phage therapy may be limited by evolving bacterial resistance.[78] Recognizing that bacteria continue to evolve resistance to phage(s), investigators have developed a strategy to identify phages that target specific virulence factors on bacteria so that the result of phage therapy are surviving bacteria mutants with decreased expression or production of such virulence factors.[66] For example, phage therapy targeting P. aeruginosa antibiotic efflux pumps, responsible for resistance to multiple antibiotics, restored antibiotic susceptibility[79] and was reported in a compassionate use case to treat an infected aortic graft.[80] Compassionate use of phage therapy in patients with CF is performed by a few centers in the United States targeting MDR P. aeruginosa, A. xylosoxidans and NTM.[72] Currently a phase 2 randomized, double-blinded, single-site clinical trial studying the safety and effectiveness of single nebulized phage therapy is enrolling patients with CF with P. aeruginosa (clinicaltrials.gov NCT04684641).

Understanding bacteria and phage evolution will be essential to the development of future phage therapy. Approaches using phage cocktails may be relevant to treat pulmonary exacerbations, while single phage therapy may be an option for chronic treatment. Different approaches to phage delivery are also under investigation because of the potential for individual patient adaptive immune antibody responses to phage therapy to decrease the effectiveness of subsequent phage therapy.[81] It is hypothesized that IV administration will induce increased host adaptive immunity compared with nebulization, but this concern remains to be studied in clinical trials.

CLINICS CARE POINTS

- Gallium and phage therapy are examples of additional strategies to treat MDR bacteria.
- Continued well-designed and executed clinical trials are required to confirm initial observations.

• Compassionate treatment may be available for these types of therapies for carefully selected candidates.

SUMMARY

While MDRO infections have recently been recognized as an emerging global threat, individuals with CF, and their care teams, have been challenged with the complexities involved in the clinical care of MRSA, *P. aeruginosa*, *Burkholderia sp.*, *S. maltophilia*, *A. xylosoxidans*, and NTM for far too long. While we await the discovery and development of additional antimicrobials with novel mechanisms of action, this article summarizes approaches that have been used to: (1) optimize the PK/PD of existing antibiotics, (2) administer new antibiotic combinations, and (3) repurpose existing antibiotics into inhaled formulations. However, because MDROs continue to evolve, additional approaches are required beyond the existing antibiotic pipeline. Novel approaches include: (1) targeting the host to improve the immune response(s) to infection [for example, GM-CSF] or (2) targeting the pathogen with a completely different class of molecule(s) that have antimicrobial activity (eg, gallium or bacteriophages). These approaches require additional clinical studies before they can be considered for routine clinical use.

FINANCIAL SUPPORT

There was no financial support provided for this article.

DISCLOSURE

T.S. Murray-none. J.L. Koff is the PI for bacteriophage clinical trial NCT04684641 and a national Co-PI for bacteriophage clinical trial NCT05010577. J.L. Koff & G.L. Stanley: Colleagues at Yale University have licensed intellectual property related to bacteriophage therapy to a company although neither J.L. Koff nor G.L. Stanley has a financial interest in this process.

REFERENCES

1. Centers for disease control and prevention https://www.cdc.gov/infectioncontrol/guidelines/mdro/. updated February 2017 Accessed July 7, 2022.
2. Cystic Fibrosis Foundation Patient Registry 2020 Annual Data Report Bethesda, Maryland ©2021 Cystic Fibrosis Foundation.
3. Rogers GB, Taylor SL, Hoffman LR, et al. The impact of CFTR modulator therapies on CF airway microbiology. J Cyst Fibros 2020;19(3):359–64.
4. Saiman L. Improving outcomes of infections in cystic fibrosis in the era of CFTR modulator therapy. Pediatr Pulmonol 2019;54(Suppl 3): S18–26.
5. Hisert KB, Heltshe SL, Pope C, et al. Restoring Cystic Fibrosis Transmembrane Conductance Regulator Function Reduces Airway Bacteria and Inflammation in People with Cystic Fibrosis and Chronic Lung Infections. Am J Respir Crit Care Med 2017; 195(12):1617–28.
6. Harris JK, Wagner BD, Zemanick ET, et al. Changes in Airway Microbiome and Inflammation with Ivacaftor Treatment in Patients with Cystic Fibrosis and the G551D Mutation. Ann Am Thorac Soc 2020;17(2): 212–20.
7. Epps QJ, Epps KL, Young DC, et al. State of the art in cystic fibrosis pharmacology optimization of antimicrobials in the treatment of cystic fibrosis pulmonary exacerbations: III. Executive summary. Pediatr Pulmonol 2021;56(7):1825–37.
8. Smith S, Rowbotham NJ, Regan KH. Inhaled antipseudomonal antibiotics for long-term therapy in cystic fibrosis. Cochrane Database of Systematic Reviews 2018;(3).
9. Elborn JS, Vataire AL, Fukushima A, et al. Comparison of Inhaled Antibiotics for the Treatment of Chronic Pseudomonas aeruginosa Lung Infection in Patients With Cystic Fibrosis: Systematic Literature Review and Network Meta-analysis. Clin Ther 2016;38(10):2204–26.
10. Wenzler E, Fraidenburg DR, Scardina T, et al. Inhaled Antibiotics for Gram-Negative Respiratory Infections. Clinical microbiology reviews 2016; 29(3):581–632.
11. Yahav D, Giske CG, Grāmatniece A, et al. New β-Lactam-β-Lactamase Inhibitor Combinations. Clin Microbiol Rev 2020;34(1).
12. Parker AC, Pritchard P, Preston T, et al. Enhanced drug metabolism in young children with cystic fibrosis. Arch Dis Child 1997;77(3):239–41.
13. Kearns GL. Hepatic drug metabolism in cystic fibrosis: recent developments and future directions. Ann Pharmacother 1993;27(1):74–9.
14. Prandota J. Clinical pharmacology of antibiotics and other drugs in cystic fibrosis. Drugs 1988;35(5): 542–78.
15. Epps QJ, Epps KL, Young DC, et al. State of the art in cystic fibrosis pharmacology-Optimization of antimicrobials in the treatment of cystic fibrosis pulmonary exacerbations: I. Anti-methicillin-resistant Staphylococcus aureus (MRSA) antibiotics. Pediatr Pulmonol 2020;55(1):33–57.
16. Epps QJ, Epps KL, Zobell JT. Optimization of antipseudomonal antibiotics for cystic fibrosis pulmonary

exacerbations: II. Cephalosporins and penicillins latest update. Pediatr Pulmonol 2021;56(6):1784–8.

17. Magreault S, Roy C, Launay M, et al. Pharmacokinetic and Pharmacodynamic Optimization of Antibiotic Therapy in Cystic Fibrosis Patients: Current Evidences, Gaps in Knowledge and Future Directions. Clin Pharmacokinet 2021;60(4):409–45.

18. Prescott WA Jr, Gentile AE, Nagel JL, et al. Continuous-infusion antipseudomonal Beta-lactam therapy in patients with cystic fibrosis. P T 2011;36(11):723–63.

19. Bensman TJ, Wang J, Jayne J, et al. Pharmacokinetic-Pharmacodynamic Target Attainment Analyses To Determine Optimal Dosing of Ceftazidime-Avibactam for the Treatment of Acute Pulmonary Exacerbations in Patients with Cystic Fibrosis. Antimicrob Agents Chemother 2017;61(10).

20. Garazzino S, Altieri E, Silvestro E, et al. Ceftolozane/Tazobactam for Treating Children With Exacerbations of Cystic Fibrosis Due to Pseudomonas aeruginosa: A Review of Available Data. Front Pediatr 2020;8:173.

21. Forrester JB, Steed LL, Santevecchi BA, et al. Vitro Activity of Ceftolozane/Tazobactam vs Nonfermenting, Gram-Negative Cystic Fibrosis Isolates. Open Forum Infect Dis 2018;5(7):ofy158.

22. Nguyen TT, Condren M, Walter J. Ceftazidime-avibactam for the treatment of multidrug resistant Burkholderia cepacia complex in a pediatric cystic fibrosis patient. Pediatr Pulmonol 2020;55(2):283–4.

23. Nolan PJ, Jain R, Cohen L, et al. In vitro activity of ceftolozane-tazobactam and ceftazidime-avibactam against Pseudomonas aeruginosa isolated from patients with cystic fibrosis. Diagn Microbiol Infect Dis 2021;99(2):115204.

24. Spoletini G, Etherington C, Shaw N, et al. Use of ceftazidime/avibactam for the treatment of MDR Pseudomonas aeruginosa and Burkholderia cepacia complex infections in cystic fibrosis: a case series. J Antimicrob Chemother 2019;74(5):1425–9.

25. Sader HS, Duncan LR, Doyle TB, et al. Antimicrobial activity of ceftazidime/avibactam, ceftolozane/tazobactam and comparator agents against Pseudomonas aeruginosa from cystic fibrosis patients. JAC Antimicrob Resist 2021;3(3):dlab126.

26. Van Dalem A, Herpol M, Echahidi F, et al. Vitro Susceptibility of Burkholderia cepacia Complex Isolated from Cystic Fibrosis Patients to Ceftazidime-Avibactam and Ceftolozane-Tazobactam. Antimicrob Agents Chemother 2018;62(9).

27. Haidar G, Philips NJ, Shields RK, et al. Ceftolozane-Tazobactam for the Treatment of Multidrug-Resistant Pseudomonas aeruginosa Infections: Clinical Effectiveness and Evolution of Resistance. Clin Infect Dis 2017;65(1):110–20.

28. Romano MT, et al. Ceftolozane/tazobactam for pulmonary exacerbation in a 63-year-old cystic fibrosis patient with renal insufficiency and an elevated MIC to Pseudomonas aeruginosa. IDCases 2020;21:e00830.

29. Stokem K, et al. Use of ceftolozane-tazobactam in a cystic fibrosis patient with multidrug-resistant pseudomonas infection and renal insufficiency. Respir Med Case Rep 2018;23:8–9.

30. Vickery SB, McClain D, Wargo KA. Successful Use of Ceftolozane-Tazobactam to Treat a Pulmonary Exacerbation of Cystic Fibrosis Caused by Multidrug-Resistant Pseudomonas aeruginosa. Pharmacotherapy 2016;36(10):e154–9.

31. Belcher R, Zobell JT. Optimization of antibiotics for cystic fibrosis pulmonary exacerbations due to highly resistant nonlactose fermenting Gram negative bacilli: Meropenem-vaborbactam and cefiderocol. Pediatr Pulmonol 2021;56(9):3059–61.

32. Zeiser ET, Becka SA, Wilson BM, et al. Switching Partners": Piperacillin-Avibactam Is a Highly Potent Combination against Multidrug-Resistant Burkholderia cepacia Complex and Burkholderia gladioli Cystic Fibrosis Isolates. J Clin Microbiol 2019;57(8).

33. Lopeman RC, Harrison J, Rathbone DL, et al. Effect of Amoxicillin in combination with Imipenem-Relebactam against Mycobacterium abscessus. Sci Rep 2020;10(1):928.

34. Zhanel GG, Golden AR, Zelenitsky S, et al. Cefiderocol: A Siderophore Cephalosporin with Activity Against Carbapenem-Resistant and Multidrug-Resistant Gram-Negative Bacilli. Drugs 2019;79(3):271–89.

35. Gavioli EM, Guardado N, Haniff F, et al. Does Cefiderocol Have a Potential Role in Cystic Fibrosis Pulmonary Exacerbation Management? Microb Drug Resist 2021 Dec;27(12):1726–32.

36. Warner NC, Bartelt LA, Lachiewicz AM, et al. Cefiderocol for the Treatment of Adult and Pediatric Patients With Cystic Fibrosis and Achromobacter xylosoxidans Infections. Clin Infect Dis 2021;73(7):e1754–7.

37. Hurley MN, Ariff AH, Bertenshaw C, et al. Results of antibiotic susceptibility testing do not influence clinical outcome in children with cystic fibrosis. J Cyst Fibros 2012;11(4):288–92.

38. Aaron SD, Vandemheen KL, Ferris W, et al. Combination antibiotic susceptibility testing to treat exacerbations of cystic fibrosis associated with multiresistant bacteria: a randomised, double-blind, controlled clinical trial. Lancet 2005;366(9484):463–71.

39. Choby JE, Ozturk T, Satola SW, et al. Widespread cefiderocol heteroresistance in carbapenem-resistant Gram-negative pathogens. Lancet Infect Dis 2021;21(5):597–8.

40. Chalhoub H, Saenz Y, Nichols WW, et al. Loss of activity of ceftazidime-avibactam due to MexAB-OprM efflux and overproduction of AmpC cephalosporinase in Pseudomonas aeruginosa isolated from

patients suffering from cystic fibrosis. Int J Antimicrob Agents 2018;52(5):697–701.

41. Barsky EE, Pereira LM, Sullivan KJ, et al. Ceftaroline pharmacokinetics and pharmacodynamics in patients with cystic fibrosis. J Cyst Fibros 2018;17(3): e25–31.

42. Branstetter J, Searcy H, Benner K, et al. Ceftaroline vs vancomycin for the treatment of acute pulmonary exacerbations in pediatric patients with cystic fibrosis. Pediatr Pulmonol 2020;55(12):3337–42.

43. Molloy L, Snyder AH, Srivastava R, et al. Ceftaroline Fosamil for Methicillin-Resistant Staphylococcus aureus Pulmonary Exacerbation in a Pediatric Cystic Fibrosis Patient. J Pediatr Pharmacol Ther 2014; 19(2):135–40.

44. Varela MC, Roch M, Taglialegna A, et al. Carbapenems drive the collateral resistance to ceftaroline in cystic fibrosis patients with MRSA. Commun Biol 2020;3(1):599.

45. Nichols DP, Durmowicz AG, Field A, et al. Developing Inhaled Antibiotics in Cystic Fibrosis: Current Challenges and Opportunities. Ann Am Thorac Soc 2019;16(5):534–9.

46. Waterer G, Lord J, Hofmann T, et al. Phase I, Dose-Escalating Study of the Safety and Pharmacokinetics of Inhaled Dry-Powder Vancomycin (AeroVanc) in Volunteers and Patients with Cystic Fibrosis: a New Approach to Therapy for Methicillin-Resistant Staphylococcus aureus. Antimicrob Agents Chemother 2020;64(3).

47. Dezube R, Jennings MT, Rykiel M, et al. Eradication of persistent methicillin-resistant Staphylococcus aureus infection in cystic fibrosis. Journal of Cystic Fibrosis 2019;18(3):357–63.

48. Flume PA, VanDevanter DR, Morgan EE, Dudley MN, Loutit JS, Bell SC, et al. A phase 3, multi-center, multinational, randomized, double-blind, placebo-controlled study to evaluate the efficacy and safety of levofloxacin inhalation solution (APT-1026) in stable cystic fibrosis patients. J Cyst Fibros 2016; 15(4):495–502.

49. Cystic Fibrosis Foundation. Drug development pipeline: inhaled levofloxacin (Quinsair). 2022. Available at: https://apps.cff.org/trials/pipeline/details/9/Inhaled-Levofloxacin-Quinsair. Accessed July 7 ,2022.

50. Banaschewski B, Verma D, Pennings LJ, et al. Clofazimine inhalation suspension for the aerosol treatment of pulmonary nontuberculous mycobacterial infections. J Cyst Fibros 2019;18(5):714–20.

51. Waterer G. Beyond antibiotics for pulmonary nontuberculous mycobacterial disease. Curr Opin Pulm Med 2020;26(3):260–6.

52. Bogdan C. Nitric oxide synthase in innate and adaptive immunity: an update. Trends Immunol 2015; 36(3):161–78.

53. Meng QH, Springall DR, Bishop AE, et al. Lack of inducible nitric oxide synthase in bronchial epithelium:

a possible mechanism of susceptibility to infection in cystic fibrosis. J Pathol 1998;184(3):323–31.

54. Zheng S, De BP, Choudhary S, et al. Impaired innate host defense causes susceptibility to respiratory virus infections in cystic fibrosis. Immunity 2003; 18(5):619–30.

55. Bogdanovski K, Chau T, Robinson CJ, et al. Antibacterial activity of high-dose nitric oxide against pulmonary Mycobacterium abscessus disease. Access Microbiol 2020;2(9). acmi000154.

56. Goldbart A, Gatt D, Golan Tripto I. Non-nuberculous mycobacteria infection treated with intermittently inhaled high-dose nitric oxide. BMJ Case Rep 2021;14(10).

57. Yaacoby-Bianu K, Gur M, Toukan Y, et al. Compassionate Nitric Oxide Adjuvant Treatment of Persistent Mycobacterium Infection in Cystic Fibrosis Patients. Pediatr Infect Dis J 2018;37(4):336–8.

58. Bentur L, Gur M, Ashkenazi M, et al. Pilot study to test inhaled nitric oxide in cystic fibrosis patients with refractory Mycobacterium abscessus lung infection. J Cyst Fibros 2020;19(2):225–31.

59. Cystic Fibrosis Foundation https://apps.cff.org/Trials/Pipeline/details/10122/Inhaled-Nitric-Oxide-Thiolanox. Accessed July 7, 2022.

60. Scott JP, Ji Y, Kannan M, et al. Inhaled granulocyte-macrophage colony-stimulating factor for Mycobacterium abscessus in cystic fibrosis. Eur Respir J 2018;51(4).

61. Cystic Fibrosis Foundation. https://apps.cff.org/Trials/Pipeline/details/10165/Inhaled-Molgramostim. Accessed July 7, 2022.

62. Chitambar CR, Narasimhan J. Targeting iron-dependent DNA synthesis with gallium and transferrin-gallium. Pathobiology 1991;59(1):3–10.

63. Goss CH, Kaneko Y, Khuu L, et al. Gallium disrupts bacterial iron metabolism and has therapeutic effects in mice and humans with lung infections. Sci Transl Med 2018;10(460).

64. Kaneko Y, Thoendel M, Olakanmi O, et al. The transition metal gallium disrupts Pseudomonas aeruginosa iron metabolism and has antimicrobial and antibiofilm activity. J Clin Invest 2007;117(4):877–88.

65. Abdalla MY, Switzer BL, Goss CH, et al. Gallium Compounds Exhibit Potential as New Therapeutic Agents against Mycobacterium abscessus. Antimicrob Agents Chemother 2015;59(8):4826–34.

66. Kortright KE, Chan BK, Koff JL, et al. Phage Therapy: A Renewed Approach to Combat Antibiotic-Resistant Bacteria. Cell Host & Microbe 2019; 25(2):219–32.

67. Wommack KE, Colwell RR. Virioplankton: viruses in aquatic ecosystems. Microbiology and molecular biology reviews : MMBR 2000;64(1):69–114.

68. Oh J, Byrd AL, Deming C, et al. Biogeography and individuality shape function in the human skin metagenome. Nature 2014;514(7520):59–64.

69. Reyes A, Haynes M, Hanson N, et al. Viruses in the faecal microbiota of monozygotic twins and their mothers. Nature 2010;466(7304):334–8.

70. Abedon ST. Bacteriophage Clinical Use as Antibacterial "Drugs": Utility and Precedent. Microbiol Spectr 2017;5(4).

71. Abdelkader K, Gerstmans H, Saafan A, et al. The Preclinical and Clinical Progress of Bacteriophages and Their Lytic Enzymes: The Parts are Easier than the Whole. Viruses 2019;11(2).

72. Dedrick RM, Guerrero-Bustamante CA, Garlena RA, Russell DA, et al. Engineered bacteriophages for treatment of a patient with a disseminated drug-resistant Mycobacterium abscessus. Nat Med 2019;25(5):730–3.

73. Luong T, Salabarria A-C, Roach DR. Phage Therapy in the Resistance Era: Where Do We Stand and Where Are We Going? Clinical Therapeutics 2020; 42(9):1659–80.

74. Dufour N, Delattre R, Ricard JD, et al. The Lysis of Pathogenic Escherichia coli by Bacteriophages Releases Less Endotoxin Than by β-Lactams. Clin Infect Dis 2017;64(11):1582–8.

75. Chan BK, Stanley G, Modak M, et al. Bacteriophage therapy for infections in CF. Pediatr Pulmonol 2021; 56(Suppl 1). S4–s9.

76. Wright RCT, Friman VP, Smith MCM, et al. Resistance Evolution against Phage Combinations Depends on the Timing and Order of Exposure. mBio 2019 Sep 24;10(5). e01652–19.

77. Dennehy JJ, Turner PE. Reduced fecundity is the cost of cheating in RNA virus phi6. Proc Biol Sci 2004;271(1554):2275–82.

78. Labrie SJ, Samson JE, Moineau S. Bacteriophage resistance mechanisms. Nat Rev Microbiol 2010; 8(5):317–27.

79. Chan BK, Sistrom M, Wertz JE, et al. Phage selection restores antibiotic sensitivity in MDR Pseudomonas aeruginosa. Sci Rep 2016;6:26717.

80. Chan BK, Turner PE, Kim S, et al. Phage treatment of an aortic graft infected with Pseudomonas aeruginosa. Evol Med Public Health 2018;2018(1):60–6.

81. Dedrick RM, Freeman KG, Nguyen JA, et al. Potent antibody-mediated neutralization limits bacteriophage treatment of a pulmonary Mycobacterium abscessus infection. Nat Med 2021;27(8):1357–61.

Update on Clinical Outcomes of Highly Effective Modulator Therapy

Alex H. Gifford, MD, FCCP[a,b,]*, Jennifer L. Taylor-Cousar, MD, MSCS, ATSF[c,d],
Jane C. Davies, MD, MB, ChB, MRCP, MRCPCH[e,f],
Paul McNally, MD, MB, BCh, BAO[g,h]

KEYWORDS

- Cystic fibrosis • CFTR modulator • HEMT • Clinical trials

KEY POINTS

- Oral medications that significantly restore cystic fibrosis transmembrane conductance regulator (CFTR) function and improve multiple clinical measures of the health of people with cystic fibrosis (pwCF) are known as highly effective CFTR modulator therapy (HEMT).
- Ivacaftor and the triple combination of elexacaftor-tezacaftor-ivacaftor, are indicated for approximately 90% of pwCF based on the CFTR genotype.
- HEMT-mediated improvements in lung function and nutritional status demonstrated in clinical trials have been confirmed in observations from postmarketing studies.
- There are multiple challenges to evaluating the safety and efficacy of HEMT at increasingly earlier stages of CFTR-mediated pathophysiology.

INTRODUCTION

Tremendous progress has been made toward achieving pharmacologic restoration of cystic fibrosis transmembrane conductance regulator (CFTR) function in people with CF (pwCF) over the last 11 years (**Fig. 1**). Today, approximately 90% of pwCF can be treated with one or more drugs collectively known as CFTR modulators that restore CFTR function to within approximately 25% to 80% threshold of wild-type activity.[1,2] For reference, a normal clinical phenotype would be expected in the setting of $\geq$50% CFTR activity.[3] However, in pwCF, CFTR modulators are considered unlikely to reverse existing organ damage,

have not yet been shown to prevent organ damage from occurring when started very early in life, and do not improve the health of all users uniformly.

Contemporary management of pwCF using CFTR modulators has been informed by clinical trials and observational studies designed to evaluate their safety, tolerability, and clinical efficacy as well as analyses of registry data supporting their use. In this review, we focus on those modulator combinations that are considered highly effective based on their substantial impact on CFTR activity and clinical improvement [highly effective modulator therapy (HEMT)]. Ivacaftor (IVA) and the triple combination of elexacaftor (ELX), tezacaftor (TEZ), and IVA (collectively, ETI) are considered to be HEMT

[a] Division of Pulmonary, Critical Care, and Sleep Medicine, University Hospitals Cleveland Medical Center, 11100 Euclid Avenue, Bolwell Building 6174, Cleveland, OH 44106, USA; [b] Rainbow Babies and Children's Hospital, Cleveland, OH, USA; [c] Department of Internal Medicine, National Jewish Medical Center, Denver, CO, USA; [d] Department of Pediatrics, National Jewish Medical Center, Denver, CO, USA; [e] National Heart and Lung Institute, Imperial College London, England, United Kingdom; [f] Royal Brompton & Harefield Hospital, Guys & St Thomas' Trust, London, United Kingdom; [g] Department of Paediatrics, RCSI University of Medicine and Health Sciences, Dublin, Ireland; [h] Cystic Fibrosis Center, Children's Health Ireland, Dublin, Ireland
* Corresponding author. Division of Pulmonary, Critical Care, and Sleep Medicine, University Hospitals Cleveland Medical Center, 11100 Euclid Avenue, Bolwell Building 6174, Cleveland, OH 44106.
E-mail address: Alex.Gifford@UHhospitals.org

Clin Chest Med 43 (2022) 677–695
https://doi.org/10.1016/j.ccm.2022.06.009
0272-5231/22/© 2022 Elsevier Inc. All rights reserved.

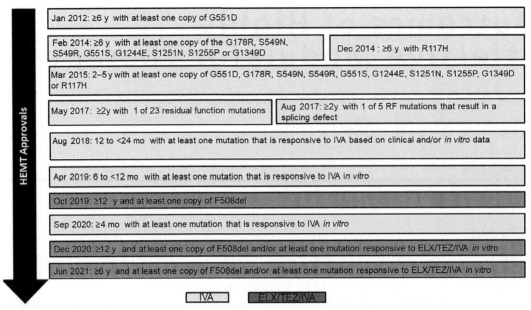

Fig. 1. Timeline of key CFTR modulator approvals by the US FDA. Date/label indications vary by region.

because their efficacy in clinical trials and post-marketing reports are far superior to that of dual modulator combinations of lumacaftor (LUM) and IVA or TEZ-IVA. We will discuss data on the use of HEMT in both clinical trials and the real-world setting, firstly in adults and adolescents (≥12 years) and then in children (≤11 years). We will also discuss variability in responses to HEMT and examine possible future trends in modulator use, especially in pregnancy and young asymptomatic children.

SUMMARY OF CONTROLLED TRIALS OF IVACAFTOR IN ADULTS AND ADOLESCENTS WITH CYSTIC FIBROSIS

IVA was the first CFTR modulator identified by high-throughput screening of small molecules that increased chloride conductance in Fischer rat thyroid cells expressing various *CFTR* gene mutations.[4] IVA noncovalently binds to specific sites on CFTR protein present in the epithelial plasma membrane, thus reversibly potentiating chloride conductance.[5] It was first approved for use by pwCF with the class III Gly551Asp (*G551D*)-CFTR mutation.[6] Based on clinical trials demonstrating safety and efficacy, the label was then expanded for use by pwCF with CFTR gating mutations that impair chloride conductance similarly to G551D-CFTR.[7,8] Finally, based on the unprecedented use of supportive *in vitro* data in human bronchial epithelial cells, the label was expanded subsequently to pwCF in the United

States (US) with additional mutations that confer varying amounts of residual CFTR function.[9]

The seminal phase 3 double-blind, placebo-controlled RCT of IVA in adolescents and adults[6] was conducted at 65 locations in 8 countries from June 2009 to July 2010. The STRIVE trial[6] enrolled 167 PwCF who were ≥12 years of age and had at least one G551D-*CFTR* allele and baseline percent-predicted forced expiratory volume in 1 second (ppFEV$_1$) between 40% and 90%. Subjects were randomized in a 1:1 ratio to receive IVA 150 mg PO BID (n = 83) or placebo (n = 78) for 48 weeks. The primary efficacy endpoint was changed from baseline through week 24 in ppFEV$_1$. Secondary endpoints included change from baseline in ppFEV$_1$ through week 48, time to first pulmonary exacerbation (PEX) through weeks 24 and 48, changes from baseline in CFQ-R RSS, weight, and sweat chloride through weeks 24 and 48. Safety was also assessed.

Primary and secondary endpoints of the STRIVE trial[6] are provided in **Table 1**. Improvements in lung function were observed as early as 2 weeks after the initiation of IVA. Through week 24, there was an average increase in ppFEV$_1$ of 10.6% among IVA-treated subjects. This degree of lung function improvement from baseline was sustained at week 48 (10.5%). At weeks 24 and 48, the rate ratios for PEX between placebo- and IVA-treated cohorts were 0.38 and 0.43, respectively. The mean reduction from baseline in sweat chloride attributed to IVA at week 48 was 48.1 mmol/L, nearly identical to that which was

Table 1
Summary of clinical trials evaluating the safety and efficacy of IVA in pwCF

Study	Phase	Age[a]	Treatment	Primary Outcome Measure	Secondary Endpoints
Ramsey et al,[6] 2011 (STRIVE)	3	≥12	IVA 150 mg BID x 48 wk	ΔppFEV$_1$: +10.6%[d,e] (24 wk)[f] ΔppFEV$_1$: +10.5%[d] (48 wk)[f]	Risk of PEX: −55%[d] (48 wk)[f] Δweight: +2.7 kg[d] (48 wk)[f] ΔCFQ-R RDS: +8.6 points[d] (48 wk)[f] Δ[Cl$_{sw}$]: −48.1 mmol[d] (48 wk)[f]
Davies et al,[40] 2013 (ENVISION)	3	6–11	IVA 150 mg BID x 48 wk	ΔppFEV$_1$: +12.5%[d] (24 wk)[f] ΔppFEV$_1$: +10.0%[d] (48 wk)[f]	Δweight: +2.8 kg[d] (48 wk)[f] ΔCFQ-R RDS: +5.1 points (48 wk)[f] Δ[Cl$_{sw}$]: −53.5 mmol[d] (48 wk)[f]
McKone et al,[10] 2014 (PERSIST)	3	≥6	IVA 150 mg BID x 144 wk[g, h]	ΔppFEV$_1$: +9.4%[b,c] (144 wk)[g] ΔppFEV$_1$: +10.3%[b] (144 wk)[h]	Δweight: +4.1 kg[b] (144 wk)[g] Δweight: +14.8 kg[b] (144 wk)[h] ΔCFQ-R RDS: +6.8 points[b] (144 wk)[g] ΔCFQ-R RDS: +10.6 points[b] (144 wk)[h]
Pilewski et al,[68] 2020 (OLE)	3	≥6	IVA 150 mg BID x 104 wk	ALT/AST >8x ULN: 0 subjects (0%)[g] ALT/AST >8x ULN: 1 subject (2.9%)[j] AST/ALT >8x ULN: 1 subject (4.8%)[k]	ΔppFEV$_1$: +3.0%[b] (104 wk)[i, l] ΔppFEV$_1$: +4.3%[b] (104 wk)[j, l] ΔppFEV$_1$: +6.5%[b] (104 wk)[k, l]
Davies et al,[41] 2016 (KIWI)	3	2–5	IVA 50 mg BID (<14 kg) or IVA 75 mg BID (≥14 kg) x 24 wk	IVA PK: similar AUC and C$_{min}$ to higher doses in adults Safety: 5 of 34 subjects (15%) had ALT or ALT increase ≥8x ULN	Δ[Cl$_{sw}$]: −46.9 mmol[d] (24 wk)[l] Δweight z-score: 0.2[d] (24 wk)[l] ΔBMI z-score: +0.4[d] (24 wk)[l]

(continued on next page)

Table 1
(continued)

Study	Phase	Age[a]	Treatment	Primary Outcome Measure	Secondary Endpoints
Rosenfeld et al,[42] 2019 (KLIMB)	3	2–5	IVA 50 mg BID (<14 kg) or IVA 75 mg BID (≥14 kg) x 84 wk	Safety: 10 of 33 subjects (30%) had ALT or AST increase >3x ULN	$\Delta[Cl_{sw}]$: −54.7 mmol[d] (108 wk)[m] Δweight z-score: 0.2 (108 wk)[m] ΔBMI z-score: +0.27[b] (108 wk)[m]
Rosenfeld et al,[43] 2018 (ARRIVAL Cohort)	3	12 to <24 mo	IVA 50 mg BID (7 to <14 kg) or IVA 75 mg BID (≥14 to <25 kg) x 24 wk	IVA PK: similar to studies of older children and adults Safety: No cataracts; 5 of 18 subjects (28%) had ALT >3x ULN	$\Delta[Cl_{sw}]$: −73.5 mmol[d] (24 wk)[l] Δweight-for-age z-score: 0.15 (24 wk)[l]
Davies et al,[44] 2020 (ARRIVAL Cohort)	3	4 to <12 mo	IVA 25 mg BID (5 to <7 kg) or IVA 50 mg BID (7 to <14 kg) x 24 wk	IVA PK: similar to studies of children aged 2 to <6 y Safety: No cataracts; 1 of 17 subjects (6%) had ALT >3x to ≤5x ULN	$\Delta[Cl_{sw}]$: −55.7 mmol[b] (24 wk)[l] Δweight-for-age z-score: 0.2 (24 wk)[l]

Abbreviations: $[Cl_{sw}]$, sweat chloride concentration; ALT, alanine aminotransferase; AST, aspartate aminotransferase; AUC, area under the curve; BID, twice daily; BMI, body mass index; CFQ-R RDS, CF Questionnaire-Revised Respiratory Domain Score; C_{min}, minimum plasma IVA concentration; PK, pharmacokinetics; ppFEV1, percent-predicted forced expiratory volume in 1 second; ULN, upper limit of normal.

a Years except when otherwise indicated.
b $P <.05$.
c $p<.01$.
d <0.001.
e Median within-subject difference from baseline.
f Mean difference from baseline between IVA- and placebo-treated cohorts.
g STRIVE participants.
h ENVISION participants.
i Study VX11 to 770 to 110 (R117H-CFTR).
j Study VX12 to 770 to 111 (non-G551D gating).
k Study VX12 to 770 to 113 (n-of-1 residual function).
l Mean within-subject difference from baseline.
m Mean absolute change from KIWI study baseline.

seen at week 24. On average, IVA-treated subjects gained 2.7 kg after 48 weeks of treatment.

The incidence of AEs was similar between IVA- and placebo-treated groups, but those that prompted treatment interruption occurred more frequently in the IVA-treated group (13% vs 6%). The SAE rate, most commonly PEXs, was lower in the IVA-treated group than in the placebo-treated group (24% vs 42%). The frequency of abnormal LFTs was similar between IVA- and placebo-treated groups.

An open-label extension (OLE) study called PERSIST[10] examined the long-term safety and efficacy of IVA in 144 adults and adolescents from the STRIVE trial.[6] After 144 weeks of IVA, the mean absolute increase in ppFEV$_1$ and body weight was 9.4% and 4.1 kg, respectively. Adolescents and adults who received open-label IVA during PERSIST had a lower PEX rate than adolescents and adults who received placebo during the controlled trial.[6] The most common adverse events (AEs) during long-term IVA use were PEX, cough, and upper respiratory tract infection (URTI). The incidence and severity of abnormal liver function tests (LFTs) were low. IVA was rarely discontinued.

REAL-WORLD OBSERVATIONAL STUDIES OF IVACAFTOR IN ADULTS AND ADOLESCENTS WITH CYSTIC FIBROSIS

Given that more than a decade has passed as IVA was first approved for use in pwCF, multiple reports of long-term treatment benefits have been published (**Table 2**). Here, we review selected broader studies. The BRIO study[11] conducted at 35 French CF centers enrolled 129 IVA users, 59% of whom were less than 18 years old and 64% of whom had a G551D-CFTR allele. Mean age and ppFEV$_1$ at IVA initiation were 19.1 years and 75.2%, respectively. BRIO authors accounted for variability in the duration of IVA treatment before enrollment and compared event rates during the 12-month period before and after IVA initiation. Lung function and body mass index (BMI) increased significantly within 6 to 12 months, and health care utilization rates were roughly halved (see **Table 2**). SAEs, most of which were PEXs, occurred in 19.4% of BRIO subjects, similar to the proportion of IVA-treated subjects who had SAEs during the STRIVE trial (24%).[6]

Volkova and colleagues[12] examined disease progression in IVA-treated pwCF using data from the US and UK registries (see **Table 2**). For each of 5 years in the US registry and 4 years in the UK registry, these authors identified cohorts that

matched 5:1 with IVA users by sex, age, and disease severity determined by CFTR genotype class. The magnitude of improvement in ppFEV$_1$ and BMI and reduction in PEX risk was similar between US and UK registries. In both registries, the prevalence of CF-related diabetes and *Pseudomonas aeruginosa* infection also decreased over time in IVA-treated cohorts. Sawicki and colleagues[13] showed that the rate of lung function decline in a cohort of 189 G551D-CFTR IVA users was nearly half as slow as that of a propensity-score matched cohort of 886 F508del-CFTR pwCF for whom CFTR modulators were not yet available, suggesting that IVA favorably modified disease progression.

Two reports from CF Foundation Therapeutics Development Network investigators provided important knowledge about the clinical mechanism and durability of health improvements associated with IVA therapy in pwCF and a G551D-CFTR mutation (see **Table 2**). The G551D Observational Study (GOAL) study[14] followed 151 IVA users ≥6 years old from their pretreatment baseline to 6 months after IVA initiation. In this cohort, ppFEV$_1$ and health-related quality of life (HRQoL) increased and sweat chloride concentrations and health care utilization declined to an extent seen in clinical trials. Additionally, IVA use was associated with increased mucociliary clearance and intestinal pH, decreased sinus and nasal symptoms, and decreased prevalence of *P aeruginosa* infection.

The G551D observational study – expanded to additional genotypes and extended for long-term follow up (GOAL-e2)[15] reported data from 5.5 years of follow-up on 78 IVA-treated pwCF (81% of original cohort). In GOAL-e2, sustained improvements in ppFEV$_1$ and CF Questionnaire-Revised Respiratory Domain Score (CFQ-R RDS), an instrument used to describe HRQoL in pwCF,[16] were only noted for adults. Sustained increases in BMI and reductions in sweat chloride concentrations were noted in children and adults (see **Table 2**). Contrasting observations were made in a cohort of 80 pwCF aged 6 to 56 years who were registered with the CF Registry of Ireland and had 36 months of pre- and post-IVA treatment data. In that study, Kirwan and colleagues[17] found that after initial acute IVA-related improvements in ppFEV$_1$, in the 3 years subsequently, ppFEV$_1$ improved by 2.26% per year for pwCF aged younger than 12 years, remained unchanged for those 12 to less than 18 year old, and declined in adults by 1.74% per year. BMI increased in IVA-treated adults by 0.28 kg/m^2, but BMI z-score was not significantly increased in children.

Table 2
Summary of selected real-world observational studies of pwCF treated with IVA

Study	Age (Years)	Subjects (n)	Country	Duration (Months)	Outcome Measure
Hubert et al,[11] 2021(BRIO)	≥18	129	France	24	ΔppFEV$_1$: +8.49%[a] (by 6 mo) [d] ΔBMI: +1.01 kg/m^2 [a] (by 12 mo) [d] Rate ratio for PEX: 0.57[a] (±12 mo of initiation) [e] Rate ratio for all hospitalizations: 0.48[a] (±12 mo of initiation) [e] Rate ratio for antibiotic courses per person-year: 0.55[a] (±12 mo of initiation) [e]
Volkova et al,[12] 2020 (Registry)	≥6	635 (US) 247 (UK)	US UK	60 (US) 48 (UK)	ΔppFEV$_1$: +7.6%[a] (US) [f] ΔppFEV$_1$: +9.2%[a] (UK) [f] ΔBMI: +0.8 kg/m^2 [a] (US) [f] ΔBMI: +0.9 kg/m^2 [a] (UK) [f] Relative risk of PEX: 0.58[a] (US) [f] Relative risk of PEX: 0.57[a] (UK) [f]
Rowe et al,[14] 2014(GOAL)	≥6	133	US	6	ΔppFEV$_1$: +6.7%[c, d] ΔBMI: +0.8 kg/m^2 [c, d] Δ[Cl$_{sw}$]: −53.8 mmol[c, d] ΔCFQ-R RDS: +7.4 points[c, d] ΔCFRSD: −9.0 points[c, d] ΔSNOT-20: −0.2 points[c, d] ΔIntestinal pH: +1.46 points[c, d] ΔMCC: >100% increase[c, d]
Guimbellot et al,[15] 2021 (GOAL-e2)	≥6	78	US	66	ΔppFEV$_1$: −2.0% (<18 year old) [d] ΔppFEV$_1$: +4.3%[a] (≥18 year old) [d] ΔBMI: +3.6 kg/m^2 [c] (<18 year old) [d] ΔBMI: +1.2 kg/m^2 [b] (≥18 year old) [d] ΔCFQ-R RDS: +3.9 points (<18 year old) [d] ΔCFQ-R RDS: +10.5 points[b] (≥18 year old) [d] Δ[Cl$_{sw}$]: −47.3 mmol[c] (<18 year old) [d] Δ[Cl$_{sw}$]: −52.4 mmol[c] (≥18 year old) [d]

Abbreviations: BMI, body mass index; CFQ-R RDS, CF Questionnaire-Revised Respiratory Domain Score; CFRSD, CF respiratory symptom diary; MCC, mucociliary clearance; ppFEV$_1$, percent-predicted forced expiratory volume in 1 second; SNOT-20, 20-item Sino-Nasal Outcome Score.

[a] $P < .05$.
[b] $p < .01$.
[c] < 0.001.
[d] Mean difference from baseline within-subjects.
[e] Adjusted for treatment duration and continuous baseline ppFEV$_1$.
[f] Mean difference between IVA-treated cohort and comparators matched 5:1 by sex, age, and disease severity assessed by CFTR genotype.

SUMMARY OF CONTROLLED TRIALS OF ELEXACAFTOR, TEZACAFTOR, AND IVACAFTOR IN ADULTS AND ADOLESCENTS WITH CYSTIC FIBROSIS

Like IVA, ELX, and TEZ are CFTR modulators identified by high-throughput screening,[18] but each has different mechanisms of action. ELX and TEZ correct CFTR function by facilitating intracellular CFTR maturation and promoting stability in the epithelial plasma membrane.[19] The triple combination ETI is currently approved for use in the US by pwCF ≥6 years old (in Europe ≥12 year old) with at least one copy of the F508del-CFTR mutation,[20–22] and in the US, those with an in vitro ETI-responsive non-F508del-CFTR mutation.[23]

TEZ-IVA was approved by the US Food and Drug Administration in February 2018 for pwCF ≥12 years of age with 2 copies of the F508del-CFTR mutation (hereafter, F/F)[24] or one copy of F508del-CFTR and a class IV–V residual function mutation (hereafter, F/RF)[25] and was considered the standard of care (SOC) at the time of the pivotal randomized phase 3 trial of ETI in the F/F population.[21] Thus, TEZ-IVA was included as an active comparator in the study. The VX17 to 445 to 103 study[21] enrolled F/F individuals in stable health who were ≥12 years of age with baseline ppFEV$_1$ 40% to 90%. After a 4-week run-in period of treatment with TEZ 100 mg daily and IVA 150 mg BID, 52 subjects were randomized 1:1 to continue this treatment, and 55 subjects were randomized to receive ELX 200 mg daily, TEZ 100 mg daily, and IVA 150 mg BID for 4 weeks.

Key findings of the VX17 to 445 to 103 study[21] are presented in **Table 3**. Compared with TEZ-IVA, ETI treatment in F/F individuals was associated with statistically and clinically significant improvements in lung function and HRQoL and a marked reduction in sweat chloride, attesting to further treatment-associated enhancement of CFTR function. Similar biomarker and clinical results were seen in individuals heterozygous for the F508del-CFTR mutation and a minimal function mutation [1 that results in no protein function/one that is unresponsive in vitro to ETI (F/MF)] who were treated with ETI in the VX17 to 445 to 102 placebo-controlled study[20] (see **Table 3**).

Although the original US FDA approval of ETI allowed use in anyone with at least one copy of F508del-CFTR regardless of the second mutation,[23] it was expected that a study would be completed in those heterozygous for F508del-CFTR and a gating or RF mutation. As in the case of those homozygous for F508del-CFTR, TEZ-IVA was SOC in the US at the time, meaning a placebo-controlled trial could not be conducted ethically. Barry and colleagues[26] conducted an 8-week study evaluating the use of ETI versus TEZ-IVA in pwCF ≥12 years of age who were heterozygous for F508del-CFTR and a gating or RF mutation (see **Table 3**). After 8 weeks of therapy, ETI use conferred an additional 3.5% improvement in ppFEV$_1$ over TEZ-IVA or IVA alone. Moreover, there were improvements in CFTR function, as evidenced by a decrease in sweat chloride concentration (−23.1 mmol/L vs active control) and improvement in the CFQ-R RSD (+8.7 points vs active control). These observations supported the use of ETI in pwCF carrying ≥1 copy of the F508del-CFTR mutation, regardless of the mutation on the second allele.

REAL-WORLD OBSERVATIONAL STUDIES OF ELEXACAFTOR, TEZACAFTOR, AND IVACAFTOR IN ADULTS AND ADOLESCENTS WITH CYSTIC FIBROSIS

As in the case of IVA, phase 3 trials of ETI provided the data necessary for approval of ETI.[20–22,26] However, prospective and retrospective studies are providing data in larger groups including those excluded from pivotal trials, providing additional safety and tolerability data as well as data on outcomes not measured in those trials (**Table 4**). For example, pwCF with advanced lung disease (ALD), defined in part by ppFEV$_1$ less than 40%,[27] were not included in phase 3 trials. Investigators have subsequently shown that even in those with ALD, treatment with ETI improved lung function, BMI, and HRQoL[28,29] and in some cases delayed referral for lung transplant evaluation.[30] Another population excluded from phase 3 clinical trials was pregnant pwCF. Although animal reproduction models revealed no untoward effects of ETI administration on fetal development at normal human doses, there is a paucity of data on humans. Taylor-Cousar and Jain[31] surveyed CF care providers regarding pwCF who used ETI during all or part of pregnancy and/or lactation. In their study, the miscarriage rate was lower than that of the general US population, and no alarming safety signals were apparent. A prospective, observational, multicenter study to evaluate Maternal and Fetal Outcomes in the Era of Modulators (MAYFLOWERS) is ongoing (NCT04828382). Furthermore, although in vitro data permitted expansion of approval for ETI to those with ETI-responsive mutations without a copy of F508del-CFTR, clinical trials in this group were not performed. Finally, although Black, Indigenous, and people of color (BIPOC) with CF were not excluded from clinical trials, representation was quite low compared

Table 3
Summary of clinical trials evaluating the safety and efficacy of ETI in pwCF

Study	Phase	Age (Years)	Treatment	Primary Outcome Measure	Secondary Endpoints
Heijerman et al,[21] 2019 (F/F)	3	≥12	ELX 200 mg daily + TEZ 100 mg daily + IVA 150 mg BID vs TEZ 100 mg daily + IVA 150 mg BID	ΔppFEV$_1$: +10.0%[c,d,e] (4 wk)[f]	ΔCFQ-R RDS: +17.4 points[c] (4 wk)[f]; Δ[Cl$_{sw}$]: −45.1 mmol[c] (4 wk)[f]
Middleton et al,[20] 2019 (F/MF)	3	≥12	ELX 200 mg daily + TEZ 100 mg daily + IVA 150 mg BID vs placebo	ΔppFEV$_1$: +13.8%[c] (4 wk)[g]	ΔppFEV$_1$: +14.3%[c] (24 wk)[g]; ΔCFQ-R RDS: +20.2 points[c] (24 wk)[g]; Δ[Cl$_{sw}$]: −41.8 mmol[c] (24 wk)[g]; ΔBMI: +1.04 kg/m^2 [c] (24 wk)[g]; ΔPEX event rate: 0.37[c] (24 wk)[g]
Griese et al,[69] 2021 (OLE)	3	≥12	ELX 200 mg daily + TEZ 100 mg daily + IVA 150 mg BID	ΔppFEV$_1$: +12.8%[a,b] (36 wk)[h]; ΔppFEV$_1$: +11.9%[a] (36 wk)[i]; ΔppFEV$_1$: +14.9%[a] (24 wk)[j]; ΔppFEV$_1$: +14.3%[a] (24 wk)[k]	ΔCFQ-R RDS: +13.8 points[a] (24 wk)[h]; ΔCFQ-R RDS: +14.3 points[a] (24 wk)[i]; ΔCFQ-R RDS: +19.2 points[a] (24 wk)[j]; ΔCFQ-R RDS: +20.1 points[a] (24 wk)[k]; Δ[Cl$_{sw}$]: −49.4 mmol[a] (24 wk)[h]; Δ[Cl$_{sw}$]: −47.2 mmol[a] (24 wk)[i]; Δ[Cl$_{sw}$]: −49.0 mmol[a] (24 wk)[j]; Δ[Cl$_{sw}$]: −50.3 mmol[a] (24 wk)[k]; ΔBMI: +1.18 kg/m^{2a} (36 wk)[h]; ΔBMI: +1.30 kg/m^{2a} (36 wk)[i]; ΔBMI: +1.21 kg/m^{2a} (24 wk)[j]; ΔBMI: +1.28 kg/m^{2a} (24 wk)[k]
Zemanick et al,[22] 2021	3	6–11	ELX 100 mg daily (<30 kg) or ELX 200 mg daily (≥30 kg) + TEZ 50 mg daily (<30 kg) or TEZ 100 mg daily (≥30 kg) + IVA 75 mg BID (<30 kg) or IVA 150 mg BID (≥30 kg)	IVA PK: 30 kg was the optimal weight for transition from 50% to 100% of the daily adult dose; Safety: Incidence of abnormal LFTs similar to other studies[20]. 16 of 66 subjects (24.2%) had rash events	ΔppFEV$_1$: +10.2%[c] (24 wk)[l]; ΔCFQ-R RDS: +7.0 points[c] (24 wk)[l]; Δ[Cl$_{sw}$]: −60.9 mmol[c] (24 wk)[l,i]; ΔLCl$_{2.5}$: −1.71[c] (24 wk)[l]

| Barry et al,[26] 2021 | 3 | ≥12 | ELX 200 mg daily + TEZ 100 mg daily + IVA 150 mg BID or TEZ 100 mg daily + TEZ 100 mg daily + IVA 150 mg BID or IVA 150 mg BID | ΔppFEV$_1$: +3.7% (8 wk)[m] | ΔppFEV$_1$: +3.5% (8 wk)[n] |

Abbreviations: [Cl$_{sw}$], sweat chloride concentration; BID, twice daily; BMI, body mass index; CFQ-R RDS, CF Questionnaire-Revised Respiratory Domain Score; ELX, elexacaftor; F/F, *F508del*-CFTR homozygotes; F/MF, *F508del*-CFTR/minimal function mutation; IVA, ivacaftor; LCI$_{2.5}$, lung clearance index; LSM, least-squares mean; ppFEV$_1$, percent-predicted forced expiratory volume in 1 second; TEZ, tezacaftor.

[a] $P < .05$.
[b] $P < .01$.
[c] $< .001$.
[d] LSM difference from baseline in F/F cohort treated with ELX 200 mg daily.
[e] LSM difference from baseline in F/MF cohort treated with ELX 200 mg daily.
[f] LSM difference between ETI- and TEZ-IVA-treated cohorts.
[g] LSM difference from baseline between ETI- and placebo-treated cohorts.
[h] LSM difference from baseline in TEZ/IVA cohort in F/F trial.
[i] LSM difference from baseline in ETI cohort in F/F trial.
[j] LSM difference from baseline in the placebo-treated cohort in F/MF trial.
[k] LSM difference from baseline in ETI-treated cohort in F/MF trial.
[l] LSM difference from baseline.
[m] LSM difference in ETI-treated cohort.
[n] LSM difference versus active control.

Table 4
Summary of selected real-world observational studies of pwCF treated with ETI

Study	Age (Years) [a]	Subjects (n)	Country	Duration [i]	Outcome Measure
Burgel et al,[11] 2021 (ALD cohort)	≥12	245	France	3	ΔppFEV$_1$: +15.1%[g] Δbody weight: +4.2 kg[g] 46% reduction in the proportion of ETI-treated subjects on oxygen[g] 45% reduction in the proportion of ETI-treated subjects on enteral tube feeding[g] 29% reduction in the proportion of ETI-treated subjects on noninvasive ventilation[g]
Taylor-Cousar and Jain,[31] 2021	21–41	45	US	3 [b]	First trimester miscarriages in 6/45 ETI-exposed pregnancies (8.9%) Pregnancy complications (n = 28) in 21 women deemed unrelated to ETI 26 infants exposed to ETI through breastfeeding had no complications
Safirstein et al,[36] 2021	26–40	7	US	−1 d to 27 d [c]	Seven cases of biliary colic developing in association with ETI initiation Days on ETI before symptoms (range): −1 to 27 Four out of 7 cases had a history of asymptomatic cholelithiasis on CT scan Six out of 7 cases required operative intervention
Rotolo et al,[35] 2020	17–39	7	US	2–12 d [c]	Seven men developed testicular discomfort within 2-wk of ETI initiation Testicular physical examination unremarkable in 5/7 cases (71%) OTC analgesics or no specific treatment in 6/7 cases (86%) Pain resolved in all cases within 3 wk irrespective of treatment
O'Connor et al,[37] 2021	22–37	14	US	8 wk [d,e,f]	pwCF became pregnant within 8 wk of starting ETI 7 pwCF reported that they were not attempting to conceive 4 pwCF reported a history of infertility

(continued on next page)

Study	Age (Years) [a]	Subjects (n)	Country	Duration [i]	Outcome Measure
Table 4 *(continued)*					
Beswick et al,[38] 2021	≥18	25	US	6	% sinus opacification (by quantitative CT scan) %SO improved by mean 22.9% after 6 mo[g] Mean SNOT-22 scores improved by 15.3 points [h] Health utility improved by 0.068 [6.8%] [h]

Abbreviations: ALD, advanced lung disease; OTC, over-the-counter; SNOT-22, 22-item Sino-Nasal Outcome Test.

[a] For retrospective studies, the age of participants included is shown; for prospective studies, age inclusion criteria are shown.

[b] Median duration of ETI use before pregnancy.

[c] Range for the duration of ETI exposure before events.

[d] Median time to conception while taking ETI.

[e] $P < .05$.

[f] $P < .01$.

[g] $p < .001$.

[h] $P < .007$.

[i] Months unless otherwise indicated.

with the prevalence of CF in these communities.[32,33] Thus, our understanding of the impact of ETI in people with variable genetic ancestry is limited.

Safety and tolerability are assessed in all phases of clinical trials. However, the number of people exposed during a trial is relatively limited compared with the entirety of the treated population. In clinical trials of ETI, the most common side effects associated with the drug were headache, URTI, abdominal pain, rash, and abnormal LFTs.[20–22,26] Very few participants discontinued therapy because of side effects. Sponsors are required to continue to collect data on safety after approval, and some of this data is used to change prescribing information, such as the recent change recommending against the use of ETI in people with end-stage liver disease based on the requirement of liver transplant in one patient.[34]

Retrospective data collection can also inform providers of side effects not observed during trials or formal real-world studies. As an example, Rotolo and colleagues[35] reported on 7 men with CF who experienced testicular pain following the initiation of ETI. Saferstein and colleagues[36] described 7 cases of pwCF who experienced biliary colic, 6 of which required surgery. Finally, O'Connor and colleagues[37] reported that 14 women with CF became pregnant after an average of 8 weeks of starting ETI. Only half of these women had previously been trying to conceive, supporting previous literature suggesting that HEMT likely increases fertility in women with CF.

Prospective observational studies often provide data on outcomes not measured in trials as well as longer-term data. Beswick and colleagues[38] sought to determine whether ETI treatment improved objective and subjective measures of a common CF complication, chronic sinus disease. Investigators studied 25 adults with CF who received 6 months of ETI prescribed by their care team. Before and after 6 months of ETI, participants underwent sinus computed tomography (CT) scans to which software was applied to quantitatively measure sinus opacification. Participants completed surveys assessing sinus-specific HRQoL and measures of work/school productivity. Statistically and clinically significant improvements following treatment were demonstrated in sinus opacification, HRQoL, and productivity, showing that ETI improved measures beyond those studied in the phase 3 trials. Similarly, investigators leading the PROMISE study, a postapproval evaluation of the efficacy of ETI in pwCF ≥12 years of age with at least one copy of *F508del*-CFTR, demonstrated that 6 months of therapy with ETI improved sweat chloride, ppFEV$_1$, BMI, and HRQOL in the real-world,[39] similar to its effects during phase 3 clinical trials. Both PROMISE and a comparable study being conducted in Ireland and the UK in children and adults, RECOVER, will generate detailed information regarding the impact of ETI on microbiology, airway inflammation, chest CT pathology, lung clearance index (LCI), glucose metabolism, and growth velocity, among others. (PROMISE, NCT04038047; RECOVER, NCT04602468)

The sequential introduction of newer generations of CFTR modulator drugs into clinical practice has followed a similar pathway, starting with the evaluation and approval of compounds in children aged ≥12 years (as part of licensing trials in adults and adolescents), followed by trials in children aged 6 to 11 years, children aged 2 to 5 years, and subsequently children between birth and 2 years of age. In the following sections, we will review the outcomes of HEMT in children up to 11 years of age.

STUDYING CYSTIC FIBROSIS TRANSMEMBRANE CONDUCTANCE REGULATOR MODULATORS IN YOUNG CHILDREN AND INFANTS WITH CYSTIC FIBROSIS

Studies in young children, whether interventional or observational, pose ethical and design challenges that may differ from those in older pwCF. Once efficacy has been demonstrated in older groups, some would question the need for and ethics of a placebo group for pediatric trials; this concern has led to some studies being single-arm and open-label, particularly in the youngest cohorts. While providing reassurance for parents that their child is not "missing out" or undergoing unpleasant tests such as blood sampling with no chance of benefit, there may be a lost opportunity in terms of AE assessment. For example, there is a paucity of data on fluctuations in liver function tests as they are not normally assessed frequently, which makes determining the causality of changes observed with drugs more complex. In terms of efficacy, there is a recognition that standard lung function testing by spirometry may be insufficiently sensitive in this relatively healthy population; the use of LCI is increasing, as is, in very young children, a focus on CFTR modulator pharmacokinetics (PK) and the pharmacodynamic (PD) biomarker of sweat chloride in lieu of clinical efficacy outcomes. Later in discussion, we review the data from trials and observational studies in children under the age of 12 and infants and consider further the challenges of studying these age groups.

SUMMARY OF CONTROLLED TRIALS OF IVACAFTOR IN YOUNG CHILDREN WITH CYSTIC FIBROSIS

Following approval in children more than 12 years of age, the placebo-controlled RCT of IVA in children aged 6 to 11 years with the *G551D*-CFTR

mutation[40] demonstrated improvements in ppFEV$_1$ (+12.5%), weight (+2.8 kg), BMI z-score (+0.45) and sweat chloride (−53.5 mmol/L) over 48 weeks compared with placebo (see **Table 1**). The results were comparable to the older cohort despite the milder disease present in this younger population. The incidence of AEs was similar between the groups.[40] Similar findings were confirmed in children greater than 6 years old with non-*G551D* gating mutations.[7]

Bsed on these reproducible efficacy data in children 6 years and above, the subsequent clinical trial was designed as a single-arm open-label study in children aged 2 to 5 years with CF and CFTR gating mutations with safety, PK, and PD properties as primary endpoints[41] (see **Table 1**). The safety profile was similar to that seen in older children with CF. Similar improvements from baseline were seen in this age group in sweat chloride and BMI z-score over 24 weeks of IVA treatment. Two exploratory endpoints relating to pancreatic function were, however, some of the most noteworthy findings of this study. IVA was associated with significant changes from baseline in fecal elastase (increase of 99.8 mcg/ml) and immunoreactive trypsinogen (IRT) (reduction of 20.7 ng/ml), suggesting a positive impact on exocrine pancreatic function. Of particular interest was the fact that 23% of children who were pancreatic insufficient at baseline had evidence of pancreatic sufficiency (fecal elastase >200 mcg/g) at 24 weeks. An OLE study to this trial[42] (see **Table 1**) found no changes to the AE profile and confirmed the maintenance of improvements in sweat chloride, fecal elastase, IRT, and BMI at 84 weeks compared with the parent study baseline. By 84 weeks, 35% of children starting the parent study with pancreatic insufficiency had fecal elastase levels greater than 200 mcg/g.

Following on from this study, a trial of IVA in 3 sequential, decreasing age groups of infants with CF and gating mutations was launched: 12 to 24 months, 4 to 12 months, and subsequently children from 1 to 4 months (see **Table 1**). In all 3 cohorts, the primary endpoints were safety, PK, and PD properties. In the first cohort,[43] IVA was found to be safe and effective in 19 children aged 12 to 24 months, and again demonstrated improvements from baseline in sweat chloride, fecal elastase, IRT, and weight z-score. Sustained reductions in levels of amylase and lipase, performed as part of the safety assessment, were seen, reinforcing the idea that early use of IVA could rescue, at least temporarily, pancreatic dysfunction in young children with CF. In the second cohort of children aged 4 to 12 months,[44] safety was consistent with IVA use in older children[43] and again demonstrated similar improvements in sweat chloride, weight z-score, fecal elastase, IRT, amylase, and lipase. The trial in children from 1 to 4 months is ongoing at the time of writing of this article.

REAL-WORLD OBSERVATIONAL STUDIES OF IVACAFTOR IN YOUNG CHILDREN WITH CYSTIC FIBROSIS

Improvements in sweat chloride, pulmonary function, and nutritional indices have been confirmed in children aged 6 to 11 in real-world data.[11,14,17,45,46] However, LCI is a more sensitive marker of early CF lung disease than spirometry and can be performed in younger children. IVA is associated with improvements in LCI in children aged 6 to 11 years[47] and children aged 2 to 5 years.[48] Despite improvements in sweat chloride and lung function, improvements in lower airway infection and inflammation were not found in a study of preschool children on IVA.[49]

A number of small studies reporting individual cases or case series have confirmed real-world improvements in pancreatic exocrine function in children using IVA,[50–56] and in some cases successful discontinuation of enzyme replacement therapy, although this improvement may not always be permanent.[56] Although data on this topic are sparse, findings from these studies suggest that factors associated with the restoration of pancreatic function include younger age and milder CFTR dysfunction at baseline.

SUMMARY OF CONTROLLED CLINICAL TRIALS OF ELEXACAFTOR, TEZACAFTOR, AND IVACAFTOR IN YOUNG CHILDREN WITH CYSTIC FIBROSIS

In the first clinical trial of ETI in children aged 6 to 11 years,[22] F/F subjects and those heterozygous for *F508del*-CFTR and a minimum function mutation were included in an open-label study design (see **Table 3**). After a washout period of 28 days before the first study drug dosing, the trial lasted for 24 weeks. The safety and PK of ETI were consistent with the results from the previous trial. Improvements over baseline, similar in magnitude to the previous study,[20] were seen for pulmonary function, sweat chloride, HRQoL, and nutritional outcomes. An improvement from baseline in LCI of 1.7 units was seen in the trial participants. Of interest in this study was the overall magnitude of the sweat chloride improvement (−60.9 mmol/L), particularly in those homozygous for *F508del*-CFTR (−70.4 mmol/L), in whom 100% had a sweat chloride measurement less than 60 mmol/L and

42.9% had a sweat chloride measurement less than 30 mmol/L at 24 weeks—a level typically seen in asymptomatic carriers.[57] A double-blind controlled trial of ETI in this age group has recently been completed (NCT04353817), although at the time of writing, data have not yet been published. An open-label study in 2 to 5 year olds has recently commenced (NCT04537793).

REAL-WORLD OBSERVATIONAL STUDIES OF ELEXACAFTOR, TEZACAFTOR, AND IVACAFTOR IN YOUNG CHILDREN WITH CYSTIC FIBROSIS

With the approval of ETI for clinical use in children aged 6 to 11 only occurring in June 2021 in the US and still awaited in Europe, at the time of writing, published real-world data in this age group are lacking. A number of ongoing studies will be collecting this real-world data as children commence on ETI clinically, including the PROMISE Pediatric Study (NCT04613128), BEGIN (NCT040509050), and RECOVER (NCT04602468).

BROADER CONSIDERATIONS PROMPTED BY CYSTIC FIBROSIS TRANSMEMBRANE CONDUCTANCE REGULATOR MODULATOR TRIAL RESULTS
Challenges to Evaluating Clinical Trial Outcomes in Younger Children with Cystic Fibrosis

Outcomes in children have been improving steadily over the last 20 years to the point that lung function in teenagers in most cases is close to the normal range.[58] This improvement is a positive consequence of many different factors, even before the introduction of CFTR modulators. However, this development poses a challenge when considering the conduct of clinical trials for new CFTR modulators, given that individuals with the worse disease are likely to have a more obvious short-term benefit in a clinical trial. Therefore, clinical trials of CFTR modulators have tended to exclude groups of children with milder lung disease. This approach is likely to further skew selection for clinical trials and lead to a selection bias.

Regulatory approval for CFTR modulator trials tends to include the presumption that the efficacy demonstrated in older pwCF can be extrapolated to some extent to younger pwCF. Thus, CFTR modulator trials in children with CF increasingly focus on safety and PK; in CF there is the added benefit of the useful PD assessment of sweat chloride concentration. The focus on safety and use of an effective biomarker allows the enrollment of smaller numbers of young children and babies in

CFTR modulator trials and make efficacy measures secondary in such trial designs. Taken together, these factors mean that the volume of efficacy data in young children is significantly less than in older children and adults, underlining the importance of the collection of registry and real-world data.

Importance of Mixed Sources of Outcome Data

Although data from controlled trials are essential to conclusively demonstrate that new CFTR modulators are safe and clinically effective, to ultimately understand outcomes and impact of relevance to people with CF, we cannot rely on data from clinical trials alone. There are several important reasons for this: First, trials will select endpoints that meet regulatory approval and are easily measurable in trial settings, and although some might include exploratory endpoints, the more likely treatments are to meet primary outcomes, the less they drive to select potentially useful secondary or exploratory outcomes. These outcomes may not be the primary concern, or reflect all of the concerns, of people living with CF. Secondly, trial participants are likely to have less complex disease and have greater motivation and adherence to therapies, something that the process of being in a trial may well further encourage. Finally, real-world studies can produce data over longer durations and in settings that reflect the reality of the people in whose outcomes we are ultimately interested.

Variable Clinical Responses to Highly Effective Modulator Therapy

Considerable variability can be seen in individual ppFEV$_1$ responses in clinical trials of HEMT. This variability may be influenced by the severity of baseline lung disease, frequency of exacerbations, and adherence to conventional treatments. There are in vitro data showing a blunting of the chloride secretory response to LUM and LUM-IVA by P aeruginosa,[59] although, to date, there is little evidence to support this being a clinical issue. Second-hand tobacco smoke exposure in children was associated not only with the expected (but tragic) lower baseline ppFEV$_1$ but also with a reduced clinical response to TEZ-IVA.[60] However, variability is not only seen in the context of organ disease; indeed, wide differences were seen in individual sweat chloride responses in phase 3 clinical trials of both IVA and ETI. This finding is true within groups with similar mutation types/classes[6,22,43] and with the same compound between different mutation groups.[22] The degree of

variability is significant, with fold-differences seen in some studies between the highest and lowest responders, well outside of the expected natural variability which can affect sweat chloride testing.[61] Although this variability has been noted in trial data, little in the way of systematic insights have been gathered on the reasons for, or consequences of, this finding. Pharmacogenomics is an area of increasing interest, with the potential for impacts on drug absorption and metabolism. Ongoing real-world studies will hopefully address these issues in the case of ETI.

Of interest, particularly to pediatricians, is the apparent increase in the degree of sweat chloride responses to some modulators seen in younger subjects compared with older subjects taking the same compound. **Fig. 2** shows the different sweat chloride responses to both highly effective and dual combination modulators in different age groups. It is important to point out that these were not head-to-head comparisons; the studies were not standardized in terms of PK, included smaller numbers as age decreases, and occurred at different times. Notwithstanding these trial differences, and particularly when looking at compounds used in subjects homozygous for F508del-CFTR, it seems that for each compound, use in younger cohorts has thus far been associated with sequentially improved sweat chloride responses. Time will determine whether this pattern is sustained, and long-term real-world monitoring will be required to determine whether sweat chloride responses in younger people change with the age and duration of modulator used.

Moving Toward an Ethos of "Prevention" Rather than Treatment: a Realistic Goal of Highly Effective Modulator Therapy Initiated Early in Life?

The data presented above begin to raise the question of whether the benefits of starting HEMT early in life, when disease is either not yet apparent or is reversible, could actually be preventative. Any drug commenced in pwCF who already have substantial organ damage is likely, at best, to halt or slow disease progression. Although most infants with CF are born with pancreatic exocrine insufficiency, the fact that function can be restored for some by IVA treatment early in life[41–43] confirms that this damage is not totally irreversible. More favorably, most evidence would suggest that the lungs at birth are largely normal,[62] with subsequent mucus accumulation, infection, and inflammation ensuing over the next months and years.[63] Data from the G551D-CFTR ferret model demonstrate substantial disease prevention with

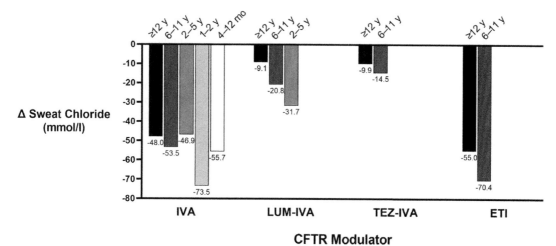

CFTR Modulator

Fig. 2. Summary of sweat chloride changes observed in age-defined cohorts during CFTR modulator clinical trials.

the immediate postnatal administration of IVA.[64] It would seem at least plausible that this could be achieved in humans: early restoration of airway surface liquid volume and pH leading to the normalization of host defenses (mucociliary clearance and pathogen killing) could either extend the period until lung disease commences or even prevent it completely. Non-CF lungs encounter environmental insults constantly—particulate pollutants, bacteria, and viruses—without becoming either inflamed or chronically infected; perhaps CFTR function restored by HEMT could render CF lungs equally well-defended.

Data supporting this hypothesis will likely not arise from clinical trials; indeed, there will need to be many years of monitoring, either in OLE or real-world observational studies, to fully understand this phenomenon. Well-developed patient registries will be of enormous benefit, but could be enhanced to capture additional outcomes. Clinicians will be understandably cautious about prescribing fewer symptom-directed treatments to these children, in part as monitoring is so challenging. Sensitive outcome measures will be needed, for example, LCI and imaging, and surveillance of lower airway infection also requires optimized methods for this group that generally does not expectorate sputum.

The data arising from babies under a year of age receiving IVA are encouraging, both in terms of safety and efficacy. While long-term safety data are undoubtedly required, this would support the cautious trialing of ETI in due course in these very young infants. However, some CF-related organ damage may never be reversed by postnatal CFTR restoration: pancreatic disease in some, likely CBAVD in most men. A question arises increasingly of whether antenatal treatment should

be considered. The same ferret study mentioned earlier did in fact show the preservation of vas deferens patency in G551D-CFTR homozygous but not compound heterozygous male offspring of mothers treated with IVA during pregnancy,[64] confirming the placental passage reported in reproductive animal testing performed as part of labeling requirements.[34,65] Furthermore, a case report[66] describing a negative newborn screen and pancreatic sufficiency in an F/F female infant born to a mother with CF treated with ETI throughout pregnancy demonstrates the potential opportunity to prevent some consequences of CFTR dysfunction. However, there is no precedent of which we are aware for treating a healthy pregnant woman with a systemic drug purely to benefit the fetus. Presuming most of these pregnant women will not have CF, the use of the drug may be prevented by licensing and reimbursement constraints in this context. Outcomes in non-CF infants exposed to these drugs administered to their CF mother *in utero* are, to date, encouraging,[31,67] but very little data are currently available and safety will remain of paramount importance as noted above. Finally, the vast majority of CF newborns are not known to have CF until postnatal presentation or screening, so while this may be an option for parents whose genetic status is already known, for example, from a previous CF child, it is unlikely to be relevant to the majority.

SUMMARY

Data from phase 3 clinical trials and real-world observational studies have demonstrated substantial and sustainable objective and subjective health improvements conferred by HEMT in children and adults. Data from observational and registry studies will continue to guide our understanding of long-term safety and organ function preservation in years to come. Although data from the first HEMT, IVA, have suggested that early life intervention with HEMT might reverse some complications of CF, such as pancreatic insufficiency, considerable further trial, and real-world data will be required to establish this comprehensively for all types of HEMT. As we move forward with the use of HEMT, we must consider not only which outcome measures are most meaningful in a generally healthier population that benefits from highly effective CFTR modulators, but also the etiology of variability in outcomes in genetically and phenotypically similar groups of pwCF. Finally, we must continue to explore the potential risk and health benefits of ETI in populations not originally or adequately enrolled in labeling trials, including pregnant and lactating women, pwCF with ALD, BIPOC with CF, and/or those with ultra-rare mutations.

CLINICS CARE POINTS

- Over the short and intermediate term, oral therapy with HEMT safely improves lung function, nutritional status, and health-related quality of life in most of the people with indicated CFTR mutations.

- Variable clinical responses to HEMT are to be expected even among pwCF with the same CFTR mutation profile.

- Additional research is needed to evaluate the safety and efficacy of HEMT in people with CF who were underrepresented or excluded from clinical trials including those with rare CFTR mutations, pregnant people with CF, and those with advanced lung or liver disease.

- Although the prevalence of drug-induced liver injury in HEMT clinical trials was generally low, liver function tests (LFTs) should be monitored in pwCF taking HEMT.

- Early treatment with HEMT may prevent permanent organ damage in some individuals with CF.

AUTHOR DISCLOSURES

A.H. Gifford has received research grants from the CF Foundation and fees from ImmuNext related to consultation on clinical research design and from Insmed and Grifols related to participation on advisory boards. J.L. Taylor-Cousar has received grants to her institution from the CF Foundation, and from Vertex Pharmaceuticals Incorporated, Gilead, N30, Celtaxsys, Proteostasis, and Bayer; has received fees from Vertex Pharmaceuticals Incorporated related to consultation on clinical research design, participation on advisory boards, and speaking engagements; has received speaking fees from Celtaxsys; and has served on advisory boards and/or provided clinical trial design consultation for Novartis, Genentech, Gilead, Protalix, Santhera, 4DMT, AbbVie, and Proteostasis. She serves on a DMC for AbbVie. She serves as an advisor to the CFF Board of Trustees, and on the CF Foundation's Clinical Research Executive Committee, Clinical Research Advisory Board, and as chair of the CF TDN's Women's Health Research-Working Group, on the scientific advisory board for Emily's Entourage, and on the ATS Scientific Grant Review and Clinical Problems Assembly Programming Committees. J.C. Davies has performed clinical trial leadership roles, educational and/or advisory activities for the following: AbbVie, Algipharma AS, Bayer AG, Boehringer Ingelheim Pharma GmbH & Co. KG, Eloxx, Enterprise, Galapagos NV, ImevaX GmbH, Ionis, Nivalis Therapeutics, Inc., Novartis, ProQR Therapeutics III B.V., Proteostasis Therapeutics, INC., Pulmocide Raptor Pharmaceuticals, Inc, Vertex Pharmaceuticals. P. McNally has received grants from the CF Foundation, CF Ireland, CF Trust, and from Vertex Pharmaceuticals; has received fees from Vertex Pharmaceuticals-related participation on advisory boards and speaking engagements; He has served on a DMC for Gilead.

REFERENCES

1. Keating D, Marigowda G, Burr L, et al. VX-445–Tezacaftor–Ivacaftor in Patients with Cystic Fibrosis and One or Two Phe508del Alleles. N Engl J Med 2018;379(17):1612–20.
2. Graeber SY, Dopfer C, Naehrlich L, et al. Effects of Lumacaftor-Ivacaftor Therapy on Cystic Fibrosis Transmembrane Conductance Regulator Function in Phe508del Homozygous Patients with Cystic Fibrosis. Am J Respir Crit Care Med 2018;197(11):1433–42.
3. Rowe SM, Accurso F, Clancy JP. Detection of cystic fibrosis transmembrane conductance regulator activity in early-phase clinical trials. Proc Am Thorac Soc 2007;4(4):387–98.
4. Hadida S, Van Goor F, Zhou J, et al. Discovery of N-(2,4-Di-tert-butyl-5-hydroxyphenyl)-4-oxo-1,4-dihydroquinoline-3-carboxamide (VX-770, ivacaftor),

a potent and orally Bioavailable CFTR potentiator. J Med Chem 2014;57(23):9776–95.

5. Laselva O, Qureshi Z, Zeng ZW, et al. Identification of binding sites for ivacaftor on the cystic fibrosis transmembrane conductance regulator. iScience 2021;24(6):102542.

6. Ramsey BW, Davies J, McElvaney NG, et al. A CFTR potentiator in patients with cystic fibrosis and the G551D mutation. N Engl J Med 2011;365(18): 1663–72.

7. De Boeck K, Munck A, Walker S, et al. Efficacy and safety of ivacaftor in patients with cystic fibrosis and a non-G551D gating mutation. J Cyst Fibros 2014; 13(6):674–80.

8. Moss RB, Flume PA, Elborn JS, et al. Efficacy and safety of ivacaftor in patients with cystic fibrosis who have an Arg117His-CFTR mutation: a double-blind, randomised controlled trial. Lancet Respir Med 2015;3(7):524–33.

9. Van Goor F, Yu H, Burton B, et al. Effect of ivacaftor on CFTR forms with missense mutations associated with defects in protein processing or function. J Cyst Fibros 2014;13(1):29–36.

10. McKone EF, Borowitz D, Drevinek P, et al. Long-term safety and efficacy of ivacaftor in patients with cystic fibrosis who have the Gly551Asp-CFTR mutation: a phase 3, open-label extension study (PERSIST). Lancet Respir Med 2014;2(11):902–10.

11. Hubert D, Marguet C, Benichou J, et al. Real-world long-term ivacaftor for cystic fibrosis in France: clinical effectiveness and healthcare resource utilization. Pulm Ther 2021. https://doi.org/10.1007/s41030-021-00158-5.

12. Volkova N, Moy K, Evans J, et al. Disease progression in patients with cystic fibrosis treated with ivacaftor: data from national US and UK registries. J Cyst Fibros 2020;19(1):68–79.

13. Sawicki GS, McKone EF, Pasta DJ, et al. Sustained Benefit from ivacaftor demonstrated by combining clinical trial and cystic fibrosis patient registry data. Am J Respir Crit Care Med 2015;192(7):836–42.

14. Rowe SM, Heltshe SL, Gonska T, et al. Clinical mechanism of the cystic fibrosis transmembrane conductance regulator potentiator ivacaftor in G551D-mediated cystic fibrosis. Am J Respir Crit Care Med 2014;190(2):175–84.

15. Guimbellot JS, Baines A, Paynter A, et al. Long term clinical effectiveness of ivacaftor in people with the G551D CFTR mutation. J cystic fibrosis 2021;20(2): 213–9.

16. Quittner AL, Modi AC, Wainwright C, et al. Determination of the minimal clinically important difference scores for the cystic fibrosis questionnaire-revised respiratory symptom scale in two populations of patients with cystic fibrosis and chronic Pseudomonas aeruginosa airway infection. Chest 2009;135(6): 1610–8.

17. Kirwan L, Fletcher G, Harrington M, et al. Longitudinal trends in real-world outcomes after initiation of ivacaftor. A cohort study from the cystic fibrosis registry of Ireland. Ann Am Thorac Soc 2019;16(2): 209–16.

18. Pinto MC, Silva IA, Figueira MF, et al. Pharmacological modulation of ion channels for the treatment of cystic fibrosis. J Exp Pharmacol 2021;13:693–723.

19. Veit G, Roldan A, Hancock MA, et al. Allosteric folding correction of F508del and rare CFTR mutants by elexacaftor-tezacaftor-ivacaftor (Trikafta) combination. JCI Insight 2020;5(18). https://doi.org/10.1172/jci.insight.139983.

20. Middleton PG, Mall MA, Drevinek P, et al. Elexacaftor-Tezacaftor-Ivacaftor for Cystic Fibrosis with a Single Phe508del Allele. N Engl J Med 2019;381(19): 1809–19.

21. Heijerman HGM, McKone EF, Downey DG, et al. Efficacy and safety of the elexacaftor plus tezacaftor plus ivacaftor combination regimen in people with cystic fibrosis homozygous for the F508del mutation: a double-blind, randomised, phase 3 trial. Lancet 2019. https://doi.org/10.1016/S0140-6736(19)32597-8.

22. Zemanick ET, Taylor-Cousar JL, Davies J, et al. A Phase 3 Open-Label Study of Elexacaftor/Tezacaftor/Ivacaftor in Children 6 through 11 Years of Age with Cystic Fibrosis and at Least One F508del Allele. Am J Respir Crit Care Med 2021;203(12):1522–32.

23. Elexacaftor-tezacaftor-ivacaftor (Trikafta) prescribing information. Vertex Pharmaceuticals, Incorporated; 2019.

24. Taylor-Cousar JL, Munck A, McKone EF, et al. Tezacaftor-Ivacaftor in Patients with Cystic Fibrosis Homozygous for Phe508del. N Engl J Med 2017; 377(21):2013–23.

25. Rowe SM, Daines C, Ringshausen FC, et al. Tezacaftor-ivacaftor in residual-function heterozygotes with cystic fibrosis. N Engl J Med 2017;377(21): 2024–35.

26. Barry PJ, Mall MA, Álvarez A, et al. Triple therapy for cystic fibrosis Phe508del–gating and –residual function genotypes. N Engl J Med 2021;385(9):815–25.

27. Kapnadak SG, Dimango E, Hadjiliadis D, et al. Cystic Fibrosis Foundation consensus guidelines for the care of individuals with advanced cystic fibrosis lung disease. J Cystic Fibrosis 2020;19(3): 344–54.

28. Burgel PR, Durieu I, Chiron R, et al. Rapid improvement after starting elexacaftor-tezacaftor-ivacaftor in patients with cystic fibrosis and advanced pulmonary disease. Am J Respir Crit Care Med 2021; 204(1):64–73.

29. O'Shea KM, O'Carroll OM, Carroll C, et al. Efficacy of elexacaftor/tezacaftor/ivacaftor in patients with cystic fibrosis and advanced lung disease. Eur Respir J 2021;57(2):2003079.

30. Bermingham B, Rueschhoff A, Ratti G, et al. Short-term effect of elexacaftor-tezacaftor-ivacaftor on lung function and transplant planning in cystic fibrosis patients with advanced lung disease. J Cyst Fibros 2021;20(5):768–71.

31. Taylor-Cousar JL, Jain R. Maternal and fetal outcomes following elexacaftor-tezacaftor-ivacaftor use during pregnancy and lactation. J Cyst Fibros 2021;20(3):402–6.

32. McGarry ME. Triple Therapy for Cystic Fibrosis with a Phe508del CFTR Mutation. N Engl J Med 2020; 382(7):684.

33. McGarry M. Transparency and diversity in cystic fibrosis research. Lancet 2020;396(10251):601.

34. Elexacaftor-tezacaftor-ivacaftor (Trikafta) prescribing information. Vertex Pharmaceuticals, Incorporated; 2021.

35. Rotolo SM, Duehlmeyer S, Slack SM, et al. Testicular pain following initiation of elexacaftor/tezacaftor/ivacaftor in males with cystic fibrosis. J Cystic Fibrosis 2020;19(5):e39–41.

36. Safirstein J, Grant JJ, Clausen E, et al. Biliary disease and cholecystectomy after initiation of elexacaftor/ivacaftor/tezacaftor in adults with cystic fibrosis. J Cystic Fibrosis 2021;20(3):506–10.

37. O'Connor KE, Goodwin DL, NeSmith A, et al. Elexacafator/tezacaftor/ivacaftor resolves subfertility in females with CF: a two center case series. J Cyst Fibros 2021;20(3):399–401.

38. Beswick DM, Humphries SM, Balkissoon CD, et al. Impact of CFTR therapy on chronic rhinosinusitis and health status: Deep Learning CT Analysis and patient reported outcomes. Ann Am Thorac Soc 2021. https://doi.org/10.1513/AnnalsATS.202101-057OC.

39. Nichols DP, Paynter AC, Heltshe SL, et al. Clinical effectiveness of elexacaftor/Tezacftor/ivacaftor in people with cystic fibrosis. Am J Respir Crit Care Med 2021. https://doi.org/10.1164/rccm.202108-1986OC.

40. Davies JC, Wainwright CE, Canny GJ, et al. Efficacy and safety of ivacaftor in patients aged 6 to 11 years with cystic fibrosis with a G551D mutation. Am J Respir Crit Care Med 2013;187(11):1219–25.

41. Davies JC, Cunningham S, Harris WT, et al. Safety, pharmacokinetics, and pharmacodynamics of ivacaftor in patients aged 2-5 years with cystic fibrosis and a CFTR gating mutation (KIWI): an open-label, single-arm study. Lancet Respir Med 2016;4(2): 107–15.

42. Rosenfeld M, Cunningham S, Harris WT, et al. An open-label extension study of ivacaftor in children with CF and a CFTR gating mutation initiating treatment at age 2-5years (KLIMB). J cystic fibrosis 2019;18(6):838–43.

43. Rosenfeld M, Wainwright CE, Higgins M, et al. Ivacaftor treatment of cystic fibrosis in children aged 12 to <24 months and with a CFTR gating mutation (ARRIVAL): a phase 3 single-arm study. Lancet Respir Med 2018;6(7):545–53.

44. Davies JC, Wainwright CE, Sawicki GS, et al. Ivacaftor in infants aged 4 to <12 Months with cystic fibrosis and a gating mutation: results of a 2-Part Phase 3 clinical trial. Am J Respir Crit Care Med 2020. https://doi.org/10.1164/rccm.202008-3177OC.

45. Dryden C, Wilkinson J, Young D, et al. The impact of 12 months treatment with ivacaftor on Scottish paediatric patients with cystic fibrosis with the G551D mutation: a review. Arch Dis Child 2018;103(1): 68–70.

46. Stalvey MS, Pace J, Niknian M, et al. Growth in Prepubertal children with cystic fibrosis treated with ivacaftor. Pediatrics 2017;139(2). https://doi.org/10.1542/peds.2016-2522.

47. Davies J, Sheridan H, Bell N, et al. Assessment of clinical response to ivacaftor with lung clearance index in cystic fibrosis patients with a G551D-CFTR mutation and preserved spirometry: a randomised controlled trial. Lancet Respir Med 2013;1(8):630–8.

48. Ratjen F, Klingel M, Black P, et al. Changes in lung clearance index in preschool-aged patients with cystic fibrosis treated with ivacaftor (GOAL): a clinical trial. Am J Respir Crit Care Med 2018;198(4): 526–8.

49. McNally P, Butler D, Karpievitch YV, et al. Ivacaftor and airway inflammation in preschool children with cystic fibrosis. Am J Respir Crit Care Med 2021; 204(5):605–8.

50. Nichols AL, Davies JC, Jones D, et al. Restoration of exocrine pancreatic function in older children with cystic fibrosis on ivacaftor. Paediatr Respir Rev 2020. https://doi.org/10.1016/j.prrv.2020.04.003.

51. Hamilton JL, Zobell JT, Robson J. Pancreatic insufficiency converted to pancreatic sufficiency with ivacaftor. Pediatr Pulmonol 2019;54(11):1654.

52. Megalaa R, Gopalareddy V, Champion E, et al. Time for a gut check: pancreatic sufficiency resulting from CFTR modulator use. Pediatr Pulmonol 2019;54(8): E16–8.

53. Munce D, Lim M, Akong K. Persistent recovery of pancreatic function in patients with cystic fibrosis after ivacaftor. Pediatr Pulmonol 2020;55(12):3381–3.

54. Smith H, Rayment JH. Sustained recovery of exocrine pancreatic function in a teenager with cystic fibrosis treated with ivacaftor. Pediatr Pulmonol 2020;55(10):2493–4.

55. Howlett C, Ronan NJ, NiChroinin M, et al. Partial restoration of pancreatic function in a child with cystic fibrosis. Lancet Respir Med 2016;4(5):e21–2.

56. Hutchinson I, McNally P. Appearance of pancreatic sufficiency and discontinuation of pancreatic enzyme replacement therapy in children with cystic fibrosis on ivacaftor. Ann Am Thorac Soc 2021;18(1): 182–3.

57. Wilschanski M, Dupuis A, Ellis L, et al. Mutations in the cystic fibrosis transmembrane regulator gene and in vivo transepithelial potentials. Am J Respir Crit Care Med 2006;174(7):787–94.

58. Goss CH, MacNeill SJ, Quinton HB, et al. Children and young adults with CF in the USA have better lung function compared with the UK. Thorax 2015; 70(3):229–36.

59. Stanton BA, Coutermarsh B, Barnaby R, et al. Pseudomonas aeruginosa reduces VX-809 stimulated F508del-CFTR chloride secretion by airway epithelial cells. PLoS One 2015;10(5):e0127742.

60. Baker E, Harris WT, Rowe SM, et al. Tobacco smoke exposure limits the therapeutic benefit of tezacaftor/ivacaftor in pediatric patients with cystic fibrosis. J Cyst Fibros 2021;20(4):612–7.

61. Vermeulen F, Le Camus C, Davies JC, et al. Variability of sweat chloride concentration in subjects with cystic fibrosis and G551D mutations. J Cyst Fibros 2017;16(1):36–40.

62. Linnane BM, Hall GL, Nolan G, et al. Lung function in infants with cystic fibrosis Diagnosed by newborn screening. Am J Respir Crit Care Med 2008; 178(12):1238–44.

63. Pillarisetti N, Williamson E, Linnane B, et al. Infection, inflammation, and lung function decline in infants with cystic fibrosis. Am J Respir Crit Care Med 2011;184(1):75–81.

64. Sun X, Yi Y, Yan Z, et al. In Utero and postnatal VX-770 administration rescues multiorgan disease in a ferret model of cystic fibrosis. Sci translational Med 2019;11(485):eaau7531.

65. Ivacaftor (Kalydeco) prescribing information. Vertex Pharmaceuticals; 2020.

66. Fortner CN, Seguin JM, Kay DM. Normal pancreatic function and false-negative CF newborn screen in a child born to a mother taking CFTR modulator therapy during pregnancy. J Cyst Fibros 2021;20(5): 835–6.

67. Nash EF, Middleton PG, Taylor-Cousar JL. Outcomes of pregnancy in women with cystic fibrosis (CF) taking CFTR modulators - an international survey. J Cyst Fibros 2020;19(4):521–6.

68. Pilewski JM, De Boeck K, Nick JA, et al. Long-term ivacaftor in people aged 6 Years and older with cystic fibrosis with ivacaftor-responsive mutations. Pulm Ther 2020;6(2):303–13.

69. Griese M, Costa S, Linnemann RW, et al. Safety and Efficacy of Elexacaftor/Tezacaftor/Ivacaftor for 24 Weeks or Longer in People with Cystic Fibrosis and One or More F508del Alleles: interim Results of an Open-Label Phase 3 Clinical Trial. Am J Respir Crit Care Med 2021;203(3):381–5.

Nontuberculous Mycobacterial Infections in Cystic Fibrosis

Stacey L. Martiniano, MD[a],*, Jerry A. Nick, MD[b,c], Charles L. Daley, MD[b,c]

KEYWORDS

- Cystic fibrosis • Nontuberculous mycobacteria • *Mycobacterium avium* complex
- *Mycobacterium abscessus*

KEY POINTS

- Mycobacterium avium complex (MAC) and Mycobacterium *abscessus* and its subspecies are the most frequently encountered nontuberculous mycobacteria (NTM) respiratory pathogens in people with cystic fibrosis (CF) in most regions.
- Diagnosis of NTM lung disease in people with CF follows international guidelines, with an emphasis on evaluating and treating all known comorbidities.
- Guidelines-based treatment of NTM in people with CF depends on the species, resistance pattern, and extent of disease.
- Optimal management of people with CF and NTM lung disease requires carefully considered treatment of both conditions.

INTRODUCTION

Nontuberculous mycobacteria (NTM) are recognized as important pathogens in the cystic fibrosis (CF) population. While historically CF was considered a fatal disease of childhood, incremental improvements in therapy had gradually improved the expected survival and the median age of the population. Now with the widespread adoption of highly effective modulator treatment (HEMT) the clinical features of CF have abruptly changed, and there are little data regarding the diagnosis and treatment of NTM within this new disease phenotype. This article will review the epidemiology, diagnosis, treatment, and prevention of NTM lung disease in people with CF (pwCF) based on available reports, with the acknowledgment that many aspects of NTM infection may be significantly impacted by the effective restoration of CFTR function.

Epidemiology

The CF population has historically suffered an especially high risk for NTM infection and presents unique challenges with regards to diagnosis, treatment, and prevention.[1] While the NTM isolation rate in the general North American population ranges from 6 to 22 per 100,000 and the NTM disease rate from 5 to 10 per 100,000,[2] there is a 1000-fold greater prevalence of NTM in respiratory cultures from pwCF. The largest available data sets come from the US CF Foundation Patient Registry (CFFPR) and from other national CF registries.[3] Since 2010 the CFFPR has tracked both positive and negative results from participants with NTM cultures, which allows for the calculation of annual prevalence among those tested, and detection of long-term trends. In the decade from 2010 to 2019 there was a significant increase in the percentage of pwCF with one or more NTM

[a] Department of Pediatrics, Children's Hospital Colorado, University of Colorado Denver School of Medicine, 13123 East 16th Avenue, Box B-395, Aurora, CO 80045, USA; [b] Department of Medicine, National Jewish Health, 1400 Jackson Street, Denver, CO 80206, USA; [c] Department of Medicine, University of Colorado Denver School of Medicine, 12631 East 17th Avenue, Box 860, Aurora, CO 80045, USA
* Corresponding author.
E-mail address: Stacey.Martiniano@childrenscolorado.org

Clin Chest Med 43 (2022) 697–716
https://doi.org/10.1016/j.ccm.2022.06.010
0272-5231/22/© 2022 Elsevier Inc. All rights reserved.

positive cultures among those tested each year, as well as an increase in the proportion of participants who were tested (**Fig. 1**). In 2019 the annual prevalence reached 13.9% among the 53% of registry participants tested, excluding those who had undergone lung transplant. Over a 5-year period, 20% of individuals tested have one or more positive NTM culture in the CFFPR.[4,5] This increase in annual prevalence of NTM within the CF population has been reported in a variety of CF cohorts worldwide[6–14] and mirrors trends reported in other forms of obstructive lung disease at risk for NTM infection.[15–18] Factors contributing to this increase in the prevalence of NTM infection likely include improved culture techniques, increased physician awareness, an aging CF population, and climate change favoring NTM survival in the environment.[19,20]

With the increasing use of HEMT in pwCF, there are reports of decreased frequency of pathogens in sputum cultures[21,22] and global shifts in the CF airway microbiome.[23] In many cases it is unclear if these findings represent a true decline in infection, or a reduced sensitivity of cultures,[22,24] and in some longitudinal analysis early declines in pathogen burden or prevalence have generally not been sustained.[25] CFFPR data from 2020 represent the first year of data collection since the 2019 approval of elexacaftor/tezacaftor/ivacaftor (E/T/I) within the US, and a dramatic reduction in the prevalence of one or more NTM sputum cultures among those tested is observed[26] (see **Fig. 1**). A similar decrease in the percentage of positive cultures for NTM following the initiation of HEMT has been reported anecdotally[27] and observed among participants with a history of NTM infection enrolled on the CFF-sponsored PREDICT Trial (NCT0207340).[28] However, it is not known if these findings reflect a reduction in infectious burden and/or prevalence of infection, or rather a decrease in the sensitivity of traditional cultures to detect the presence of NTM infection. In addition, the COVID-19 pandemic disrupted many aspects of care, including the collection of sputum samples, and may have impacted these data.

The overwhelming majority of NTM species detected in pwCF are from either the *M. avium* complex (MAC) or *Mycobacterium abscessus* (MAB).[29] MAC has historically been the most common NTM isolated from respiratory specimens in the continental US and Australia[5,7,30] in contrast to many European countries[8,31–34] and tropical locations[35,36] whereby MAB is the most commonly reported NTM. Other NTM species have been recovered sporadically, including *Mycobacterium kansasii*[37–40] and *Mycobacterium*

fortuitum.[6,39,41–44] *Mycobacterium simiae* and MAB are the most common species isolated in Israel.[13,45] Compared with the US CFFPR other national registries have reported a substantially lower annual prevalence of positive NTM cultures[30,46,47] (**Fig. 2**). The mean annual prevalence of NTM among nontransplanted participants was 4.2% in the 2019 European CF Society Patient Registry (ECFSPR) which included data on more than 50,000 pwCF from 38 countries.[48] A common limitation to registry data is the number of individuals without available NTM cultures, especially among children and healthier adults. The 2019 ECFSPR included cultures from 87% of the nontransplanted population, compared with only 53% in the CFFPR. The high proportion of untested pwCF in the US may contribute to the much higher annual prevalence seen in the CFFPR. There are also dramatic regional differences in NTM prevalence and species predominance. In a 5-year US CFFPR analysis the highest NTM prevalence was detected in Hawaii (50%), followed by Florida and North Dakota (31%). Hawaii had the highest prevalence of MAB (50%) and Nevada had the highest prevalence of MAC (24%).[5] Within a region, various CF centers or specific cohorts (eg, late-diagnosed pwCF) have reported much higher prevalence, reflecting localized variation in both exposure and testing.[49,50]

Population Genomics of Nontuberculous Mycobacteria Worldwide

Over the past decade, a series of reports have used whole-genome sequencing (WGS) of clinical isolates to describe the genetic diversity of NTM within the CF population. A highly similar clone of *M. abscessus* subsp. *massiliense* was identified by WGS in geographically distinct CF and non-CF outbreaks on 3 continents.[51–53] A large-scale population genomics study of MAB isolates from CF Centers in the UK, Europe, Australia, and US confirmed the presence of dominant circulating clones (DCC) of *M. abscessus* subsp. *abscessus* and *M. abscessus* subsp. *massiliense* in all locations sampled.[54] The same DCC have since been identified in several non-US CF isolate cohorts.[55–58] In the US, a population genomics study of more than 550 MAB isolates from CF Centers in 28 states found that over half of CF subjects with *M. abscessus* subsp. *abscessus* had the predominant DCC.[59] The US population included 2 other DCC that were previously observed in other populations, as well as a highly prevalent clone of *M. abscessus* subsp. *massiliense* that is genetically distinct from the "transmissible" clone described

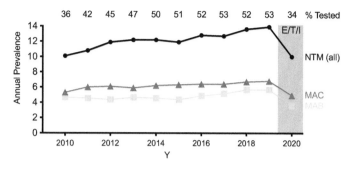

Fig. 1. Annual prevalence of NTM in the US CF population 2010–2020. The percent of participants (excluding those posttransplant) tested for NTM each year has steadily increased (*top row*). The percent of pwCF with one or more positive cultures for any species of NTM (*black circles*) increased significantly from 2010 to 2019 (linear regression of slope greater than zero, *P* < .0001). In the first full year of elexacaftor/tezacaftor/ivacaftor (E/T/I) use, the percent of pwCF with positive NTM cultures decreased dramatically, as did the percentage of subjects tested. The prevalence of pwCF with 1 or more positive cultures for MAC (*green triangles*) or *M. abscessus* (MAB, *blue squares*) also increased from 2010 to 2019 (MAC *P* = .0001, MAB: *P* < .006), and declined in 2020.

in the widely separated outbreaks.[51–53,60] The clinical implications of infection with DCC remain uncertain. DCC isolates from non-US CF isolate cohorts were reported to more frequently acquire antimicrobial resistance mutations compared with unclustered isolates,[54] which was not observed in the analysis of isolates from US CF Centers.[59] DCC in the US were also not associated with the diagnosis of NTM pulmonary disease or antibiotic treatment failure.[59] Interestingly, DCC of MAB have now been identified in additional non-CF cohorts, including pulmonary and extrapulmonary infections,[61,62] and there is some suggestion that non-CF individuals may have facilitated long-distance transmission of DCC lineages.[63]

More recently, the first study of population genomics of MAC has been reported, with an analysis of 364 MAC isolates from 186 pwCF from 42 US Care Centers across 23 states.[64] Unexpectedly, clusters of highly similar isolates of MAC were found to be shared among pwCF at the same CF Center, and between Centers, although at a much lower prevalence than seen with MAB.

This is consistent with a smaller US study of CF and non-CF MAC isolates in which subjects from different hospital cohorts shared highly similar *M. avium* isolates.[65] A Korean study of MAC pulmonary isolates from 3 pairs of cohabiting family members with NTM pulmonary disease found that clinical isolates were not genetically similar to each other, but in some cases showed similarity to household-derived isolates.[66] A WGS study in Philadelphia, PA, found a high proportion of *M. avium* isolates from household plumbing biofilms that matched isolates from patient respiratory specimens.[67] Finally, genomic analyses of colony sweeps[68] and longitudinal MAC isolates[64,65] suggest that a considerable portion of patients with MAC have polymicrobial infections of different species or divergent strain types. Together these results suggest differing exposure sources and acquisition for MAC versus MAB, without the contribution of DCC.[64]

Beyond population analyses, recent MAB investigations have used WGS to study subclone variation, genomic adaptation during infection, and mechanisms of antimicrobial resistance. A

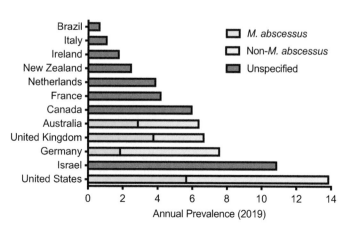

Fig. 2. Annual prevalence of NTM from 2019 national CF registries. The reported annual percent of individuals with 1 or more positive culture for NTM among those tested, excluding transplanted pwCF, are shown for the respective countries. When reported the proportion of *M. abscessus* (*blue bar*) or NTM other than *M. abscessus* (*gray bar*) is depicted.

longitudinal examination of MAB colony sweeps from 18 pwCF revealed the evolutionary trajectories of subclones including potential hypermutator phenotypes in 11% of subjects.[69] This study also identified parallel evolution of mutations across multiple subjects including candidate "adaptation" genes under selection during chronic infection.[69] WGS of MAB isolates from multiple body sites of 2 pwCF pre and postlung transplant identified subpopulations with differing macrolide resistance genotypes, suggesting that sputum isolates do not always reflect intra-patient diversity.[70] Finally, WGS data from MAB isolates with corresponding *in vitro* susceptibility data resulted in a predictive algorithm that identified 8 potential new mutations for macrolide resistance in clinical isolates.[71,72]

Individual Risk Factors for Nontuberculous Mycobacteria in Cystic Fibrosis

Given that the vast majority of pwCF do not have chronic infection with NTM, there is intense interest in identifying features that may predispose them to this complication. Our understanding of individual risk factors for NTM in pwCF is incomplete. Most reports have studied relatively small cohorts from single CF Centers or specific geographic areas, often leading to contradictory conclusions. These divergent findings may relate in part to differences in study methodology, as many reports do not distinguish between a positive NTM culture and the presence of NTM pulmonary disease, and often individuals with MAC and MAB are combined. Nearly every study has reported a strong association with older age and the increased prevalence of NTM isolation[5,7,9,32,44,45,73,74] and NTM disease.[41,45] A very high prevalence has been reported in pwCF with an adult diagnosis,[5,49,75] which is typically associated with a delayed presentation due to less severe mutations[49,76] and relatively milder lung disease.[5,7] CFTR-related genotypes associated with partial CFTR function, such as D1152H, R75Q and the 5T allele, have been specifically correlated with an increased frequency of NTM positive cultures,[77,78] and in non-CF population, the presence of a single Q1352H allele has been linked to an increased prevalence of NTM disease.[79] It is worth noting, however, that other studies have reported the opposite conclusions, in particular that NTM is common in severe lung disease.[41,45,73,80] For example, in Israel, NTM infection was associated with a known "severe" CFTR genotype and pancreatic insufficiency.[13] These differences may arise from relative differences in the prevalence of MAC and MAB, and

to the age of the cohorts studied, as MAC is more often associated with older pwCF, while MAB is frequently seen in younger patients and those with more severe lung disease.[5,11,32,81]

The presence of *Aspergillus fumigatus*[9,13,45,74,82–85] and allergic bronchopulmonary aspergillosis (ABPA)[13,86,87] have been frequently associated with increased risk for NTM. A significant association between NTM positive cultures and coinfection with *S. aureus* and/or *S. maltophilia* was identified in a recent meta-analysis.[74] *Pseudomonas aeruginosa* has been associated with decreased prevalence of NTM in some studies,[7,38] and higher rates in others,[45,85] especially in adult cohorts.[74] A small study of airway microbiota in subjects before and after their first positive culture identified positive correlations between *Pseudomonas, Streptococcus, Veillonella, Prevotella,* and *Rothia* with the diagnosis of NTM pulmonary disease and with persistent NTM infection.[88]

While increased survival may indirectly result in greater NTM prevalence through longer cumulative exposure,[89] a greater concern is the possibility that various medications and CF treatment strategies have contributed to the apparent increase in NTM prevalence. While these reports are for the most part retrospective and their conclusions are not entirely consistent, they have served to heighten awareness of the potential for unforeseen consequences of many therapies in common use. In particular, the administration of systemic steroids, often in the context of ABPA treatment, has been associated with increased prevalence of NTM.[45,74,83,86,87] Vitamin D deficiency has been associated with a higher risk of incident NTM respiratory isolation in adults within a large US Care Center.[90] Use of azithromycin, an antibiotic with antiinflammatory properties, has also been associated with an increased prevalence of NTM,[45,91] although others have reported a decreased[92–94] or unchanged prevalence[74,95–97] in patients treated with the medication. Finally, attending a CF Center may pose a risk, as some, but not all single-center outbreak investigations have identified patient-to-patient transmission (discussed later in discussion).

Environmental Risk Factors

For most pwCF, the source of NTM infection is the natural or home environment. Given the well-recognized regional variability in prevalence and species predominance, several studies have sought to define environmental niches and subsequent risk for infection by vulnerable populations. Atmospheric conditions have been linked to variation in NTM prevalence in pwCF the US.[98] Among pwCF at 21 geographically diverse CF Centers in the US, average annual atmospheric water vapor content was significantly predictive of Center prevalence ($P = .0019$). The only individual risk factor associated with incident infection was indoor swimming. In a review of the prevalence of NTM in the US CFFPR, high saturated vapor pressure was associated with an increased risk for NTM.[29] This is supported by a small study in Florida which identified close household proximity to water (<500 m) as a significant risk factor for presentation with NTM positive cultures in children with CF.[85] Various soil conditions and the presence or absence of trace minerals have also been associated with increased prevalence of NTM positive cultures. In a population-based nested case–control study of pwCF living in Colorado, a consistent association with molybdenum in the source water and MAB infection was detected.[99] Other investigations have identified associations with annual precipitation, soil sodium levels, and levels of soil manganese.[100,101] These findings are consistent with studies in non-CF populations infected with NTM.[102,103] Together, these reports and others point to conditions in the soil which lead to greater abundance of NTM, combined with factors related to greater persistence of moisture droplets in the air, as the additive components that help determine the relative risk for NTM in a particular region.[5]

Diagnosis of Nontuberculous Mycobacteria Lung Disease in Cystic Fibrosis

Given the ubiquitous nature of NTM, the isolation of an NTM from a respiratory specimen is not synonymous with disease nor is it necessarily an indication to initiate treatment. Current criteria for the diagnosis of NTM pulmonary disease call for the presence of ≥2 positive cultures, in the setting of characteristic clinical symptoms and radiographic findings, and the exclusion of other diseases.[1] These criteria have not been validated in any patient population, and are particularly challenging in the setting of CF, whereby radiographic signs suggestive of NTM are common, and identical clinical symptoms can occur due to coinfections with virulent pathogens such as *P. aeruginosa* and *S. aureus*.[19]

The primary clinical question for a patient who has cultured positive for a species of NTM on more than one occasion is whether this represents an indolent infection or NTM pulmonary disease that may benefit from treatment. Patients who are smear positive for NTM are more likely to have NTM pulmonary disease,[38,45] as well as those who demonstrate the progression of findings on high-resolution chest computed tomography (HRCT) associated with NTM, such as tree-in-bud opacities, nodules, and cavitary lesions.[104] Unexpectedly rapid decline in pulmonary function is frequently associated with NTM pulmonary disease in pwCF with positive cultures for NTM.[41,105,106] Further, in pwCF and NTM pulmonary disease, decline in pulmonary function measured by forced exhaled volume in 1 second (FEV_1) has been shown to decline in the year before initial recovery of NTM compared with those with transient or indolent infection who demonstrate a stable FEV_1 in the year before initial NTM infection.[107] Suggested criteria for the diagnosis of NTM pulmonary disease pwCF, adapted from expert guidelines,[1,108] is outlined in **Box 1**.

Laboratory Identification of Nontuberculous Mycobacteria in the Cystic Fibrosis Sputum

Recovery of NTM from CF sputum samples can be difficult due to coinfection with *P. aeruginosa* and other microbes, which frequently overgrow the culture before the slower growing mycobacteria can be detected.[109–112] Development of effective sample decontamination protocols to remove conventional bacteria and fungi has allowed for improved culture-based detection of mycobacteria in CF samples.[113–115] Currently, the standard approach to decontamination involves 2 steps,[110] to avoid excessive decontamination which can reduce NTM viability in samples.[116] Decontamination is first performed with N-acetyl L-cysteine-NaOH, before mycobacterial culture.[110,113,114] Samples that remain contaminated can then be treated with 5% oxalic acid or alternatively 1% chlorhexidine, which may permit recovery of NTM, albeit with reduced sensitivity.[109,117,118] Recent studies reported the use of a novel culture media for rapidly growing mycobacteria (RGM) in pwCF that does not require decontamination.[119,120]

Both liquid and solid media are recommended for culturing NTM with incubation for at least 6 weeks.[1] Once an NTM has been detected in culture, it is critical that the organism be speciated, as treatment varies depending on the species and presence or absence of a functional macrolide resistance (*erm*) gene. New methods of rapid specification are available including line probe assays, partial gene sequencing, multi-locus sequencing, and matrix-assisted laser desorption ionization-time-of-flight (MALDI-TOF) mass spectrometry. Line probe assays are easy to perform and allow the identification of the most frequently encountered NTM. Partial sequencing allows a

> **Box 1**
> **Suggested criteria for the diagnosis of NTM disease in the setting of CF**
>
> 1. Pulmonary or systemic symptoms. For example, increased respiratory symptoms (cough, sputum production, dyspnea, hemoptysis) or constitutional symptoms such as fever, night sweats, or weight loss.
>
> 2. Radiologic findings consistent with NTM infection, such as nodular or cavitary opacities on a chest radiograph or a high-resolution computed tomography scan that shows bronchiectasis with multiple small nodules.
>
> 3. Microbiologic criteria including a positive AFB culture results from at least 2 sputum samples; or one positive bronchial wash or lavage culture; or a lung biopsy with mycobacterial histologic features and positive culture for NTM; or a biopsy showing mycobacterial histologic features plus a sputum or bronchial wash or lavage culture positive for NTM
>
> 4. Exclusion of other comorbidities common in CF, including adequate treatment of:
>
>   - Coinfections such as *P. aeruginosa* and *S. aureus*
>   - Inadequate airway clearance regimens
>   - Nutritional deficiencies
>   - CF-related diabetes (CFRD)
>   - Asthma and allergic bronchopulmonary aspergillosis
>   - CF sinus disease
>
> All 4 criteria should be met before treatment.

higher level of discrimination than line probe assays but requires access to sequencing facilities: 16S rRNA allows discrimination to species level for most species, whereas *hsp*65, *rpo*B genes, and the 16S-23S internal transcribed spacer (ITS) allow discrimination to the subspecies level. Sequencing of multiple loci allows excellent discrimination of the various MAB subspecies. MALDI-TOF mass spectrometry cannot provide the level of subspecies discrimination given by sequencing.[121]

Drug Susceptibility Testing

The American Thoracic Society (ATS) led multisociety NTM guidelines and the Clinical and Laboratory Standards Institute (CLSI) have published recommendations for drug susceptibility testing of the most commonly encountered NTM.[122,123]

Laboratory-defined cutoffs for resistance have not been associated with clinical outcomes in the treatment of MAC except for macrolides and amikacin.[1] Resistance to macrolides has been associated with poor clinical outcomes so current recommendations are to perform testing on all initial isolates.[1,122] Resistance is defined as a clarithromycin minimal inhibitory concentration of $\geq$ 32 µg/ml. Repeat susceptibility testing should also be performed in the following situations:

1. Failure to convert the culture to negative after 6 months of treatment (treatment refractory)
2. When MAC is recultured after conversion while on treatment (failure)
3. When MAC is recultured after the completion of treatment (recurrence)

MAC and MAB isolates should also be tested against amikacin and there are 2 resistance cutpoints for MAC. For the parenteral formulation, resistance is considered present when the MIC is $\geq$ 64 µg/mL but for the liposomal (inhaled) formulation, the resistance cut-point is $\geq$ 128 µg/ml.[122] For MAB and other RGM, microdilution methods are recommended although there are no studies that have associated MIC breakpoints with clinical outcomes in the setting of NTM pulmonary infections.[122] A recent study from Korea reported no association between the currently recommended laboratory-derived cut-points for resistance for imipenem, cefoxitin, or amikacin and treatment outcomes.[124] Antimicrobials that should be tested against RGM are amikacin, tobramycin (for *Mycobacterium chelonae*), cefoxitin, ciprofloxacin, clarithromycin, doxycycline (or minocycline), imipenem, linezolid, moxifloxacin, and trimethoprim-sulfamethoxazole.[122]

Some RGM (*Mycobacterium fortuitum*, *M. abscessus* subspecies *abscessus*, and *M. abscessus* subspecies *bolettii*) contain an *erm* gene, *erm*(41), which causes inducible resistance to macrolides.[125] It is currently recommended that the final reading for macrolide resistance be at least 14 days after inoculation unless resistance (MIC $\geq$8 ug/mL) is noted earlier.[122] Alternatively, molecular methods can be used to detect a normal sequence *erm*(41) gene.

Screening for Nontuberculous Mycobacteria in the Cystic Fibrosis Population

NTM are often first detected in pwCF in the absence of clinical suspicion, as part of routine infection screening. CF consensus guidelines recommend that NTM surveillance cultures be obtained in sputum-producing pwCF annually.[108] Additional screening for NTM is also recommended before the initiation of chronic macrolide therapy to avoid exposing an undiagnosed NTM infection to azithromycin as a single agent.[19,104] Attempted treatment of NTM with a single macrolide antibiotic has been associated with increased development of resistance to the antibiotic,[126,127] which is a mainstay of treatment of MAC and other NTM. More frequent screening should be considered during an unexpected clinical decline and in those deemed to be at higher risk for acquiring the infection, or in those with that infection could have more severe consequences. In particular, more frequent screening may be justified in older patients, those with advanced lung disease awaiting transplant, and those with previous NTM positive cultures. Conversely, in small children and individuals not capable of producing a sputum sample, and with no recognized risk factors or clinical symptoms, NTM screening can be deferred.[108] After a pwCF has been identified as having a positive NTM culture, close surveillance is warranted, with repeat sputum cultures obtained regularly at all subsequent clinical encounters.[108] However, a substantial proportion of pwCF are not routinely screened. Analysis of the CFFPR from 2010 to 2014 determined that while 79% of pwCF greater than 12 years had at least one NTM culture during that interval, only 20% had annual cultures,[5] and over the same interval only 20% of US Care Centers performed routine annual screening of NTM independent of clinical status.[128]

Nearly all studies reporting the prevalence of NTM in the CF population have used acid-fast bacillus (AFB) smear and culture from spontaneously expectorated sputum, induced sputum, or bronchial wash or bronchoalveolar lavage (BAL) fluid. No other methods have been validated for NTM detection in this setting, although NTM can on occasion be detected through laryngeal suction, oropharyngeal swabs, or gastric aspirate.[37,41,83,129–131] In the future, it seems likely that culture-independent methods of NTM detection will be used. In particular, molecular techniques can be performed rapidly and are extremely sensitive and specific for the detection of NTM in sputum,[132–134] although not yet validated in the setting of CF. Given the dramatic decline in the percent of pwCF able to produce sputum regularly due to HEMT, there is also intense interest in identifying sputum-independent markers for NTM infection, disease, and response to treatment. Skin testing for delayed-type hypersensitivity against NTM antigens does not appear sufficiently sensitive or specific to use for screening.[37,42,135] Serologic assays, such as IgG against mycobacterium antigen A60 for NTM surveillance appear promising[112,136] but currently lack validation in the CF population. A recent study from Sweden reported that anti-MAB IgG ELISA was 6-fold higher in pwCF with MAB pulmonary disease compared with those without diseases (sensitivity 95%, specificity 73%).[137] Testing for NTM infection with commercially available urine lipoarabinomannan (LAM) immunologic assays developed for *Mycobacterium tuberculosis* lack sensitivity in pwCF.[138] However, in a pilot study urine LAM analysis using gas chromatography-mass spectrometry proved very sensitive in identifying pwCF with a history of positive cultures,[139] and a trial is underway to test urine LAM as a screen for pwCF at low risk for infection (NCT04579211).

Treatment of Nontuberculous Mycobacteria Lung Disease

Treatment of NTM pulmonary disease in pwCF should be based on international guidelines sponsored by the ATS, European Respiratory Society, European Society for Microbiology and Infectious Diseases, and the Infectious Disease Society of America that were developed for the general population[1] as well as guidelines developed under the sponsorship of the CFF and the ECFS specific to individuals with CF.[108] Standard treatment regimens typically include at least 3 drugs directed against the specific NTM pathogen, in the oral, inhaled and/or intravenous form.

Treatment of Mycobacterium avium Complex Pulmonary Disease

Initial treatment of noncavitary NTM pulmonary disease due to MAC uses a macrolide, rifamycin, and ethambutol.[1] Azithromycin is the preferred macrolide due to better tolerance, single daily dosing, lower pill burden, and less interaction with HEMT, rifampicin and other drugs metabolized through the CYP3A enzyme system compared with clarithromycin.[140] Additionally, chronic azithromycin therapy has been shown to have benefits in pwCF felt to be due to immunomodulatory properties of the drug, in particular, those with *P. aeruginosa*.[141–144] Intermittent oral antibiotic therapy (*i.e.* three times weekly) is recommended for non–CF-related MAC pulmonary disease with less extensive disease and recent studies have demonstrated success rates similar to daily therapy but with less drug intolerance.[145,146] However, intermittent therapy is not recommended in CF due to the presence of underlying lung disease and concerns of the abnormal absorption of antimycobacterials and altered pharmacokinetics (PK) in CF.[147] In pwCF with macrolide-resistant MAC or who are systemically ill, are AFB smear positive, or have evidence of a cavitary lesion on chest imaging, a 1- to 3-month course of intravenous daily amikacin may be added at the beginning of the treatment course along with the standard 3 oral antibiotics. Patients within this category should generally be managed in collaboration with an expert in the treatment of NTM and CF.

Treatment of Mycobacterium abscessus Pulmonary Disease

Typically, treatment regimens for MAB are divided into an initial intensive phase followed by a continuation phase.[1] The intensive phase consists of 3 to 12 weeks of 3 antibiotics, including intravenous amikacin, cefoxitin, imipenem, or tigecycline, in addition to oral antibiotics. After intravenous therapy, patients usually continue on prolonged chronic suppressive therapy with oral and inhaled treatments with adjustments of therapy based on microbiologic, clinical and radiographic responses.[148] In some patients, intermittent courses of intravenous antibiotics are required to control the infection. Changes in the drug regimen are common, due to intolerance, side effects, and lack of efficacy. These patients should also be generally managed in collaboration with an expert in the treatment of NTM and CF.

MAB can be divided into 3 subspecies including *M. abscessus*, *Mycobacterium bolettii*, and *M. massiliense*.[149] *M. abscessus* subspecies *abscessus* and subspecies *M. bolletii* contain an *erm*(41) gene which can result in inducible macrolide resistance. *Mycobacterium massiliense* has a truncated nonfunctional gene so the organism does not develop inducible macrolide resistance. There are significant differences in treatment outcomes for *M. abscessus* subspecies *abscessus* and subspecies *massiliense* in both patients with CF and non-CF.[150] In a study from France, clarithromycin-based regimens led to mycobacterial eradication in 100% of patients with *M massiliense* but only 27% of *M. abscessus* ($P = .009$).[151] These differences are presumably related to the development of inducible macrolide resistance in most strains of subspecies *abscessus* but not in *massiliense*. Whether a macrolide should be continued in the face of potential inducible resistance is not known but given the potential benefits of macrolides in the setting of CF lung disease most providers maintain the macrolide in the treatment regimen. However, the macrolide should not be considered an active drug in the setting of mutational or inducible macrolide resistance.

Monitoring of Clinical Response and Drug Toxicity

Clinical, radiographic, and microbiologic data should be collected regularly to assess whether or not a patient is responding to therapy.[1] To monitor the time of conversion to negative cultures, expectorated or induced sputum AFB cultures should be collected every 1 to 2 months while on treatment. Routine monitoring of drug toxicity is also essential, and a plan for monitoring should be established at the initiation of treatment. PwCF are commonly treated with aminoglycosides for other lung pathogens, and therefore prone to auditory-vestibular toxicity and renal injury, making baseline and regular audiology evaluations and monitoring of renal function essential. Even among oral agents, the potential for drug-related side effects and toxicity is considerable, including bone marrow suppression and hepatitis. Of particular concern is a change in visual acuity due to ethambutol. Patients are recommended to monitor their vision daily and ethambutol should be discontinued immediately at the first sign of visual disturbance.

Therapeutic Drug Monitoring

Currently, recommended dosages of antimycobacterials are based on PK and pharmacodynamic data from healthy volunteers and patients with tuberculosis. Though there are no randomized trials showing the clinical utility of performing therapeutic drug monitoring (TDM) routinely, it is recommended that TDM be considered in situations in which drug malabsorption or drug underdosing or nonadherence are expected or suspected.[1] TDM should also be considered in the setting of treatment failure or when multiple drug interactions are possible.[1,108,152] TDM may be more beneficial in pwCF as optimal drug dosing is particularly challenging due to the potential for drug malabsorption, impaired gastric motility, larger volume of distribution, increased metabolic rate, and potentially increased elimination.[153–155] Currently, it is standard practice to monitor amikacin serum levels when administered intravenously to reduce nephrotoxicity and ototoxicity.[1] Recent data suggest that TDM may be beneficial in all pwCF to prevent the possibility of treatment failure due to abnormal drug concentrations.[156] A single-dose pharmacokinetic evaluation of azithromycin, rifampin, and ethambutol in pwCF showed that peak concentrations of azithromycin in pwCF was higher and rifampin peak concentrations were significantly lower compared with healthy controls.[156] Addition of food and enzymes in pwCF did not improve PK parameters of the 3 drugs. Importantly, at the individual level, 95% of pwCF had one or more abnormal peak concentration z-scores when compared with healthy controls. Serum concentrations of antimycobacterial have been associated with treatment outcomes in pwCF as well. In one small case series, researchers demonstrated that serum levels of oral agents for the treatment of NTM are usually far below the target range in pwCF and in one case whereby treatment was failing, increasing the dose to achieve therapeutic levels was associated with the eradication of the organism.[147] In patients with non-CF NTM disease, another series reported 48% of patients had low serum concentrations of ethambutol, 56% for clarithromycin, and 35% for azithromycin, despite using ATS/IDSA recommended doses.[140] Based on these studies and others, it seems that the dosing of patients with both CF and non-CF NTM disease may in some cases be subtherapeutic, possibly contributing to poor response to treatment.[147]

Nonpharmacologic Treatment Options

In addition to the pharmacologic treatment of NTM infection, nonpharmacologic therapies for underlying CF lung disease that primarily target clearance of airway mucus obstruction are essential. All NTM treatment regimens need to be part of a comprehensive CF care plan that includes effective airway clearance, nutrition management, and treatment of CF comorbidities such as sinus disease and CF-related diabetes. This care is most effectively delivered at a CF Center, which uses a multidisciplinary and interdisciplinary approach, providing access to a respiratory therapist, dietitian, and social worker, in addition to nurses and physicians experienced in CF care. A list of CF Foundation-accredited CF Care Centers can be located at http://www.cff.org/LivingWithCF/Care CenterNetwork/CFFoundation-accreditedCare Centers/.

In addition to antibiotics, a variety of agents are being considered for the treatment of NTM,[157] often in combination with conventional therapy. Based primarily on case reports or preclinical studies[158–160] recent or current trials have tested inhaled GM-CSF (NCT03597347), intravenous gallium, inhaled nitric oxide (NCT03208764, NCT04685720), and various cytokines. Considerable interest has been raised by the report of effective suppression by engineered bacteriophages of disseminated MAB in a pwCF posttransplant,[161] although the development of neutralizing antibodies against the phage may limit the duration of therapy in the absence of immunosuppression.[162]

Surgical Treatment Options

Surgical resection (pneumonectomy, lobectomy, or segmentectomy) may be a consideration as adjuvant therapy to medical treatment in selected patients with NTM pulmonary disease.[1] Non-CF patients with MAB pulmonary disease have been reported to have a higher rate of sustained culture conversion after surgery than with antimicrobial therapy alone.[163,164] In pwCF, often there is a lobe with a greater burden of disease; however, disease is generally diffuse and bronchiectasis eventually will involve all lobes. It is difficult to identify, with certainty, a focus of NTM infection in the setting of coinfection with typical CF pathogens such as *P. aeruginosa* and *S. aureus*, and pwCF with a history of NTM are at a very high risk to acquire a second NTM in their lifetime.[107] In rare circumstances a pwCF with NTM disease may be identified who is a good candidate to benefit from lung resection, but only in combination with intensive pre and postoperative antibiotic treatment, and in the hands of surgeon experienced in mycobacterial surgery.[1,165]

Treatment Outcomes and Impact of Nontuberculous Mycobacteria Pulmonary Disease

Currently, treatment success is generally defined by sustained culture conversion for at least 12 months.[1,164] Rates of successful therapy seem to vary based on NTM species and subspecies, patterns of antibiotic resistance, and severity of disease. In a retrospective review of pwCF from Colorado, the rate of sustained culture conversion in response to the initial treatment of MAB was 45%, and response to the treatment of MAC was 60%.[107] Similarly, a study from the U.K. reported treatment success in 80% of 10 patients with MAC lung disease and 48% of 60 patients with MAB infection.[166] The issue of treatment failure is particularly problematic in the context of CF. General considerations in the evaluation of treatment failure include antibiotic resistance, inadequate dosing and/or poor absorption of antibiotics, suboptimal airway clearance, lack of adherence to the prescribed medications, and the contribution of other comorbidities, including exacerbations of other chronic infections, chronic aspiration, and CF-related diabetes.

After a pwCF has been treated for NTM pulmonary disease, close surveillance is still warranted. In patients previously infected with an NTM or treated for NTM pulmonary disease, the presence of a second NTM is a relatively common occurrence. Many previous trials have noted the presence of individuals with more than one species of

NTM recovered from their sputum.[7–9,32,44,45,81,167] In patients from the Colorado CF Center with NTM, MAC was typically the first identified NTM, but a subsequent positive culture for MAB was common, while subjects who first cultured MAB also had a high rate of secondary positive cultures for MAC.[107] Remarkably 26% of subjects were identified with a second NTM species at 5 years and 36% at 10 years. These findings support the need for lifelong strategies for NTM surveillance and management in pwCF that present a positive NTM culture.

Lung Transplant in Cystic Fibrosis and Nontuberculous Mycobacteria

Bilateral lung transplant is often indicated in the setting of advanced CF lung disease, and pwCF referred for lung transplant have an especially high prevalence of NTM positive cultures and/or NTM pulmonary disease.[80,168] Lung transplant in the context of infection with MAB remains controversial. A series of reports from single centers have documented significant morbidity associated with lung transplant for pwCF infected with MAB. The most significant complications are local wound infection or disseminated MAB infection post-transplant in those with pretransplant infection, which results in prolonged antibiotic treatment and in some cases death[168–174] Dissemination of MAB may include the infection of the transplanted lung, pleural space, incision site, skin, bones, soft tissue, and morbidity is compounded by the often severe side effects and toxicities from multi-drug antibiotic treatment.[168,174] Several patients have been described in which preexisting NTM was not detected but posttransplant was a source of posttransplant morbidity and mortality.[172,173,175] In some individuals, NTM present pretransplant is not recovered posttransplant.[168,174,176–178]

In most case series, the authors have concluded that despite greater morbidity, long-term survival is not reduced.[80,174,176–178] However, in some series, increased mortality has been reported both in CF[168,179] and non-CF cohorts.[180] Investigators at Great Ormond Street Hospital for Children (U.K.) reported decreased survival among a series of children with CF receiving lung transplant, Deaths attributed to infection were confined to those infected with *M. abscessus* subsp. *abscessus*, compared with favorable outcomes in those infected with *M. abscessus* subsp. *massiliense* or *bolletii*.[168,179] Of interest, all of the *M. abscessus* subsp. *abscessus* infections resulting in death post-transplant were identified within the DCCs.[168] Based on expert opinion, "*chronic infection with highly virulent and/or resistant microbes that are poorly controlled pre-transplant*" has been listed as an absolute contraindication for lung transplant by the International Society for Heart and Lung Transplantation,[181] while infection with multi-drug-resistant MAB is listed as a relative contraindication "*if the infection is sufficiently treated preoperatively and there is a reasonable expectation for adequate control postoperatively.*"[181] The CFF and ECFS recommend that individuals with CF receiving NTM treatment with sequential negative cultures may be eligible for transplant listing.[108] Consensus opinion within the available literature is that all pwCF referred for transplant should be evaluated for NTM disease, and if present aggressive and prolonged courses of multiple antimycobacterial agents before transplant, perioperatively and posttransplant are critical to improving outcomes.[168,172,174,178,181,182] In one case the addition of bacteriophage to intensive antibiotics achieved long-term suppression of disseminated MAB infection posttransplant,[161] without the development of neutralizing antibodies despite a prolonged treatment course.[162] In a recent survey of 37 pediatric and adult lung transplant centers across Europe, North America and Australia, 57% of responding centers reported that they consider persistence of MAB despite optimal therapy as an absolute contraindication to transplant, and 76% of centers reported MAB combined with another relative contraindication was an absolute contraindication to transplant.[183] Few lung transplant programs report that they have a clear written policy regarding the assessment and listing of pwCF and NTM infection[183]; however, the Great Ormond Street Hospital for Children has stated as of 2020 they are not considering *M. abscessus* subsp. *abscessus*-infected patients for lung transplantation at their center.[168] The CFF Consensus Guideline for Lung Transplant Referral recommends consultation with at least 2 transplant centers before determining whether an individual is not a transplant candidate, as criteria may differ widely between centers based on institutional experience, resources, and risk thresholds.[184]

INFECTION PREVENTION

Infections with NTM were historically believed to only occur from environmental sources.[39,185] However, over the past decade the potential for patient-to-patient spread within CF Centers has been reported.[53,167,186,187] Most prominently is the report from the Adult CF Center at Papworth Hospital, U.K. whereby WGS, analysis of antibiotic resistance patterns, and epidemiologic investigation within the clinic and hospital identified two clusters of *M. abscessus* subsp. *massiliense* infecting 11 individuals with many shared exposures within the health care setting.[53] Several other CF Centers have also reported results from the analysis of MAB isolates collected within their patient cohorts. Many outbreak investigations have relied heavily on similarities or differences in single nucleotide polymorphism (SNP) numbers and location within the core genome of isolates tested by WGS, and to various extents on epidemiologic tracking and testing for environmental reservoirs. Several centers worldwide have concluded that direct or indirect person-to-person transmission of MAB likely occurred within their facilities[53,58,167,186,187] while others have determined that transmission of MAB was either very rare or did not occur.[56,188,189] Based on the reports of transmission, the CFF recommends that all health care personnel implement contact precautions (i.e. wear a gown and gloves) when caring for all pwCF, regardless of respiratory culture results, in both ambulatory and inpatient settings.[190] Additionally, they recommend that the molecular typing of all NTM isolates be performed if there is a suspected patient-to-patient transmission event. In Centers whereby transmission seemed to occur, the adoption of various preventative measures has reduced the incidence of new infections.[191]

The identification of 2 or more pwCF within a CF Center who share isolates with highly similar core genomes is not sufficient evidence for patient-to-patient transmission, as the highly conserved DCC within MAB comprise most of infections in CF and non-CF cohorts, with nearly identical isolates identified in different continents.[54,69] A systematic approach is being used by several US CF Centers to investigate healthcare-associated links in transmission of NTM among pwCF (HALT NTM study, NCT04024423).[192] The stepwise approach starts with WGS analysis of NTM isolates to determine relatedness at the core genome level followed by an epidemiologic investigation of pwCF with genetically similar NTM isolates in the health care system. Epidemiologic investigation includes thorough health record review, accessory genome analysis to determine relatedness at the pan-genome level, health care environmental sampling for NTM by microbiological culture, WGS comparison to respiratory isolates from pwCF, and finally, watershed mapping of home residences to assess the likelihood of shared acquisition from the home environment. Analysis of 11 clusters involving 27 individuals at the Colorado Adult CF Program was able to rule out patient-to-patient transmission in all but 3 pwCF infected with MAC. One cluster of M. abscessus subspecies abscessus with very high similarity in both the core genome and pan genome had no healthcare-associated exposure but were found to all reside in the same watershed.[193] A large outbreak investigation at Duke University Hospital including both patients with CF and non-CF likewise used pan-genome analysis and environmental sampling to confirm the environmental acquisition of the infection.[194]

SUMMARY

With the widespread adoption of HEMT, NTM is being recovered less frequently from the sputum of pwCF, but the true prevalence of pulmonary NTM infections is not known. Current trends in all at-risk populations (excluding CF) have shown a steady increase in prevalence. The improvement in survival achieved through HEMT may ultimately lead to a greater proportion of the CF population resembling the phenotype most often associated with NTM infection, including those with greater age[7,41,44,45,73] and less severe CFTR mutations[49,77,78] in the context of natural and engineered environments that seem increasingly favorable toward NTM survival.

Diagnosis of NTM disease in the setting of CF can be difficult given the overlapping clinical and radiographic findings caused by common CF pathogens, and the fact that the isolation of NTM may or may not be associated with progressive disease. As treatment may not be necessary in all cases, CF-specific diagnostic criteria are greatly needed. With the vast majority of pwCF expected to benefit from HEMT, clinical and radiographic signs and symptoms seem less reliable, and sputum cultures are less sensitive or unavailable. While in some individuals, improved airway function afforded by HEMT may prevent NTM disease, in others it may conceivably delay diagnosis. Through the CFF-sponsored PREDICT trial (NCT02073409), the diagnostic criteria for NTM disease in pwCF are being assessed, and potentially redefined to reflect the new CF phenotype, and to test culture-independent markers of infection. Treatment presents a significant burden on the patient and health care system[195] requiring a prolonged multi-drug regimen, often including several months of multiple continuous intravenous antibiotics and associated with frequent drug-related toxicities. For pwCF this treatment burden comes in addition to existing time- and cost-intensive regimens of medications and airway clearance. Longitudinal NTM treatment outcome data in pwCF are being collected through the CFF-sponsored PATIENCE (NCT02419989) and FORMaT (ACTRN12618001831279p) trials. Primarily through the repurposing of available antibiotics, there are a greater number of options, although failure to eradicate the infection remains common despite intensive treatment.

CLINICS CARE POINTS

- The CF population is at high risk for NTM infection and routine screening should be performed.

- Infection most commonly occurs from environmental sources, however, direct or indirect patient-to-patient spread is possible.

- As the majority of people with CF who are infected with NTM may not require treatment, CF-specific NTM pulmonary disease diagnostic criteria are needed.

- Treatment of NTM pulmonary disease in people with CF should be based on international consensus guidelines.

ACKNOWLEDGMENTS

The authors would like to thank Rebecca M. Davidson, PhD for critical reading of the article. Funding provided by the National Institutes of Health (NIH): R01HL146228 and the Cystic Fibrosis Foundation: NICK20Y2-SVC, NICK20Y2-OUT, NICK17K0, NICK18P0, and MARTIN17K0.

DISCLOSURE

Dr. Daley: Research Grants - AN2, Bugworks, Insmed, Paratek and Advisory Committees: AN2, Aztrazeneca, Genentech, Insmed, Matinas, Paratek, Pfizer, Spero. Dr. Martiniano: Data Safety Monitoring Board: Beyond Air. Dr. Nick: No disclosures.

REFERENCES

1. Daley CL, Iaccarino JM, Lange C, et al. Treatment of nontuberculous mycobacterial pulmonary disease: an official ATS/ERS/ESCMID/IDSA clinical practice guideline. Clin Infect Dis 2020;71(4): 905–13.

2. Prevots DR, Marras TK. Epidemiology of human pulmonary infection with nontuberculous mycobacteria: a review. Clin Chest Med 2015;36(1):13–34.

3. Jackson AD, Goss CH. Epidemiology of CF: How registries can be used to advance our understanding of the CF population. J cystic fibrosis : official J Eur Cystic Fibrosis Soc 2018;17(3):297–305.

4. Cystic_Fibrosis_Foundation_Patient_Registry. 2020 Annual Data Report, Bethesda, MD. 2021. Available at: https://www.cff.org/sites/default/files/2021-11/Patient-Registry-Annual-Data-Report.pdf

5. Adjemian J, Olivier KN, Prevots DR. Epidemiology of pulmonary nontuberculous mycobacterial sputum positivity in patients with cystic fibrosis in the United States, 2010-2014. Ann Am Thorac Soc 2018;15(7):817–26.

6. Smith MJ, Efthimiou J, Hodson ME, et al. Mycobacterial isolations in young adults with cystic fibrosis. Thorax 1984;39(5):369–75.

7. Olivier KN, Weber DJ, Wallace RJ Jr, et al. Nontuberculous mycobacteria. I: multicenter prevalence study in cystic fibrosis. Research Support, Non-U.S. Gov'tResearch Support, U.S. Gov't, P.H.S. Am J Respir Crit Care Med 2003;167(6):828–34.

8. Roux A-L, Catherinot E, Ripoll F, et al. Multicenter study of prevalence of nontuberculous mycobacteria in patients with cystic fibrosis in France. Multicenter Study Support, 2009 Research Support, Non-U.S. Gov't. J Clin Microbiol 2009;47(12):4124–8.

9. Esther CR Jr, Esserman DA, Gilligan P, et al. Chronic Mycobacterium abscessus infection and lung function decline in cystic fibrosis. Research Support, N.I.H., Extramural. J Cystic Fibrosis 2010;9(2):117–23.

10. Leung JM, Olivier KN. Nontuberculous mycobacteria: the changing epidemiology and treatment challenges in cystic fibrosis. Curr Opin Pulm Med 2013; 19(6):662–9.

11. Qvist T, Gilljam M, Jonsson B, et al. Epidemiology of nontuberculous mycobacteria among patients with cystic fibrosis in Scandinavia. J cystic fibrosis 2014;14:S1569–993.

12. Qvist T, Pressler T, Hoiby N, et al. Shifting paradigms of nontuberculous mycobacteria in cystic fibrosis. Respir Res 2014;15:41. https://doi.org/10.1186/1465-9921-15-41.

13. Bar-On O, Mussaffi H, Mei-Zahav M, et al. Increasing nontuberculous mycobacteria infection in cystic fibrosis. J cystic fibrosis : official J Eur Cystic Fibrosis Soc 2015;14(1):53–62.

14. Raidt L, Idelevich EA, Dubbers A, et al. Increased prevalence and resistance of important pathogens recovered from respiratory specimens of cystic fibrosis patients during a decade. Pediatr Infect Dis J 2015;34(7):700–5.

15. Adjemian J, Olivier KN, Seitz AE, et al. Prevalence of nontuberculous mycobacterial lung disease in U.S. Medicare beneficiaries. Am J Respir Crit Care Med 2012;185(8):881–6.

16. Prevots DR, Shaw PA, Strickland D, et al. Nontuberculous mycobacterial lung disease prevalence at four integrated health care delivery systems. Am J Respir Crit Care Med 2010;182(7):970–6.

17. Dean SG, Ricotta EE, Fintzi J, et al. Mycobacterial testing trends, United States, 2009-2015(1). Emerg Infect Dis 2020;26(9):2243–6.

18. Winthrop KL, Marras TK, Adjemian J, et al. Incidence and prevalence of nontuberculous mycobacterial lung disease in a large U.S. Managed care health plan, 2008-2015. Ann Am Thorac Soc 2020;17(2):178–85.

19. Leung JM, Olivier KN. Nontuberculous mycobacteria in patients with cystic fibrosis. Semin Respir Crit Care Med 2013;34(1):124–34.

20. Ramsay KA, Stockwell RE, Bell SC, et al. Infection in cystic fibrosis: impact of the environment and climate. Expert Rev Respir Med 2016;10(5):505–19.

21. Heltshe SL, Mayer-Hamblett N, Burns JL, et al. Pseudomonas aeruginosa in cystic fibrosis patients with G551D-CFTR treated with ivacaftor. Clin Infect Dis 2015;60(5):703–12.

22. Rowe SM, Heltshe SL, Gonska T, et al. Clinical mechanism of the cystic fibrosis transmembrane conductance regulator potentiator ivacaftor in G551D-mediated cystic fibrosis. Am J Respir Crit Care Med 2014;190(2):175–84.

23. Yi B, Dalpke AH, Boutin S. Changes in the cystic fibrosis airway Microbiome in response to CFTR modulator therapy. Front Cell Infect Microbiol 2021;11:548613. https://doi.org/10.3389/fcimb.2021.548613.

24. Rogers GB, Taylor SL, Hoffman LR, et al. The impact of CFTR modulator therapies on CF airway microbiology. J cystic fibrosis 2020; 19(3):359–64.

25. Hisert KB, Heltshe SL, Pope C, et al. Restoring cystic fibrosis transmembrane conductance regulator function reduces airway bacteria and inflammation in people with cystic fibrosis and chronic lung infections. Am J Respir Crit Care Med 2017; 195(12):1617–28.

26. Cystic fibrosis Foundation (U.S.) patient registry. 2019 annual data report. Available at: https://www.cff.org/medical-professionals/patient-registry.

27. Gur M, Bar-Yoseph R, Toukan Y, et al. Twelve years of progressive Mycobacterium abscessus lung disease in CF-Response to Trikafta. Pediatr Pulmonol 2021;56(12):4048–50.

28. Nick JA, Khan U, Vu PT, et al. Prospective analysis of the effect of highly effective modulator therapy on prevalence of positive cultures for nontuberculous mycobacterial infection in the PREDICT trial. J Cystic Fibrosis 2021;(Suppl).

29. Adjemian J, Olivier KN, Prevots DR. Nontuberculous mycobacteria among cystic fibrosis patients in the United States: screening practices and environmental risk. Am J Respir Crit Care Med 2014. https://doi.org/10.1164/rccm.201405-0884OC.

30. Cystic Fibrosis Australia. Australian Cystic Fibrosis Registry: Annual Report 2019. Available at: https://www.cysticfibrosis.org.au/CysticFibrosis/media/CFQ/Media%20Releases/CFQ-Annual-Report-2019.pdf

31. Abidin NZ, Gardner AI, Robinson HL, et al. Trends in nontuberculous mycobacteria infection in children and young people with cystic fibrosis. J cystic fibrosis 2020. https://doi.org/10.1016/j.jcf.2020.09.007.

32. Pierre-Audigier C, Ferroni A, Sermet-Gaudelus I, et al. Age-related prevalence and distribution of nontuberculous mycobacterial species among patients with cystic fibrosis. Research Support, Non-U.S. Gov't. J Clin Microbiol 2005;43(7):3467–70.

33. Satana D, Erkose-Genc G, Tamay Z, et al. Prevalence and drug resistance of mycobacteria in Turkish cystic fibrosis patients. Ann Clin Microbiol Antimicrob 2014;13:28. https://doi.org/10.1186/1476-0711-13-28.

34. Qvist T, Gilljam M, Jonsson B, et al. Epidemiology of nontuberculous mycobacteria among patients with cystic fibrosis in Scandinavia. J cystic fibrosis 2015;14(1):46–52.

35. Ho D, Belmonte O, Andre M, et al. High prevalence of nontuberculous mycobacteria in cystic fibrosis patients in tropical French Reunion Island. Pediatr Infect Dis J 2021;40(3):e120–2.

36. Aiello TB, Levy CE, Zaccariotto TR, et al. Prevalence and clinical outcomes of nontuberculous mycobacteria in a Brazilian cystic fibrosis reference center. Pathog Dis 2018;76(5). https://doi.org/10.1093/femspd/fty051.

37. Hjelte L, Petrini B, Kallenius G, et al. Prospective study of mycobacterial infections in patients with cystic fibrosis. Thorax 1990;45(5):397–400.

38. Esther CR Jr, Henry MM, Molina PL, et al. Nontuberculous mycobacterial infection in young children with cystic fibrosis. Research Support, N.I.H., Extramural Support and AuthorAnonymous, Research Support, Non-U.S. Gov't Research Support, U.S. Gov't, P.H.S. Pediatr Pulmonology 2005;40(1):39–44.

39. Sermet-Gaudelus I, Le Bourgeois M, Pierre-Audigier C, et al. Mycobacterium abscessus and children with cystic fibrosis. Research Support, Non-U.S. Gov't. Emerging Infect Dis 2003;9(12):1587–91.

40. Torrens JK, Dawkins P, Conway SP, et al. Nontuberculous mycobacteria in cystic fibrosis. Thorax 1998;53(3):182–5.

41. Fauroux B, Delaisi B, Clement A, et al. Mycobacterial lung disease in cystic fibrosis: a prospective study. Pediatr Infect Dis J 1997;16(4):354–8.

42. Hjelt K, Hojlyng N, Howitz P, et al. The role of Mycobacteria Other than Tuberculosis (MOTT) in patients with cystic fibrosis. Research Support, Non-U.S. Gov't. Scand J Infect Dis 1994;26(5):569–76.

43. Aitken ML, Moss RB, Waltz DA, et al. A phase I study of aerosolized administration of tgAAVCF to cystic fibrosis subjects with mild lung disease. Hum Gene Ther 2001;12(15):1907–16.

44. Kilby JM, Gilligan PH, Yankaskas JR, et al. Nontuberculous mycobacteria in adult patients with cystic fibrosis. Case Reports Research Support, U.S. Gov't, P.H.S. Chest 1992;102(1):70–5.

45. Levy I, Grisaru-Soen G, Lerner-Geva L, et al. Multicenter cross-sectional study of nontuberculous mycobacterial infections among cystic fibrosis patients, Israel. Multicenter Study. Emerging Infect Dis 2008;14(3):378–84.

46. Registro Brasileiro de Fibrose Cística (REBRAFC). 2019 Patient Registry. Available at: http://rebrafc.org.br.

47. CF Registry of Ireland. 2019 Annual Report. 2020. Available at: https://cfri.ie/annual-reports/

48. European cystic fibrosis society. ECFS patient Regsitry annual data report. 2019. Available at: https://www.ecfs.eu/projects/ecfs-patient-Registry/annual-reports.

49. Rodman DM, Polis JM, Heltshe SL, et al. Late diagnosis defines a unique population of long-term survivors of cystic fibrosis. Research Support, Non-U.S. Gov't Research Support, U.S. Gov't, P.H.S. Am J Respir Crit Care Med 2005;171(6):621–6.

50. Campos-Herrero MI, Chamizo FJ, Caminero JA, et al. Nontuberculous mycobacteria in cystic fibrosis patients on the Island of Gran Canaria. A population study. J Infect Chemother : official J Jpn Soc Chemother 2016;22(8):526–31.

51. Davidson RM, Hasan NA, de Moura VC, et al. Phylogenomics of Brazilian epidemic isolates of Mycobacterium abscessus subsp. bolletii reveals relationships of global outbreak strains. Infect Genet Evol : J Mol Epidemiol Evol Genet Infect Dis 2013;20:292–7.

52. Tettelin H, Davidson RM, Agrawal S, et al. High-level relatedness among Mycobacterium abscessus subsp. massiliense strains from widely separated outbreaks. Emerg Infect Dis 2014;20(3):364–71.

53. Bryant JM, Grogono DM, Greaves D, et al. Whole-genome sequencing to identify transmission of Mycobacterium abscessus between patients with cystic fibrosis: a retrospective cohort study. Lancet 2013;381(9877):1551–60.

54. Bryant JM, Grogono DM, Rodriguez-Rincon D, et al. Emergence and spread of a human-transmissible multidrug-resistant nontuberculous mycobacterium. Science 2016;354(6313):751–7.

55. Tortoli E, Kohl TA, Trovato A, et al. Mycobacterium abscessus in patients with cystic fibrosis: low impact of inter-human transmission in Italy. Eur Respir J 2017;50(1). https://doi.org/10.1183/13993003.02525-2016.

56. Doyle RM, Rubio M, Dixon G, et al. Cross-transmission is not the source of new Mycobacterium abscessus infections in a multicenter cohort of cystic fibrosis patients. Clin Infect Dis 2020;70(9):1855–64.

57. Redondo N, Mok S, Montgomery L, et al. Genomic analysis of Mycobacterium abscessus complex isolates collected in Ireland between 2006 and 2017. J Clin Microbiol 2020;(7):58. https://doi.org/10.1128/JCM.00295-20.

58. Yan J, Kevat A, Martinez E, et al. Investigating transmission of Mycobacterium abscessus amongst children in an Australian cystic fibrosis centre. J cystic fibrosis 2020;19(2):219–24.

59. Davidson RM, Hasan NA, Epperson LE, et al. Population genomics of Mycobacterium abscessus from United States cystic fibrosis care centers. Ann Am Thorac Soc 2021. https://doi.org/10.1513/AnnalsATS.202009-1214OC.

60. Everall I, Nogueira CL, Bryant JM, et al. Genomic epidemiology of a national outbreak of post-surgical Mycobacterium abscessus wound infections in Brazil. Microb Genom 2017;3(5):e000111.

61. Bronson RA, Gupta C, Manson AL, et al. Global phylogenomic analyses of Mycobacterium abscessus provide context for non cystic fibrosis infections and the evolution of antibiotic resistance. Nat Commun 2021;12(1):5145.

62. Davidson RM, Benoit JB, Kammlade SM, et al. Genomic characterization of sporadic isolates of the dominant clone of Mycobacterium abscessus subspecies massiliense. Scientific Rep 2021;11(1):15336.

63. Ruis C, Bryant JM, Bell SC, et al. Dissemination of Mycobacterium abscessus via global transmission networks. Nat Microbiol 2021;6(10):1279–88.

64. Hasan NA, Davidson RM, Epperson LE, et al. Population genomics and Inference of Mycobacterium avium complex clusters in cystic fibrosis care centers, United States. Emerg Infect Dis 2021;27(11):2836–46.

65. Keen EC, Choi J, Wallace MA, et al. Comparative genomics of Mycobacterium avium complex reveals Signatures of environment-specific adaptation and Community acquisition. mSystems 2021;6(5):e0119421.

66. Yoon JK, Kim TS, Kim JI, et al. Whole genome sequencing of Nontuberculous Mycobacterium (NTM) isolates from sputum specimens of co-habiting patients with NTM pulmonary disease and NTM isolates from their environment. BMC genomics 2020;21(1):322.

67. Lande L, Alexander DC, Wallace RJ Jr, et al. Mycobacterium avium in Community and household water, Suburban Philadelphia, Pennsylvania, USA, 2010-2012. Emerg Infect Dis 2019;25(3):473–81.

68. Operario DJ, Pholwat S, Koeppel AF, et al. Mycobacterium avium complex diversity within lung disease, as revealed by whole-genome sequencing. Am J Respir Crit Care Med 2019;200(3):393–6.

69. Bryant JM, Brown KP, Burbaud S, et al. Stepwise pathogenic evolution of Mycobacterium abscessus. Science 2021;(6541):372.

70. Shaw LP, Doyle RM, Kavaliunaite E, et al. Children with cystic fibrosis are infected with multiple subpopulations of Mycobacterium abscessus with different antimicrobial resistance Profiles. Clin Infect Dis 2019;69(10):1678–86.

71. Lipworth S, Hough N, Leach L, et al. Whole-genome sequencing for predicting clarithromycin resistance in Mycobacterium abscessus. Antimicrob Agents Chemother 2019;63(1). https://doi.org/10.1128/AAC.01204-18.

72. Lipworth S, Hough N, Buchanan R, et al. Improved performance predicting clarithromycin resistance in Mycobacterium abscessus on an independent data set. Antimicrob Agents Chemother 2019;63(8). https://doi.org/10.1128/AAC.00400-19.

73. Aitken ML, Burke W, McDonald G, et al. Nontuberculous mycobacterial disease in adult cystic fibrosis patients. Research Support, U.S. Gov't, P.H.S. Chest 1993;103(4):1096–9.

74. Reynaud Q, Bricca R, Cavalli Z, et al. Risk factors for nontuberculous mycobacterial isolation in patients with cystic fibrosis: a meta-analysis. Pediatr Pulmonol 2020;55(10):2653–61.

75. Keating CL, Liu X, Dimango EA. Classic respiratory disease but atypical diagnostic testing distinguishes adult presentation of cystic fibrosis. Chest 2010;137(5):1157–63.

76. Nick JA, Chacon CS, Brayshaw SJ, et al. Effects of gender and age at diagnosis on disease progression in long-term survivors of cystic fibrosis. Am J Respir Crit Care Med 2010;182(5):614–26.

77. Ziedalski TM, Kao PN, Henig NR, et al. Prospective analysis of cystic fibrosis transmembrane regulator mutations in adults with bronchiectasis or pulmonary nontuberculous mycobacterial infection. Chest 2006;130(4):995–1002.

78. Kim JS, Tanaka N, Newell JD, et al. Nontuberculous mycobacterial infection: CT scan findings, genotype, and treatment responsiveness. Comp Study Chest. 2005;128(6):3863–9.

79. Jang MA, Kim SY, Jeong BH, et al. Association of CFTR gene variants with nontuberculous mycobacterial lung disease in a Korean population with a low prevalence of cystic fibrosis. J Hum Genet 2013;58(5):298–303.

80. Chalermskulrat W, Sood N, Neuringer IP, et al. Nontuberculous mycobacteria in end stage cystic fibrosis: implications for lung transplantation. Research Support, N.I.H., Extramural Support, 2006 Research Support, Non-U.S. Gov't. Thorax 2006;61(6):507–13.

81. Catherinot E, Roux AL, Vibet MA, et al. Mycobacterium avium and Mycobacterium abscessus complex target distinct cystic fibrosis patient subpopulations. Research Support, Non-U.S. Gov't. J cystic fibrosis 2013;12(1):74–80.

82. Burgel P, Morand P, Audureau E, et al. Azithromycin and the risk of nontuberculous mycobacteria in adults with cystic fibrosis. Conference Abstract. Pediatr Pulmonology 2011;46:328.

83. Ager S, O'Brien C, Spencer DA, et al. A retrospective review of non-tuberculous mycobacteria in paediatric cystic fibrosis patients at a regional centre. Conference Abstract. J Cystic Fibrosis 2011;10:S36.

84. Paugam A, Baixench M-T, Demazes-Dufeu N, et al. Characteristics and consequences of airway colonization by filamentous fungi in 201 adult patients with cystic fibrosis in France. Med Mycol 2010;48(Suppl 1):S32–6.

85. Bouso JM, Burns JJ, Amin R, et al. Household proximity to water and nontuberculous mycobacteria in children with cystic fibrosis. Pediatr Pulmonol 2017;52(3):324–30.

86. Mussaffi H, Rivlin J, Shalit I, et al. Nontuberculous mycobacteria in cystic fibrosis associated with allergic bronchopulmonary aspergillosis and steroid therapy. Eur Respir J 2005;25(2):324–8.

87. Evans JT, Ratnaraja N, Gardiner S, et al. Mycobacterium abscessus in cystic fibrosis: what does it all mean? Conference Abstract. Clin Microbiol Infect 2011;17:S602.

88. Caverly LJ, Zimbric M, Azar M, et al. Cystic fibrosis airway microbiota associated with outcomes of nontuberculous mycobacterial infection. ERJ Open Res 2021;7(2). https://doi.org/10.1183/23120541.00578-2020.

89. Falkinham JO 3rd. Surrounded by mycobacteria: nontuberculous mycobacteria in the human environment. J Appl Microbiol 2009;107(2):356–67.

90. Richter WJ, Sun Y, Psoter KJ, et al. Vitamin D deficiency is associated with increased nontuberculous mycobacteria risk in cystic fibrosis. Ann Am Thorac Soc 2021;18(5):913–6.

91. Renna M, Schaffner C, Brown K, et al. Azithromycin blocks autophagy and may predispose cystic fibrosis patients to mycobacterial infection. Research Support, Non-U.S. Gov't. J Clin Invest 2011;121(9):3554–63.

92. Binder AM, Adjemian J, Olivier KN, et al. Epidemiology of nontuberculous mycobacterial infections and associated chronic macrolide use among persons with cystic fibrosis. Am J Respir Crit Care Med 2013;188(7):807–12.

93. Coolen N, Morand P, Martin C, et al. Reduced risk of nontuberculous mycobacteria in cystic fibrosis adults receiving long-term azithromycin. J cystic fibrosis : official J Eur Cystic Fibrosis Soc 2015;14(5):594–9.

94. Cogen JD, Onchiri F, Emerson J, et al. Chronic azithromycin Use in cystic fibrosis and risk of

treatment-Emergent respiratory pathogens. Ann Am Thorac Soc 2018;15(6):702–9.

95. Catherinot E, Roux AL, Vibet MA, et al. Inhaled therapies, azithromycin and Mycobacterium abscessus in cystic fibrosis patients. Eur Respir J 2013; 41(5):1101–6.

96. Giron RM, Maiz L, Barrio I, et al. [Nontuberculous mycobacterial infection in patients with cystic fibrosis: a multicenter prevalence study]. Multicenter Study. Archivos de Bronconeumologia 2008;44(12):679–84. Estudio multicentrico de prevalencia de micobacterias ambientales en pacientes con fibrosis quistica.

97. Radhakrishnan DK, Yau Y, Corey M, et al. Nontuberculous mycobacteria in children with cystic fibrosis: isolation, prevalence, and predictors. Pediatr Pulmonology 2009;44(11):1100–6.

98. Prevots DR, Adjemian J, Fernandez AG, et al. Environmental risks for nontuberculous mycobacteria: individual exposures and climatic factors in the Cystic Fibrosis population. Ann Am Thorac Soc 2014. https://doi.org/10.1513/AnnalsATS.201404-184OC.

99. Lipner EM, Crooks JL, French J, et al. Nontuberculous mycobacterial infection and environmental molybdenum in persons with cystic fibrosis: a case-control study in Colorado. J Expo Sci Environ Epidemiol 2021. https://doi.org/10.1038/s41370-021-00360-2.

100. Foote SL, Lipner EM, Prevots DR, et al. Environmental predictors of pulmonary nontuberculous mycobacteria (NTM) sputum positivity among persons with cystic fibrosis in the state of Florida. PLoS One 2021;16(12):e0259964.

101. Adjemian J, Olivier KN, Seitz AE, et al. Spatial clusters of nontuberculous mycobacterial lung disease in the United States. Am J Respir Crit Care Med 2012. https://doi.org/10.1164/rccm.201205-0913OC.

102. Lipner EM, French J, Bern CR, et al. Nontuberculous mycobacterial disease and molybdenum in Colorado watersheds. Int J Environ Res Public Health 2020;17(11). https://doi.org/10.3390/ijerph17113854.

103. Lipner EM, French JP, Falkinham JO 3rd, et al. NTM infection risk and trace Metals in Surface water: a population-based Ecologic epidemiologic study in Oregon. Ann Am Thorac Soc 2021. https://doi.org/10.1513/AnnalsATS.202101-053OC.

104. Olivier KN, Weber DJ, Lee JH, et al. Nontuberculous mycobacteria. II: nested-cohort study of impact on cystic fibrosis lung disease. Research Support, Non-U.S. Gov't Research Support, U.S. Gov't, P.H.S. Am J Respir Crit Care Med 2003; 167(6):835–40.

105. Forslow U, Geborek A, Hjelte L, et al. Early chemotherapy for non-tuberculous mycobacterial infections in patients with cystic fibrosis. Acta Paediatr 2003;92(8):910–5.

106. Leitritz L, Griese M, Roggenkamp A, et al. Prospective study on nontuberculous mycobacteria in patients with and without cystic fibrosis. Comparative Study Support, 2004 Research Support, Non-U.S. Gov't. Med Microbiol Immunol 2004;193(4):209–17.

107. Martiniano SL, Sontag MK, Daley CL, et al. Clinical significance of a first positive nontuberculous mycobacteria culture in cystic fibrosis. Research Support, N.I.H., Extramural. Ann Am Thorac Soc 2014; 11(1):36–44.

108. Floto RA, Olivier KN, Saiman L, et al. US Cystic Fibrosis Foundation and European Cystic Fibrosis Society consensus recommendations for the management of non-tuberculous mycobacteria in individuals with cystic fibrosis. Thorax 2016;71(Suppl 1):i1–22.

109. Whittier S, Olivier K, Gilligan P, et al. Proficiency testing of clinical microbiology laboratories using modified decontamination procedures for detection of nontuberculous mycobacteria in sputum samples from cystic fibrosis patients. The Nontuberculous Mycobacteria in Cystic Fibrosis Study Group. Clinical Trial Multicenter, Multicenter Study Support, 1997 Research Support, Non-U.S. Gov't. J Clin Microbiol 1997;35(10):2706–8.

110. Bange FC, Bottger EC. Improved decontamination method for recovering mycobacteria from patients with cystic fibrosis. Eur J Clin Microbiol Infect Dis : official Publ Eur Soc Clin Microbiol 2002;21(7): 546–8.

111. Whittier S, Hopfer RL, Knowles MR, et al. Improved recovery of mycobacteria from respiratory secretions of patients with cystic fibrosis. J Clin Microbiol 1993;31(4):861–4.

112. Oliver A, Maiz L, Canton R, et al. Nontuberculous mycobacteria in patients with cystic fibrosis. Clin Infect Dis 2001;32(9):1298–303.

113. Steingart KR, Ng V, Henry M, et al. Sputum processing methods to improve the sensitivity of smear microscopy for tuberculosis: a systematic review. Lancet Infect Dis 2006;6(10):664–74.

114. Brown-Elliott BA, Griffith DE, Wallace RJ Jr. Diagnosis of nontuberculous mycobacterial infections. Clin Lab Med 2002;22(4):911–25, vi.

115. Wallace E, Hendrickson D, Tolli N, et al. Culturing mycobacteria. Methods Mol Biol 2021;2314:1–58.

116. Buijtels PC, Petit PL. Comparison of NaOH-N-acetyl cysteine and sulfuric acid decontamination methods for recovery of mycobacteria from clinical specimens. J Microbiol Methods 2005;62(1):83–8.

117. Bange FC, Kirschner P, Bottger EC. Recovery of mycobacteria from patients with cystic fibrosis. J Clin Microbiol 1999;37(11):3761–3.

118. Ferroni A, Vu-Thien H, Lanotte P, et al. Value of the chlorhexidine decontamination method for recovery of nontuberculous mycobacteria from sputum

samples of patients with cystic fibrosis. Eval Stud Support, Non-U.S. Gov't. J Clin Microbiol 2006; 44(6):2237–9.

119. Plongla R, Preece CL, Perry JD, et al. Evaluation of RGM medium for isolation of nontuberculous mycobacteria from respiratory samples from patients with cystic fibrosis in the United States. J Clin Microbiol 2017;55(5):1469–77.

120. Preece CL, Perry A, Gray B, et al. A novel culture medium for isolation of rapidly-growing mycobacteria from the sputum of patients with cystic fibrosis. J cystic fibrosis : official J Eur Cystic Fibrosis Soc 2016;15(2):186–91.

121. Buchan BW, Riebe KM, Timke M, et al. Comparison of MALDI-TOF MS with HPLC and nucleic acid sequencing for the identification of Mycobacterium species in cultures using solid medium and broth. Am J Clin Pathol 2014;141(1):25–34.

122. Clinical and Laboratory Standards Institute. Susceptibility testing of mycobacteria, Nocardia spp., and other aerobic actinomycetes. 3rd edition. Wayne, PA, USA: CLSI standard document M24; 2018.

123. Griffith DE, Aksamit T, Brown-Elliott BA, et al. An official ATS/IDSA statement: diagnosis, treatment, and prevention of nontuberculous mycobacterial diseases. Practice Guideline Review. Am J Respir Crit Care Med 2007;175(4):367–416.

124. Park Y, Park YE, Jhun BW, et al. Impact of susceptibility to Injectable Antibiotics on the treatment outcomes of Mycobacterium abscessus pulmonary disease. Open Forum Infect Dis 2021;8(6): ofab215. https://doi.org/10.1093/ofid/ofab215.

125. Nash KA, Brown-Elliott BA, Wallace RJ Jr. A novel gene, erm(41), confers inducible macrolide resistance to clinical isolates of Mycobacterium abscessus but is absent from Mycobacterium chelonae. Antimicrob Agents Chemother 2009;53(4): 1367–76.

126. Doucet-Populaire F, Buriankova K, Weiser J, et al. Natural and acquired macrolide resistance in mycobacteria. Curr Drug Targets Infect Disord 2002; 2(4):355–70.

127. Griffith DE, Brown-Elliott BA, Langsjoen B, et al. Clinical and molecular analysis of macrolide resistance in Mycobacterium avium complex lung disease. Am J Respir Crit Care Med 2006;174(8): 928–34.

128. Low D, Wilson DA, Flume PA. Screening practices for nontuberculous mycobacteria at US cystic fibrosis centers. J cystic fibrosis : official J Eur Cystic Fibrosis Soc 2020;19(4):569–74.

129. Verma N, Spencer D. Disseminated Mycobacterium gordonae infection in a child with cystic fibrosis. Pediatr Pulmonology 2012;47(5):517–8.

130. Segal E, Diez GS, Prokopio E, et al. [Nontuberculous mycobacteria in patients with cystic fibrosis].

131. Medicina 1998;58(3):257–61. Microbacterias no tuberculosas en pacientes con fibrosis quistica.

131. Esther CR Jr, Kerr A, Gilligan PH. Detection of Mycobacterium abscessus from deep pharyngeal swabs in cystic fibrosis. Infect Control Hosp Epidemiol 2015;36(5):618–9.

132. Ngan GJ, Ng LM, Jureen R, et al. Development of multiplex PCR assays based on the 16S-23S rRNA internal transcribed spacer for the detection of clinically relevant nontuberculous mycobacteria. Lett Appl Microbiol 2011;52(5):546–54.

133. Leung KL, Yip CW, Cheung WF, et al. Development of a simple and low-cost real-time PCR method for the identification of commonly encountered mycobacteria in a high throughput laboratory. J Appl Microbiol 2009;107(5):1433–9.

134. Devine M, Moore JE, Xu J, et al. Detection of mycobacterial DNA from sputum of patients with cystic fibrosis. Research Support, Non-U.S. Gov't. Irish J Med Sci 2004;173(2):96–8.

135. Mulherin D, Coffey MJ, Halloran DO, et al. Skin reactivity to atypical mycobacteria in cystic fibrosis. Research Support, Non-U.S. Gov't. Respir Med 1990;84(4):273–6.

136. Ferroni A, Sermet-Gaudelus I, Le Bourgeois M, et al. Measurement of immunoglobulin G against Mycobacterial antigen A60 in patients with cystic fibrosis and lung infection due to Mycobacterium abscessus. Research Support, Non-U.S. Gov't. Clin Infect Dis 2005;40(1):58–66.

137. Qvist T, Pressler T, Taylor-Robinson D, et al. Serodiagnosis of Mycobacterium abscessus complex infection in cystic fibrosis. Eur Respir J 2015; 46(3):707–16.

138. Qvist T, Johansen IS, Pressler T, et al. Urine lipoarabinomannan point-of-care testing in patients affected by pulmonary nontuberculous mycobacteria–experiences from the Danish Cystic Fibrosis cohort study. BMC Infect Dis 2014;14:655. https:// doi.org/10.1186/s12879-014-0655-4.

139. De P, Amin AG, Graham B, et al. Urine lipoarabinomannan as a marker for low-risk of NTM infection in the CF airway. J Cystic Fibrosis 2020. https://doi. org/10.1016/j.jcf.2020.06.016.

140. van Ingen J, Egelund EF, Levin A, et al. The pharmacokinetics and pharmacodynamics of pulmonary Mycobacterium avium complex disease treatment. Am J Respir Crit Care Med 2012. https://doi.org/10.1164/rccm.201204-0682OC.

141. Clement A, Tamalet A, Leroux E, et al. Long term effects of azithromycin in patients with cystic fibrosis: a double blind, placebo controlled trial. Multicenter Study. Randomized Controlled Trial. Support, 2006 Research Support, Non-U.S. Gov't. *Thorax.* 2006;61(10):895–902.

142. Equi A, Balfour-Lynn IM, Bush A, et al. Long term azithromycin in children with cystic fibrosis: a

randomised, placebo-controlled crossover trial. Clinical Trial Randomized Controlled Trial. Lancet 2002;360(9338):978–84.

143. Saiman L, Marshall BC, Mayer-Hamblett N, et al. Azithromycin in patients with cystic fibrosis chronically infected with Pseudomonas aeruginosa: a randomized controlled trial. JAMA 2003;290(13): 1749–56.

144. Wolter J, Seeney S, Bell S, et al. Effect of long term treatment with azithromycin on disease parameters in cystic fibrosis: a randomised trial. Clinical Trial Randomized Controlled Trial Support, 2002 Research Support, Non-U.S. Gov't. Thorax 2002; 57(3):212–6.

145. Wallace RJ Jr, Brown-Elliott BA, McNulty S, et al. Macrolide/Azalide therapy for nodular/bronchiectatic mycobacterium avium complex lung disease. Chest 2014;146(2):276–82.

146. Jeong BH, Jeon K, Park HY, et al. Intermittent antibiotic therapy for nodular bronchiectatic Mycobacterium avium complex lung disease. Am J Respir Crit Care Med 2015;191(1):96–103.

147. Gilljam M, Berning SE, Peloquin CA, et al. Therapeutic drug monitoring in patients with cystic fibrosis and mycobacterial disease. Case Reports Support, 1999 Research Support, Non-U.S. Gov't. Eur Respir J 1999;14(2):347–51.

148. Ebert DL, Olivier KN. Nontuberculous mycobacteria in the setting of cystic fibrosis. Review. Clin Chest Med 2002;23(3):655–63.

149. Cho YJ, Yi H, Chun J, et al. The genome sequence of 'Mycobacterium massiliense' strain CIP 108297 suggests the independent taxonomic status of the Mycobacterium abscessus complex at the subspecies level. PLoS One 2013;8(11):e81560.

150. Griffith DE, Daley CL. Treatment of Mycobacterium abscessus pulmonary disease. Chest 2022;161(1): 64–75.

151. Roux AL, Catherinot E, Soismier N, et al. Comparing Mycobacterium massiliense and Mycobacterium abscessus lung infections in cystic fibrosis patients. J cystic fibrosis : official J Eur Cystic Fibrosis Soc 2015;14(1):63–9.

152. Peloquin CA. Therapeutic drug monitoring in the treatment of tuberculosis. Drugs 2002;62(15): 2169–83.

153. Kearns GL, Trang JM. Introduction to pharmacokinetics: aminoglycosides in cystic fibrosis as a prototype. J Pediatr 1986;108(5 Pt 2):847–53.

154. de Groot R, Smith AL. Antibiotic pharmacokinetics in cystic fibrosis. Differences and clinical significance. Clin Pharmacokinet 1987;13(4):228–53.

155. Rey E, Treluyer JM, Pons G. Drug disposition in cystic fibrosis. Clin Pharmacokinet 1998;35(4): 313–29.

156. Martiniano SL, Wagner BD, Brennan L, et al. Pharmacokinetics of oral antimycobacterials and

dosing guidance for Mycobacterium avium complex treatment in cystic fibrosis. J cystic fibrosis : official J Eur Cystic Fibrosis Soc 2021. https://doi.org/10.1016/j.jcf.2021.04.011.

157. Waterer G. Beyond antibiotics for pulmonary nontuberculous mycobacterial disease. Curr Opin Pulm Med 2020;26(3):260–6.

158. Scott JP, Ji Y, Kannan M, et al. Inhaled granulocyte-macrophage colony-stimulating factor for Mycobacterium abscessus in cystic fibrosis. Eur Respir J 2018;51(4). https://doi.org/10.1183/13993003.02127-2017.

159. Olakanmi O, Britigan BE, Schlesinger LS. Gallium disrupts iron metabolism of mycobacteria residing within human macrophages. *Infection and immunity.* Oct 2000;68(10):5619–27.

160. Goldbart A, Gatt D, Golan Tripto I. Non-nuberculous mycobacteria infection treated with intermittently inhaled high-dose nitric oxide. BMJ Case Rep 2021;(10):14. https://doi.org/10.1136/bcr-2021-243979.

161. Dedrick RM, Guerrero-Bustamante CA, Garlena RA, et al. Engineered bacteriophages for treatment of a patient with a disseminated drug-resistant Mycobacterium abscessus. Nat Med 2019;25(5):730–3.

162. Dedrick RM, Freeman KG, Nguyen JA, et al. Potent antibody-mediated neutralization limits bacteriophage treatment of a pulmonary Mycobacterium abscessus infection. Nat Med 2021; 27(8):1357–61.

163. Jeon K, Kwon OJ, Lee NY, et al. Antibiotic treatment of Mycobacterium abscessus lung disease: a retrospective analysis of 65 patients. Am J Respir Crit Care Med 2009;180(9):896–902.

164. Jarand J, Levin A, Zhang L, et al. Clinical and microbiologic outcomes in patients receiving treatment for Mycobacterium abscessus pulmonary disease. Clin Infect Dis 2011;52(5):565–71.

165. Mitchell JD. Surgical approach to pulmonary nontuberculous mycobacterial infections. *Clin Chest Med* Mar 2015;36(1):117–22.

166. Saint GL, Thomas MF, Zainal Abidin N, et al. Treating nontuberculous mycobacteria in children with cystic fibrosis: a multicentre retrospective study. Arch Dis Child 2022;107(5):479–85.

167. Jonsson BE, Gilljam M, Lindblad A, et al. Molecular epidemiology of Mycobacterium abscessus, with focus on cystic fibrosis. Research Support, Non-U.S. Gov't. J Clin Microbiol 2007;45(5):1497–504.

168. Kavaliunaite E, Harris KA, Aurora P, et al. Outcome according to subspecies following lung transplantation in cystic fibrosis pediatric patients infected with Mycobacterium abscessus. Transpl Infect Dis : official J Transplant Soc 2020;22(3):e13274.

169. Taylor JL, Palmer SM. Mycobacterium abscessus chest wall and pulmonary infection in a cystic

fibrosis lung transplant recipient. Case Reports. J Heart Lung Transplant 2006;25(8):985–8.

170. Zaidi S, Elidemir O, Heinle JS, et al. Mycobacterium abscessus in cystic fibrosis lung transplant recipients: report of 2 cases and risk for recurrence. Case Reports. Transpl Infect Dis 2009; 11(3):243–8.

171. Sanguinetti M, Ardito F, Fiscarelli E, et al. Fatal pulmonary infection due to multidrug-resistant Mycobacterium abscessus in a patient with cystic fibrosis. J Clin Microbiol 2001;39(2):816–9.

172. Zaidi S, Elidemir O, Heinle JS, et al. Mycobacterium abscessus in cystic fibrosis lung transplant recipients: report of 2 cases and risk for recurrence. Transpl Infect Dis : official J Transplant Soc 2009; 11(3):243–8.

173. Gilljam M, Schersten H, Silverborn M, et al. Lung transplantation in patients with cystic fibrosis and Mycobacterium abscessus infection. Case Reports Support, 2010 Research Support, Non-U.S. Gov't. J cystic fibrosis : official J Eur Cystic Fibrosis Soc 2010;9(4):272–6.

174. Perez AA, Singer JP, Schwartz BS, et al. Management and clinical outcomes after lung transplantation in patients with pre-transplant Mycobacterium abscessus infection: a single center experience. Transpl Infect Dis : official J Transplant Soc 2019; 21(3):e13084.

175. Flume PA, Egan TM, Paradowski LJ, et al. Infectious complications of lung transplantation. Impact of cystic fibrosis. Am J Respir Crit Care Med 1994; 149(6):1601–7.

176. Lobo LJ, Chang LC, Esther CR Jr, et al. Lung transplant outcomes in cystic fibrosis patients with preoperative Mycobacterium abscessus respiratory infections. Clin Transpl 2013;27(4):523–9.

177. Qvist T, Pressler T, Thomsen VO, et al. Nontuberculous mycobacterial disease is not a contraindication to lung transplantation in patients with cystic fibrosis: a retrospective analysis in a Danish patient population. Transpl Proc 2013;45(1):342–5.

178. Raats D, Lorent N, Saegeman V, et al. Successful lung transplantation for chronic Mycobacterium abscessus infection in advanced cystic fibrosis, a case series. Transpl Infect Dis 2019;21(2): e13046.

179. Robinson PD, Harris KA, Aurora P, et al. Paediatric lung transplant outcomes vary with Mycobacterium abscessus complex species. Eur Respir J 2013; 41(5):1230–2.

180. Friedman DZP, Cervera C, Halloran K, et al. Nontuberculous mycobacteria in lung transplant recipients: prevalence, risk factors, and impact on survival and chronic lung allograft dysfunction. Transpl Infect Dis 2020;22(2):e13229.

181. Weill D, Benden C, Corris PA, et al. A consensus document for the selection of lung transplant candidates: 2014–an update from the pulmonary transplantation Council of the international society for Heart and lung transplantation. J Heart Lung Transplant 2015;34(1):1–15.

182. Watkins RR, Lemonovich TL. Evaluation of infections in the lung transplant patient. Curr Opin Infect Dis 2012;25(2):193–8.

183. Tissot A, Thomas MF, Corris PA, et al. NonTuberculous Mycobacteria infection and lung transplantation in cystic fibrosis: a worldwide survey of clinical practice. BMC Pulm Med 2018;18(1):86.

184. Ramos KJ, Smith PJ, McKone EF, et al. Lung transplant referral for individuals with cystic fibrosis: cystic Fibrosis Foundation consensus guidelines. J cystic fibrosis : official J Eur Cystic Fibrosis Soc 2019;18(3):321–33.

185. Bange FC, Brown BA, Smaczny C, et al. Lack of transmission of mycobacterium abscessus among patients with cystic fibrosis attending a single clinic. Clin Infect Dis 2001;32(11):1648–50.

186. Harris KA, Kenna DTD, Blauwendraat C, et al. Molecular Fingerprinting of Mycobacterium abscessus strains in a cohort of pediatric cystic fibrosis patients. J Clin Microbiol 2012;50(5): 1758–61.

187. Aitken ML, Limaye A, Pottinger P, et al. Respiratory outbreak of Mycobacterium abscessus subspecies massiliense in a lung transplant and cystic fibrosis center. Letter. Am J Respir Crit Care Med 2012; 185(2):231–2.

188. Wetzstein N, Kohl TA, Schultze TG, et al. Antimicrobial susceptibility and Phylogenetic Relations in a German cohort infected with Mycobacterium abscessus. J Clin Microbiol 2020;58(12). https://doi.org/10.1128/JCM.01813-20.

189. Harris KA, Underwood A, Kenna DT, et al. Whole-genome sequencing and epidemiological analysis do not provide evidence for cross-transmission of mycobacterium abscessus in a cohort of pediatric cystic fibrosis patients. Clin Infect Dis 2015;60(7): 1007–16.

190. Saiman L, Siegel JD, LiPuma JJ, et al. Infection prevention and control guideline for cystic fibrosis: 2013 update. Infect Control Hosp Epidemiol 2014; 35(1 Suppl).

191. Gross JE, Nick JA, Martiniano SL. Prevention of transmission of Mycobacterium abscessus among patients with cystic fibrosis. Curr Opin Pulm Med 2019. https://doi.org/10.1097/MCP.0000000000000621.

192. Gross JE, Caceres S, Poch K, et al. Healthcare-associated links in transmission of nontuberculous mycobacteria among people with cystic fibrosis (HALT NTM) study: Rationale and study design. PLoS One 2021;16(12):e0261628.

193. Gross JE, Caceres S, Poch K, et al. Investigating nontuberculous mycobacteria transmission at the

Colorado adult cystic fibrosis program. Am J Respir Crit Care Med 2022. https://doi.org/10.1164/rccm.202108-1911OC.

194. Davidson RM, Nick SE, Kammlade SM, et al. Genomic analysis of a hospital-associated outbreak of Mycobacterium abscessus: implications on transmission. J Clin Microbiol 2021;JCM0154721. https://doi.org/10.1128/JCM.01547-21.

195. Ballarino GJ, Olivier KN, Claypool RJ, et al. Pulmonary nontuberculous mycobacterial infections: antibiotic treatment and associated costs. Respir Med 2009;103(10):1448–55.

Non-Modulator Therapies
Developing a Therapy for Every Cystic Fibrosis Patient

Marie E. Egan, MD

KEYWORDS

- Cystic fibrosis • Gene therapy • Gene editing • Messenger RNA • Premature termination codon
- Read through agents • Antisense oligonucleotide

KEY POINTS

- For patients with premature termination codon (PTC) mutations, there is hope that developing read-through agents will result in new therapeutics that will restore Cystic fibrosis transmembrane conductance regulator (CFTR) function for this group of patients.
- For cystic fibrosis (CF) patients with PTC mutations, large deletions, insertions, and frameshifts, genetic-based therapies may be needed to restore CFTR function.
- Genetic-based therapies for CF include ribonucleic acid (RNA) therapies, deoxyribonucleic acid (DNA) therapies, and gene editing technologies.
- Delivery of nucleic acid therapies to targeted tissues is a major challenge for these approaches.

INTRODUCTION

Over the last decade, the development of cystic fibrosis transmembrane conductance regulator (CFTR) modulator therapy for people with cystic fibrosis (CF) has refocused our clinical treatment plans from providing supportive care by treating the complications of living with nonfunctional CFTR to treating the underlying defect by restoring function to mutant CFTR. There is incredible hope that these new medications will improve patients' long-term outcomes.[1–3] These therapies which are composed of one to three small molecules, optimize the function of the patients' endogenous mutant CFTR, which results in restoration of CFTR channel function.[1,2,4–6] Although highly effective modulators are available for approximately 85% of individuals with CF, it is unlikely that these therapies will provide life-altering therapy for all. For approximately 10% to 12% of CF patients with premature termination codon (PTC) mutations, modulator therapies alone are unlikely to be of significant benefit because these individuals do not produce a CFTR protein to modulate, potentiate, or optimize. In addition to the PTC mutations, there are other rare CFTR mutations such as large deletions, insertions, and frameshifts that produce no CFTR protein, so they are not amenable to modulator therapy (**Fig. 1**). Clearly, there is a need to develop non-modulator therapies for these CF patient populations.

For patients with PTC mutations, there are small molecules under development that are designed to allow for read-04through of the PTC resulting in a full-length CFTR protein. This approach will be discussed briefly, but the major focus of this article is genetic-based therapies that include RNA therapies, DNA therapies, and gene editing technologies to treat mutations that are not responsive to modulator therapy. Although several of these genetic-based nucleic acid therapies are mutation agnostic so they will benefit all patients with CF, the development of nucleic acid therapies is essential for patients whose mutations are not amenable to modulator therapy and for those who do not tolerate modulator therapy due to

Division of Pulmonary Allergy Immunology Sleep Medicine, Department of Pediatrics, Pediatric Pulmonary Allergy Immunology and Sleep Medicine, Yale Cystic Fibrosis Center, School of Medicine, Yale University, 333 Cedar Street, PO Box 208064, New Haven, CT 06520, USA
E-mail address: marie.egan@yale.edu

Clin Chest Med 43 (2022) 717–725
https://doi.org/10.1016/j.ccm.2022.06.011
0272-5231/22/© 2022 Elsevier Inc. All rights reserved.

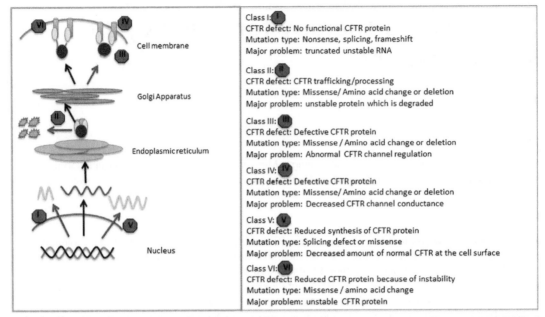

Fig. 1. CFTR mutation classes. I: Class I mutations Gly542X, Trp1282X, II: Class II mutations Phe508del, Asn1303Lys, III: Class III Gly551Asp, Gly551Ser, IV: Class IV mutations ArgR117His, Arg347Pro, V: Class V mutations 3849+10kbC>T,5T, and VI: Class VI mutations Gln1412X, 4279insA.

side effects. Currently, genetic-based therapies are in clinical use for several medical conditions such as spinal muscular atrophy (SMA) and retinal dystrophy; however, they are only in preclinical realm for CF. There are several important challenges, including delivery of these therapeutics to the cells most affected by the lack of CFTR, which will need to be addressed if we are to harness the power of these emerging therapies for the treatment of CF.[7–12] Ultimately, certain nucleic acid therapies could be given once in a lifetime and lead to a permanent cure.

Read Through Agents: Small Molecules for Premature Termination Codon Mutations

Many CF patients who do not respond to modulator therapy have Class 1 mutations where CFTR protein and function are absent. Most Class 1 mutations are PTC mutations. A PTC mutation occurs when there is point mutation in the genetic code that introduces one of three termination codons (uracil adenine adenine, uracil adenine guanine or uracil guanine adenine) into CFTR instead of coding for an amino acid. Subsequently, during translation of mRNA, the PTC signals for termination of protein synthesis resulting in a truncated nonfunctional CFTR protein that is unstable and quickly degraded. In addition, messenger RNA (mRNA) abundance and stability are markedly reduced due to nonsense-mediated RNA decay,

which eliminates abnormal transcripts that could produce truncated proteins.[13–15] The potential for "reading through" of a PTC in CFTR during translation was first shown by Bedwell and colleagues, when treating cultured CF airway epithelial cells that carried W1282X, with gentamicin, a ribosomal binding antibiotic.[16] Certain aminoglycosides such as gentamicin alter the fidelity of ribosomal translation allowing for insertion of a tRNA into the ribosomal acceptor site, thus adding an amino acid to the polypeptide chain instead of signaling for the termination complex.[13] Subsequently, Kerem and colleagues showed topical administration to the nasal epithelium of patients with PTC mutations improved nasal potential difference measurements (assessment of CFTR function in the nasal epithelium) but has no effect on those homozygous for F508del.[17] Although these studies have been instrumental for the proof of concept that pharmacologic read through for PTC mutations in CF is possible, there are significant difficulties that limit gentamicin's development as a "read through" agent due to its low-efficiency, off-target effects and potential toxicity when delivered systemically on a chronic basis.[13] However, medicinal chemists have improved the efficiency and decreased the potential toxicity and side effects of these drugs to develop the next generation of aminoglycoside-derived read through agents including ELX-02 which is in clinical trials for patients who carry the G542X mutation[18]

(NCT04135495, NCT04126473). The early results are encouraging, however it is important to interpret results cautiously as a previous non-aminoglycoside agent that was developed to treat PTC mutations, Ataluren seemed very promising in phase 2 clinical trials in both pediatric and adult patients with CF but in later studies showed that no significant differences in clinical outcomes were observed.[13,19]

The Power of RNA as a Therapeutic

RNA is a single-stranded nucleic acid that is composed of nucleotide bases with a ribose phosphate backbone, it is essential for many cell functions including regulating gene expression, protein synthesis, and the transfer of amino acids. There are several RNA molecules that are being examined for their therapeutic potential in CF including, transfer RNA (tRNA) that may benefit patients with nonsense mutations, small RNA oligonucleotides that could be most beneficial to patients with splicing mutations, and mRNA that should help all patients regardless of mutation.

Engineered tRNAs are being developed as a therapeutic approach to overcome nonsense mutations. As mentioned above, during normal protein production, mRNA is decoded by the ribosome and the message is translated into a protein. This process requires tRNAs which are specialized RNAs that couple with the mRNA and ferry the amino acids, the building blocks of proteins, the ribosome to allow for the elongation of the peptide, and the developing protein. When there is a nonsense mutation in the mRNA, instead of a tRNA delivering an amino acid to the ribosome, the termination complex is assembled to stop protein production. Engineered tRNAs are designed to introduce an amino acid to an elongating peptide overriding the signal of a stop codon[20] and the peptide continues to be made. In preclinical studies, several investigators have shown this approach can promote read through of stop codons in cultured CF airway epithelial cells leading to full-length CFTR protein.[20] A significant challenge to this approach will be delivery of the tRNAs to the targeted cell populations.

Antisense oligonucleotides (ASOs) are small pieces (30–60 nucleotides) of single strand RNA that are designed and synthesized to either block/interfere with mRNA production or enable mRNA degradation or enhance mRNA production.[11] Although there have been many clinical trials exploring the clinical potential of ASOs, only a few medications have received FDA approval, most notable for SMA and muscular dystrophy.[7,11] Eluforsen, a 33 oligonucleotide ASO, was

developed to treat the F508del CFTR mutation. This small molecule showed promise in preclinical studies demonstrating increased CFTR function, but when the efficacy of this agent was tested in a phase 2 clinical trial, there was no evidence of increased CFTR activity or clinical benefit in CF subjects.[21–24] To date, none of the FDA-approved ASO RNA drugs are designed nor efficacious for CF.

How else might ASOs be used in CF? Patients carrying splice site mutations might benefit from ASOs.[7,25,26] Splice site mutations, such as 3489C > G + 10 KB, introduce a cryptic site that leads to splicing and an aberrant mRNA and nonfunctional protein. Investigational teams are developing ASOs to block the cryptic splice site so that normal mRNA is produced and full-length CFTR protein is produced and functional. When cultured and primary airway epithelial cells were treated with these ASOs in the laboratory, CFTR is correctly spliced and normal protein is produced. In addition, CFTR function is restored to normal. Clinical trials are expected to begin within the year. A major advantage of this RNA approach is that they can be delivered without a complex delivery system.

To restore CFTR function by delivering mRNA, mRNA needs to be delivered to critical cell types. Delivery will be difficult for multiple reasons including the large size of the mRNA molecule which requires unique delivery systems that will be able to protect and facilitate its delivery.[10,27] Once mRNA is delivered, it will need to be able to be recognized by the protein assembly apparatus in the cell so that the blueprint, mRNA, will be properly deciphered resulting in full-length CFTR proteins which traffic to the cell surface. Clearly, this is a complex process with multiple check points and choke points that must be overcome. Several clinical trials investigating the potential of mRNA therapy for the treatment of CF respiratory disease have been completed recently. In the clinical trials, MRT5005 a specialized lipid nanoparticle carrying CFTR mRNA was aerosolized and inhaled into the lung and lung function was measured before and after treatment.[28] Although preliminary results demonstrated improvement in forced expiratory volume in 1 second demonstrating that mRNA may be a viable therapy for CF, subsequent studies failed to replicate the lung function improvement observed previously. This situation serves as a reminder of how difficult it is to move a promising agent across the therapeutic finish line.

To summarize, there are several RNA approaches that have potential as therapeutics in CF. However, there are challenges that will need to be overcome before these approaches become clinical treatments. The challenges include efficient delivery of the therapeutic agent to critical tissues; ensuring there is RNA stability so that there is longevity to the treatment; and understanding the potential off-target effects and toxicity.[11]

Gene Transfer: A Mutation Agnostic Approach to Treatment

Gene therapy, also known as gene transfer or addition, is not a new idea for the CF community as it was introduced in 1989, the year the gene was identified. Multiple clinical trials were undertaken to deliver CFTR to airway cells, but none led to the significant correction of CF pathology.[29–36] The last large gene therapy clinical trial for CF was conducted by the UK consortium in 2014.[12,37–39] Although the nonviral vector delivery of CFTR was safe and well tolerated, the efficacy was very modest which was likely related to inefficient delivery of the gene therapy particles to the airway cells.

Today, gene therapy fits into a larger regenerative medicine umbrella. The FDA has approved gene therapeutic agents for several diseases including certain cancers,[40,41] thalassemia,[42–44] inherited blindness,[45,46] and SMA type 1.[47–49] In many of these successes, the gene therapy vector is delivered to a single cell type or a limited body area which can be contrasted to the needs of a patient with CF in whom multiple organs tissues and cell types will need to be targeted. Delivery remains to be the biggest challenge and has been the major focus of research efforts. Developing high-efficiency vectors that can improve delivery of the CFTR gene to the necessary cells is of utmost importance.

Gene Editing: Many Approaches and Rapidly Evolving Technologies

With gene editing approaches, the endogenous CFTR mutation is repaired or corrected.[7,8] There are a variety of gene editing technologies/tools that can be used to accomplish an edit of a patient's gene to correct the CFTR mutation.[50] Gene editing technologies including clustered regularly interspaced short palindromic repeats (CRISPR)/CRISPR-associated (Cas),[51] zinc-finger nucleases (ZFNs),[52–56] transcription activator-like effector nucleases,[57] and triplex forming peptide nucleic acid (PNA)/DNA[58,59] have been applied to CFTR. All of these technologies rely on DNA repair pathways and are designed to identify the region of CFTR that contains the disease-causing mutation. Reagents are developed to target a specific

mutation of interest and then use exogenous or endogenous nucleases to trigger recombination and repair of DNA. For instance, Crane and colleagues showed ZFNs could correct F508del-CFTR and restore CFTR function in induced pluripotent stem cells.[56] Triplex-forming PNAs have been designed to correct the human CFTR mutations and murine CFTR mutations.[59–61] PNA/DNA delivered to cells via polymeric nanoparticles to CF airway epithelial cells restored CFTR function in CF-affected airway cells with a variety of disease-causing mutations including W1282X, G542X, and the F508del.[59–61] In addition, PNA/DNA nanoparticles were delivered in vivo by inhalation in mouse models of CF[60] leading to partial restoration of CFTR function in respiratory tracts.

There are many examples of CRISPR/Cas technology used to correct mutant CFTR. The first example to demonstrate the power of this approach showed restored function in intestinal organoids, cells obtained from CF patients via rectal biopsy, and grown in culture.[51] In these experiments, intestinal organoids were treated with CRISPR/Cas9 editing tools to correct the CFTR mutation, and then CFTR activity in the treated organoids was compared with that of the untreated organoids using a swelling assay. Significant CFTR function was observed in the treated organoids demonstrating restoration of CFTR function. This field of investigations is rapidly evolving and now there are CRSPR-based or derived technologies that allow for more sophisticated approaches to editing such as base editors and prime editors. Base editing allows for the modification of a single nucleotide after a small single-stranded loop is created in the double-stranded DNA with a specialized Cas9 that is enzymatically inactive.[62] Prime editors are recently developed Cas9-derived agents that allow for modification of more than a single base pair. They are highly efficient but require very specialized packaging systems to allow for the delivery of the specialized Cas9 and the engineered guide RNA with fusion to a reverse transcriptase.[62] Presently, there are ongoing clinical trials exploring the potential of these approaches for the treatment of a variety of human diseases including cancer, sickle cell disease, and inherited retinal diseases, but not for CF.

Cell-Based Therapy

Cell-based therapies correct a gene defect ex vivo, and then corrected cells are returned to the patient. This approach has been a very effective cancer therapy such as chimeric antigen receptor T cell therapy,[40,41] and for epidermolysis bullosa, a rare skin disease.[63–65] To be a viable option for CF, CF-affected basal cells or stem cells would need to be corrected using one of the gene editing or gene transfer technologies in the laboratory, ex vivo. Subsequently, the corrected cells would be delivered to the appropriate organ of interest such as the lung, where they would need to function properly.[66–69] This approach is quite powerful as it corrects mutations in stem cells which are self-renewing, thus a single treatment could result in a permanent solution. Vaidyanathan and colleagues demonstrated that his may be viable option when they treated primary CF airway basal cells with Cas9 delivered by adeno-associated viral vectors to correct the F508del CFTR gene defect ex vivo. Then, purified corrected basal cells were delivered

into the sinus cavity of a rat to see if they would engraft and grow into proper sinus cells. Results showed that they were able to engraft, differentiate, and had normal CFTR function. These data demonstrate the promise and potential of cell-based therapy.[70] However, this approach is many years away from being a CF clinical therapy. There are many questions that need to be answered such as how many stems cells will need to be generated for an effective treatment, will cells engraft into appropriate tissue niches, and will it occur without impediments. It is also unknown if these gene corrected stem cells are at risk for increased somatic mutations which could lead to unexpected consequences such as premature aging or cancer development. Also, we need to understand the

Table 1
Summary of the approaches to treat cystic fibrosis patients who are not responsive to modulator therapy

Therapy	How Does It Work	Target Audience	Challenges
Read-through agents 17,19,80-81	Addition of an amino acid instead of the premature termination of translation	Premature stop codons (nonsense mutations)	Overcoming possible consequences of nonsense-mediated decay, unclear if the amino acid substitution will lead to a fully functioning protein, daily/repeat administration needed
Engineered tRNAs[20]	A nonsense suppressing anticodon is delivered to overcome the premature termination of translation	Premature stop codons (nonsense mutations)	Effective delivery to specific cells, repeat administration needed
mRNA therapy[11,28,76]	Deliver CFTR mRNA which can lead to synthesis of functional CFTR protein	Mutation agnostic	Effective delivery to specific cells, repeat administration needed
Oligonucleotides[21–25]	Designed nucleotides delivered to restore/normalize mutant mRNA	Mutation specific	Effective delivery to specific cells, repeat administration needed
Gene transfer/addition[38,39,62,79]	Deliver a copy of the CFTR cDNA which will lead to synthesis of functional CFTR protein	Mutation agnostic	Effective delivery to specific cells, repeat administration needed
Gene editing therapies[7,51,56,57,62,79,80]	Repair the mutation via nuclease activity in conjunction with cDNA guide	Mutation specific	Effective delivery to specific cells, repeat administration needed
Cell-based therapies[54,56,67,70]	Stem cells undergo gene editing ex vivo and then are reintroduced to the patient for engraftment	Mutation specific	Effective engraftment of corrected cells to the airways in a safe and effective manner, repeat administration needed

longevity of corrected stem cells, that is, how many new generations of corrected cells will be produced and will all expected cell types be generated.

Challenges Ahead: Delivery and Beyond

There are many novel nucleic acid approaches being developed to overcome mutations in CFTR (**Table1**). Advances in the nucleic acid therapeutic field make these approaches much more feasible than they were in the past. However, high-efficiency vectors that can improve delivery of the CFTR gene, mRNA, tRNA, or gene editing components to affected cells are needed but remain elusive. Vectors or delivery systems can be derived from viruses or composed of lipids (lipid nanoparticles) or polymers (polymeric nanoparticles).[71–76] Investigators are developing high-throughput approaches that are designed to identify the best particles for topical as well as systemic delivery thus targeting all the tissues affected in CF.[77,78] There are additional challenges and questions that need to be answered before these approaches enter the clinical realm including potential off-target effects. Also, we will need to define treatment success, that is how much CFTR function needs to be restored to be clinically impactful and what are the most reliable biomarkers to track potential success. Last, what are the safety signals that should be followed .

CLINICS CARE POINTS

- Individuals with cystic fibrosis (CF) who are homozygous for premature stop codon mutations, frameshift mutations, and large deletions or insertions will not benefit from highly effective modulator therapy.

- Nucleic acid-based therapies hold promise for CF patients who are homozygous for premature stop codon mutations, frameshift mutations, and large deletions or insertions and who will not benefit from highly effective modulator therapy; however, at the present time, these approaches are not in clinical use for CF.

- Delivery of nucleic acid therapies remains a major obstacle to bringing these therapies to the clinic.

DISCLOSURE

Dr M.E. Egan has no commercial or financial conflicts. She conducts research that focuses on nucleic acid therapy for cystic fibrosis and is funded by the Cystic Fibrosis Foundation, NIH.

REFERENCES

1. Middleton PG, Mall MA, Drevinek P, et al. Elexacaftor-Tezacaftor-Ivacaftor for Cystic Fibrosis with a Single Phe508del Allele. N Engl J Med 2019;381: 1809–19.

2. Keating D, Marigowda G, Burr L, et al. VX-445-Tezacaftor-Ivacaftor in Patients with Cystic Fibrosis and One or Two Phe508del Alleles. N Engl J Med 2018;379:1612–20.

3. Heijerman HGM, McKone EF, Downey DG, et al. Efficacy and safety of the elexacaftor plus tezacaftor plus ivacaftor combination regimen in people with cystic fibrosis homozygous for the F508del mutation: a double-blind, randomised, phase 3 trial. Lancet 2019;394:1940–8.

4. Harrison MJ, Murphy DM, Plant BJ. Ivacaftor in a G551D homozygote with cystic fibrosis. N Engl J Med 2013;369:1280–2.

5. Davies JC, Moskowitz SM, Brown C, et al. VX-659-Tezacaftor-Ivacaftor in Patients with Cystic Fibrosis and One or Two Phe508del Alleles. N Engl J Med 2018;379:1599–611.

6. Rowe SM, Daines C, Ringshausen FC, et al. Tezacaftor-Ivacaftor in residual-function heterozygotes with cystic fibrosis. N Engl J Med 2017;377: 2024–35.

7. Christopher Boyd A, Guo S, Huang L, et al. Hart SL: new approaches to genetic therapies for cystic fibrosis. J Cyst Fibros 2020;19(Suppl 1):S54–9.

8. Hodges CA, Conlon RA. Delivering on the promise of gene editing for cystic fibrosis. Genes Dis 2019; 6:97–108.

9. Mention K, Santos L, Harrison PT. Gene and base editing as a therapeutic option for cystic fibrosis-learning from other diseases. Genes (Basel) 2019; 10:387.

10. Pranke I, Golec A, Hinzpeter A, et al. Emerging therapeutic approaches for cystic fibrosis. From gene editing to personalized medicine. Front Pharmacol 2019;10:121.

11. Sasaki S, Guo S. Nucleic acid therapies for cystic fibrosis. Nucleic Acid Ther 2018;28:1–9.

12. Griesenbach U, Davies JC, Alton E. Cystic fibrosis gene therapy: a mutation-independent treatment. Curr Opin Pulm Med 2016;22:602–9.

13. Sharma J, Du M, Wong E, et al. A small molecule that induces translational readthrough of CFTR nonsense mutations by eRF1 depletion. Nat Commun 2021;12:4358.

14. Linde L, Boelz S, Neu-Yilik G, et al. The efficiency of nonsense-mediated mRNA decay is an inherent character and varies among different cells. Eur J Hum Genet 2007;15:1156–62.

15. Linde L, Boelz S, Nissim-Rafinia M, et al. Nonsense-mediated mRNA decay affects nonsense transcript levels and governs response

of cystic fibrosis patients to gentamicin. J Clin Invest 2007;117:683–92.

16. Howard M, Frizzell RA, Bedwell DM. Aminoglycoside antibiotics restore CFTR function by overcoming premature stop mutations. Nat Med 1996; 2:467–9.

17. Wilschanski M, Yahav Y, Yaacov Y, et al. Gentamicin-induced correction of CFTR function in patients with cystic fibrosis and CFTR stop mutations. N Engl J Med 2003;349:1433–41.

18. Leubitz A, Frydman-Marom A, Sharpe N, et al. Safety, tolerability, and pharmacokinetics of single ascending doses of ELX-02, a potential treatment for genetic disorders caused by nonsense mutations, in healthy volunteers. Clin Pharmacol Drug Dev 2019;8:984–94.

19. Kerem E, Konstan MW, De Boeck K, et al. Ataluren for the treatment of nonsense-mutation cystic fibrosis: a randomised, double-blind, placebo-controlled phase 3 trial. Lancet Respir Med 2014; 2:539–47.

20. Lueck JD, Yoon JS, Perales-Puchalt A, et al. Engineered transfer RNAs for suppression of premature termination codons. Nat Commun 2019;10:822.

21. Beumer W, Swildens J, Leal T, et al. Evaluation of eluforsen, a novel RNA oligonucleotide for restoration of CFTR function in in vitro and murine models of p.Phe508del cystic fibrosis. PLoS One 2019;14: e0219182.

22. Brinks V, Lipinska K, de Jager M, et al. The cystic fibrosis-like airway surface layer is not a significant barrier for delivery of eluforsen to airway epithelial cells. J Aerosol Med Pulm Drug Deliv 2019;32: 303–16.

23. Drevinek P, Pressler T, Cipolli M, et al. Antisense oligonucleotide eluforsen is safe and improves respiratory symptoms in F508DEL cystic fibrosis. J Cyst Fibros 2020;19:99–107.

24. Sermet-Gaudelus I, Clancy JP, Nichols DP, et al. Antisense oligonucleotide eluforsen improves CFTR function in F508del cystic fibrosis. J Cyst Fibros 2019;18:536–42.

25. Oren YS, Pranke IM, Kerem B, et al. The suppression of premature termination codons and the repair of splicing mutations in CFTR. Curr Opin Pharmacol 2017;34:125–31.

26. Chiba-Falek O, Kerem E, Shoshani T, et al. The molecular basis of disease variability among cystic fibrosis patients carrying the 3849+10 kb C-->T mutation. Genomics 1998;53:276–83.

27. Robinson E, MacDonald KD, Slaughter K, et al. Lipid nanoparticle-delivered chemically modified mRNA restores chloride secretion in cystic fibrosis. Mol Ther 2018;26:2034–46.

28. zuckerman JMK, Schechter MS, Dorgan D, et al. Safety and tolerability of a single dose of MRT5005, an inhaled CFTR MRNA therapeutic in adult CF patients. Pediatr Pulmonology 2019;54: 350.

29. Grubb BR, Pickles RJ, Ye H, et al. Inefficient gene transfer by adenovirus vector to cystic fibrosis airway epithelia of mice and humans. Nature 1994; 371:802–6.

30. Boucher RC, Knowles MR, Johnson LG, et al. Gene therapy for cystic fibrosis using E1-deleted adenovirus: a phase I trial in the nasal cavity. The University of North Carolina at Chapel Hill. Hum Gene Ther 1994;5:615–39.

31. Fisher KJ, Choi H, Burda J, et al. Recombinant adenovirus deleted of all viral genes for gene therapy of cystic fibrosis. Virology 1996;217:11–22.

32. Engelhardt JF, Simon RH, Yang Y, et al. Adenovirus-mediated transfer of the CFTR gene to lung of nonhuman primates: biological efficacy study. Hum Gene Ther 1993;4:759–69.

33. Zabner J, Couture LA, Gregory RJ, et al. Adenovirus-mediated gene transfer transiently corrects the chloride transport defect in nasal epithelia of patients with cystic fibrosis. Cell 1993;75:207–16.

34. Welsh MJ, Smith AE, Zabner J, et al. Cystic fibrosis gene therapy using an adenovirus vector: in vivo safety and efficacy in nasal epithelium. Hum Gene Ther 1994;5:209–19.

35. Wagner JA, Nepomuceno IB, Messner AH, et al. A phase II, double-blind, randomized, placebo-controlled clinical trial of tgAAVCF using maxillary sinus delivery in patients with cystic fibrosis with antrostomies. Hum Gene Ther 2002;13:1349–59.

36. Wagner JA, Moran ML, Messner AH, et al. A phase I/II study of tgAAV-CF for the treatment of chronic sinusitis in patients with cystic fibrosis. Hum Gene Ther 1998;9:889–909.

37. Alton EW, Boyd AC, Cheng SH, et al. A randomised, double-blind, placebo-controlled phase IIB clinical trial of repeated application of gene therapy in patients with cystic fibrosis. Thorax 2013;68:1075–7.

38. Alton E, Armstrong DK, Ashby D, et al. Repeated nebulisation of non-viral CFTR gene therapy in patients with cystic fibrosis: a randomised, double-blind, placebo-controlled, phase 2b trial. Lancet Respir Med 2015;3:684–91.

39. Alton EW, Boyd AC, Porteous DJ, et al. A phase I/IIa safety and efficacy study of Nebulized liposome-mediated gene therapy for cystic fibrosis supports a Multidose trial. Am J Respir Crit Care Med 2015; 192:1389–92.

40. Yang X, Wang GX, Zhou JF. CAR T cell therapy for hematological malignancies. Curr Med Sci 2019; 39:874–82.

41. Gourd E. CAR T-cell cocktail therapy for B-cell malignancies. Lancet Oncol 2019;20:e669.

42. Karponi G, Zogas N. Gene therapy for beta-thalassemia: Updated perspectives. Appl Clin Genet 2019;12:167–80.

43. Harrison C. First gene therapy for beta-thalassemia approved. Nat Biotechnol 2019;37: 1102–3.

44. Stower H. Gene therapy for beta thalassemia. Nat Med 2018;24:1781.

45. Bennett J. Gene therapy for color blindness. N Engl J Med 2009;361:2483–4.

46. Bennett J, Wellman J, Marshall KA, et al. Safety and durability of effect of contralateral-eye administration of AAV2 gene therapy in patients with childhood-onset blindness caused by RPE65 mutations: a follow-on phase 1 trial. Lancet 2016; 388:661–72.

47. Sheridan C. Gene therapy rescues newborns with spinal muscular atrophy. Nat Biotechnol 2018;36: 669–70.

48. Mendell JR, Al-Zaidy S, Shell R, et al. Single-dose gene-replacement therapy for spinal muscular atrophy. N Engl J Med 2017;377:1713–22.

49. Nizzardo M, Simone C, Rizzo F, et al. Gene therapy rescues disease phenotype in a spinal muscular atrophy with respiratory distress type 1 (SMARD1) mouse model. Sci Adv 2015;1: e1500078.

50. Marson FAL, Bertuzzo CS, Ribeiro JD. Personalized or precision medicine? The example of cystic fibrosis. Front Pharmacol 2017;8:390.

51. Schwank G, Koo BK, Sasselli V, et al. Functional repair of CFTR by CRISPR/Cas9 in intestinal stem cell organoids of cystic fibrosis patients. Cell Stem Cell 2013;13:653–8.

52. Bednarski C, Tomczak K. Vom hovel B, Weber WM, cathomen T: targeted Integration of a super-Exon into the CFTR locus leads to functional correction of a cystic fibrosis cell line model. PLoS One 2016; 11:e0161072.

53. Lee CM, Flynn R, Hollywood JA, et al. Correction of the DeltaF508 mutation in the cystic fibrosis transmembrane conductance regulator gene by zinc-finger nuclease homology-directed repair. Biores Open Access 2012;1:99–108.

54. Suzuki S, Crane AM, Anirudhan V, et al. Highly efficient gene editing of cystic fibrosis patient-derived airway basal cells results in functional CFTR correction. Mol Ther 2020;28(7):1684–95.

55. Ramalingam S, London V, Kandavelou K, et al. Generation and genetic engineering of human induced pluripotent stem cells using designed zinc finger nucleases. Stem Cells Dev 2013;22: 595–610.

56. Crane AM, Kramer P, Bui JH, et al. Targeted correction and restored function of the CFTR gene in cystic fibrosis induced pluripotent stem cells. Stem Cell Rep 2015;4:569–77.

57. Xia E, Zhang Y, Cao H, et al. TALEN-mediated gene targeting for cystic fibrosis-gene therapy. Genes (Basel) 2019;10:39.

58. Economos NG, Oyaghire S, Quijano E, et al. Peptide nucleic acids and gene editing: perspectives on structure and repair. Molecules 2020;25:735.

59. McNeer NA, Anandalingam K, Fields RJ, et al. Nanoparticles that deliver triplex-forming peptide nucleic acid molecules correct F508del CFTR in airway epithelium. Nat Commun 2015;6:6952.

60. Oyaghire SN, Quijano E, Piotrowski-Daspit AS, et al. Poly(Lactic-co-Glycolic acid) nanoparticle delivery of peptide nucleic acids in vivo. Methods Mol Biol 2020;2105:261–81.

61. Ricciardi AS, Quijano E, Putman R, et al. Peptide nucleic acids as a tool for site-speclflc gene editing. Molecules 2018;23:632.

62. Vu A, McCray PB Jr. New directions in pulmonary gene therapy. Hum Gene Ther 2020;31:921–39.

63. Eichstadt S, Barriga M, Ponakala A, et al. Phase 1/2a clinical trial of gene-corrected autologous cell therapy for recessive dystrophic epidermolysis bullosa. JCI Insight 2019;4:e130554.

64. Lwin SM, Syed F, Di WL, et al. Safety and early efficacy outcomes for lentiviral fibroblast gene therapy in recessive dystrophic epidermolysis bullosa. JCI Insight 2019;4:e126243.

65. Marinkovich MP, Tang JY. Gene therapy for epidermolysis bullosa. J Invest Dermatol 2019;139:1221–6.

66. Lee RE, Miller SM, Mascenik TM, et al. Assessing human airway epithelial progenitor cells for cystic fibrosis cell therapy. Am J Respir Cell Mol Biol 2020;63(3):374–85.

67. Berical A, Lee RE, Randell SH, et al. Challenges facing airway epithelial cell-based therapy for cystic fibrosis. Front Pharmacol 2019;10:74.

68. Huang SX, Green MD, de Carvalho AT, et al. The in vitro generation of lung and airway progenitor cells from human pluripotent stem cells. Nat Protoc 2015;10:413–25.

69. King NE, Suzuki S, Barilla C, et al. Correction of airway stem cells: genome editing approaches for the treatment of cystic fibrosis. Hum Gene Ther 2020;31:956–72.

70. Vaidyanathan S, Salahudeen AA, Sellers ZM, et al. High-efficiency, selection-free gene repair in airway stem cells from cystic fibrosis patients rescues CFTR function in differentiated epithelia. Cell Stem Cell 2020;26:161–71.e4.

71. Farbiak L, Cheng Q, Wei T, et al. All-in-one dendrimer-based lipid nanoparticles enable precise HDR-mediated gene editing in. Vivo Adv Mater 2021;33:e2006619.

72. Kauffman AC, Piotrowski-Daspit AS, Nakazawa KH, et al. Tunability of biodegradable poly(amine- co-ester) polymers for customized nucleic acid delivery and other biomedical applications. Biomacromolecules 2018;19:3861–73.

73. Xu E, Saltzman WM, Piotrowski-Daspit AS. Escaping the endosome: assessing cellular trafficking

mechanisms of non-viral vehicles. J Control Release 2021;335:465–80.

74. Piotrowski-Daspit AS, Glaze PM, Saltzman WM. Debugging the genetic code: non-viral in vivo delivery of therapeutic genome editing technologies. Curr Opin Biomed Eng 2018;7:24–32.

75. Piotrowski-Daspit AS, Kauffman AC, Bracaglia LG, et al. Polymeric vehicles for nucleic acid delivery. Adv Drug Deliv Rev 2020;156:119–32.

76. Lee SM, Cheng Q, Yu X, et al. A systematic study of Unsaturation in lipid nanoparticles leads to improved mRNA transfection in vivo. Angew Chem Int Ed Engl 2021;60:5848–53.

77. Lokugamage MP, Sago CD, Dahlman JE. Testing thousands of nanoparticles in vivo using DNA barcodes. Curr Opin Biomed Eng 2018;7:1–8.

78. Lokugamage MP, Sago CD, Gan Z, et al. Constrained nanoparticles deliver siRNA and sgRNA to T cells in vivo without targeting ligands. Adv Mater 2019;31:e1902251.

79. Yan Z, McCray PB Jr, Engelhardt JF. Advances in gene therapy for cystic fibrosis lung disease. Hum Mol Genet 2019;28:R88–94.

80. Ensinck M, Mottais A, Detry C, et al. On the corner of models and cure: gene editing in cystic fibrosis. Front Pharmacol 2021;12:662110.

Updates in Nutrition Management of Cystic Fibrosis in the Highly Effective Modulator Era

Alexandra Wilson, MS, RDN, CDCES[a], Kimberly Altman, MS, RD, CSP, CDN[b],
Terri Schindler, MS, RDN[c], Sarah Jane Schwarzenberg, MD[d],*

KEYWORDS

- Cystic fibrosis transmembrane conductance regulator (CFTR) • Highly effective modulator therapy
- Body composition • Nutrient dense • Cardiovascular risk

KEY POINTS

- Nutrition management is a key therapy in providing the best care for people with cystic fibrosis (CF); nutrition recommendations should be individualized to optimize health.
- Advances in therapeutic treatment of CF has resulted in longer lifespan and improved nutritional status of many people with CF.
- CF providers can benefit from a review of new information in providing optimal nutrition as part of treatment and overall management.
- New research in nutritional assessment, dietary quality, impact of highly effective modulator therapy on nutritional needs of people with CF, and how new information in nutrition-related comorbid conditions, the intestinal microbiome, exercise, and micronutrients can alter our thinking in managing our patients.

INTRODUCTION

Attainment and maintenance of good nutrition has been an important aspect of management in cystic fibrosis (CF) for decades. Corey and colleagues concluded in 1988 that increased survival in a cohort of people with CF (PwCF) in Toronto compared with a similar clinic in Boston was related to improved growth and nutrition in the Toronto cohort, the main differences being a high-fat diet and higher doses of pancreatic enzyme replacement therapy (PERT) being recommended in Toronto[1]; this was corroborated by a prospective observational study using data from the Cystic Fibrosis Foundation Patient Registry (CFFPR) wherein children with CF who achieved a weight-for-age percentile (WAP) at 4 years predicted survival at age 18 years, with higher WAP at 4 years predicting higher survival.[2]

Other studies have supported and extended these findings. In a single-center study, maintaining height-for-age higher than the 50th percentile from ages 2 to 7 years correlated with better forced expiratory volume at 1 minute %predicted (FEV1pp) at age 6 to 7 years.[3,4] Children ages 2 to 7 years in the CFFPR who increased their weight-for-length and body mass index (BMI) percentiles by greater than 10 percentile points had a

a Cystic Fibrosis Clinical Research, Clinical Research Services, National Jewish Health, 1400 Jackson Street, K333, Denver, CO 80206, USA; b Gunnar Esiason Adult Cystic Fibrosis and Lung Center, Columbia University Medical Center, New York Presbyterian Hospital, New York, NY, USA; c Pediatric Pulmonology, University Hospitals Cleveland Medical Center, Rainbow Babies and Children's Hospital; d Department of Pediatrics; University of Minnesota Masonic Children's Hospital, Academic Office Building, 2450 Riverside Avenue South AO-201, Minneapolis, MN 55454, USA
* Corresponding author.
E-mail address: schwa005@umn.edu

Clin Chest Med 43 (2022) 727–742
https://doi.org/10.1016/j.ccm.2022.06.012

small but significant improvement in FEV1pp.[3] Malnutrition was a risk factor for death identified on multivariate analysis among adults with CF undergoing invasive mechanical ventilation[5] and was also associated with reduced survival among PwCF in the Canadian CF Registry.[6] In summary, survival in CF is associated with maintaining nutrition status as reflected by good growth in children and weight maintenance in adults.

A myriad of complex factors impedes the achievement and maintenance of optimal nutrition in PwCF. Individuals with CF may have disordered sense of smell resulting from nasal polyps and sinusitis, potentially affecting the taste of food and appetite. Behaviors developed during childhood can result in a lifetime of poor eating habits. Unhealthy body image, well documented in CF, may affect desire to meet estimated energy needs. Several factors affect digestion and absorption of food,[7,8] including exocrine pancreatic insufficiency (EPI), small bowel bacterial overgrowth, intestinal inflammation, reduced bile acid production, and intestinal dysmotility. Socioeconomic factors such as food insecurity may also play a role. Full reviews of these many issues have been reviewed.

Evidence-based guidelines have been published to assist clinicians in managing the nutritional needs of PwCF at different ages (**Table 1**). Although there are comprehensive CF nutrition reviews,[9–11] there are also clinical care guidelines for age- and CF-related conditions that also contain nutrition care recommendations.[12] In this publication, the authors hope to supplement these guidelines with newer information on some of the issues facing those of us who manage PwCF with respect to nutrition, including new developments in nutrition assessment, how highly effective modulator therapy (HEMT) is changing the nutritional needs of people with CF, and how new information in CF-specific comorbidities, the microbiome, exercise, and micronutrients can alter our thinking in managing our patients.

DISCUSSION
The Effects of Cystic Fibrosis Transmembrane Conductance Regulator Modulators on Nutrition in People with Cystic Fibrosis

Nutrition in PwCF is now seen through the lens of CFTR modulator therapy, which has a dramatic effect on the management of the disease in those whose mutations are compatible with the available therapies. Although designed to improve sweat chloride and pulmonary function, these modulators have some effect on nutrition in PwCF. The mechanisms of these changes are just being elucidated, so it is expected that more information will come forth in the next few years.

Improvement in weight was seen in studies of ivacaftor in G551D mutation in ages greater than 2 years.[13–15] Weight gain seemed to plateau between 16 and 24 weeks. With longer studies (48 weeks of treatment), height velocity improved as well, compared with placebo.[16] After 5.5 years of therapy with ivacaftor in PwCF and a G551D mutation, the prevalence of overweight status trended upward in both children and adults, but the status of obesity trended upward only in adults.[17]

There have been studies to understand the possible mechanisms for improvement of weight with modulators.[18] Stallings and colleagues showed significant decrease in resting energy expenditure by 5.5% ± 12% in PwCF with gating mutations on ivacaftor.[19] Gelfond and colleagues showed that ivacaftor decreased the mean time to increase and sustain intestinal pH to 5.5 from the acidic stomach; this is critical to PERT performance and bile acid solubilization.[20] Fecal elastase improved in children aged 12 to 24 months on ivacaftor, but older patients experienced little to no change.[13,19,21]

Elexacaftor/tezacaftor/ivacaftor (ETI) therapy can have a profound impact on weight gain in PwCF. Substantial increase in BMI was shown in the early adult studies.[22,23] More information is likely to come from the ongoing PROMISE observational study of the impact of triple modulator therapy across several organ systems.[24]

Defining Weight-Based Nutrition Goals

The CFFPR continues to show an association between nutrition and pulmonary outcomes in CF[25] (**Figs. 1** and **2**), reinforcing the need for PwCF to meet pediatric growth parameters and weight maintenance within a normal range as adults[9,11,26]; this is further validated in evidence-based guidelines concluding higher FEV1pp is associated with BMI and height z-score referencing CDC growth charts in children.[9]

Nutrition assessment continues to be recommended routinely, measuring weight-for-length in infants younger than 2 years, BMI percentile for children ages 2 to 20 years, and BMI for adults. Optimal nutrition results when weight-for-length reaches greater than or equal to 50th percentile in children younger than 2 years, BMI greater than or equal to 50th percentile for children ages 2 to 20 years, and BMI greater than or equal to 22 kg/m^2 for adult women and BMI greater than or equal to 23 kg/m^2 for adult men.[9,11,26] Underweight results when BMI reaches less than 10th

Table 1
Currently available nutrition care guidelines for people with cystic fibrosis

Organization	Reference	Focus	Limitations
Academy of Nutrition and Dietetics	McDonald et al[9], 2021	Evidence-based practice guideline for primary nutrition issues in CF (nutrition screening, assessment, and dietary intake)	Less focus on micronutrients; refers to other guidelines
Thoracic Society of Australia and NZ	Saxby et al,[10] 2021	Comprehensive guideline	N/A
European Society for Clinical Nutrition and Metabolism; European Society for Pediatric Gastroenterology Hepatology and Nutrition; European Cystic Fibrosis Society	Turck et al,[11] 2016	Evidence-based guideline covering most aspects of nutritional management	Limited space to expand on some aspects of nutrition; may need to supplement with other guidelines
European Cystic Fibrosis Society	Castellani et al,[91] 2018	Best practices in managing CF across many organ systems	Nutrition is a small part of a larger document
Cystic Fibrosis Foundation of North America	Schwarzenberg et al,[52] 2016	Indications for and use of enteral tube feeding	Limited evidence basis for recommendations ("evidence informed")
Cystic Fibrosis Foundation of North America	Lahiri et al,[92] 2016	Recommendations for preschoolers with CF	Nutrition is a small part of a larger document
Cystic Fibrosis Foundation of North America	Tangpricha et al,[80] 2012	Screening, diagnosis, management and treatment of vitamin D deficiency in PwCF	N/A
European Cystic Fibrosis Society	Sermet-Gaudelus et al,[93] 2010	Early management of infants diagnosed by newborn screening; substantial emphasis on nutrition	Now 11 year old; does not focus on nutrition
Cystic Fibrosis Foundation of North America	Cystic Fibrosis et al,[94] 2009	Management of infants; substantial emphasis on nutrition	Now 12 years old
Cystic Fibrosis Foundation of North America	Stallings et al,[42] 2008	—	Now 11 years old
European Cystic Fibrosis Society	Edenborough et al,[95] 2008	Pregnancy guidelines	Minimal information on nutrition; 13 years old
Cystic Fibrosis Foundation of North America	Yankaskas et al,[96] 2004	Care of adults with CF	Limited information on nutrition; 17 years old.

percentile in children, and BMI less than 18.5 kg/m² in adults is associated with a higher risk of mortality.[9]

Although growth and BMI measures are useful tools, they may be poor indicators of nutritional deficits and declining pulmonary function at an early stage.[27] King and colleagues determined that BMI fails to identify all adults with fat-free mass (FFM) depletion and that measurement of FFM was superior to BMI to detect individuals

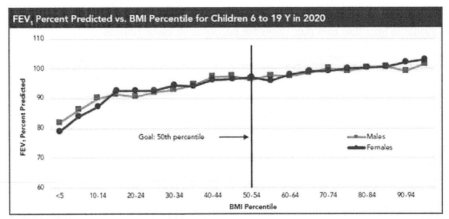

Fig. 1. In children with CF, there is an association between better nutrition and better pulmonary health. Patients with cystic fibrosis under care at CF Foundation–accredited care centers in the United States, who consented to have their data entered. (*From* Cystic Fibrosis Foundation Patient Registry 2020 Annual Data Report, Bethesda, Maryland, ©2021 Cystic Fibrosis Foundation; with permission.)

with low FEV1pp. Calella and colleagues completed a retrospective study of 69 PwCF ages 10 to 19 years who had dual-energy x-ray absorptiometry (DXA) scanning for assessment of bone mineral density (BMD).[28] This study revealed that although BMI had a positive relationship with FEV1pp (r = 0.52, $P < 0.01$), the relationship was stronger with lean body mass (LBM) (r = 0.68, $P < 0.01$). Both investigators suggest that assessment of body composition may foster early interventions, whereas reliance on BMI alone may delay recognition of malnutrition.[27,28]

Body composition assessment, depending on the method used, may provide information on distribution of adiposity, LBM, bone health, and hydration status, which may aid in management of

PwCF at risk of malnutrition.[29,30] There are several different anthropometric assessment methods (**Table 2**), each with their own advantages and disadvantages. The type of body composition measure to use will depend on whether used for clinical or research purposes and ease of use in clinical settings for purposes of nutrition assessment. DXA, long considered a gold standard for measuring body composition, is used regularly in clinical settings but requires additional time at clinical visits and may not be covered by insurance. It measures total and segmental LBM, body adiposity,[29] and bone density. Bioelectrical impedance analysis (BIA) and skin folds (SF) are more readily available in a clinical setting but rely on prediction equations and assume normal

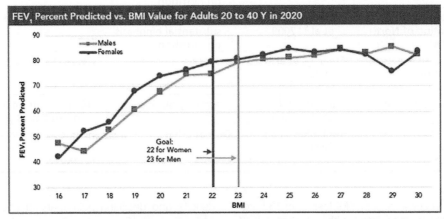

Fig. 2. In adults with CF, there is an association between better nutrition and better pulmonary health. Patients with cystic fibrosis under care at CF Foundation–accredited care centers in the United States, who consented to have their data entered. (*From* Cystic Fibrosis Foundation Patient Registry 2020 Annual Data Report, Bethesda, Maryland, ©2021 Cystic Fibrosis Foundation; with permission.)

Table 2
Methods of body composition assessment—strengths and considerations of available methods

	Strengths	Considerations
Skinfold thickness measurements	Quick and noninvasive	Prediction equations for conversion of measurements to FFM and percent fat are based on healthy populations and show variable accuracy in CF
Multifrequency bioelectrical impedance analysis (BIA) and bioelectrical impedance spectroscopy (BIS)	Quick and noninvasive Tetrapolar multifrequency BIA and BIS (newer technology) have fewer limitations than older BIA devices	Single frequency BIA (older technology)—poor accuracy compared with reference methods • Simple BIA devices such as stand-on scales with only 2 contact points (feet) are not validated in CF and not recommended, as the results may not reflect the distribution of FFM and fat mass across the whole body • Equipment is expensive to acquire • Limited validation studies in CF with tetrapolar multifrequency BIA or BIS
Whole-body dual-energy x-ray absorptiometry (DXA) scanning	Accurate reference method for body composition assessment • Provides information and regional body composition as well as total FFM, fat mass, and bone mineral content • Newer DXA scanners are much quicker than older devices • Low exposure to ionizing radiation	Whole-body DXA scanning is not routinely performed when bone density scanning is undertaken and may require additional cost • Requires individual to lie still and flat at the duration of scan, which may be difficult for young children and those with severe lung disease
Mid-arm circumference measurements	Used to assess muscle stores in conjunction with triceps skinfold • Simple, quick and non-invasive • Useful for sequential monitoring	Cannot reliably be converted to whole-body FFM stores, as arm muscle and fat stores may not reflect whole-body distribution
Abdominal circumference	Useful for monitoring abdominal/central adiposity and comparison with reference norms for metabolic risk in adults with high BMI • Simple, quick, and noninvasive	No CF-specific evidence to determine if the general population cut-offs for abdominal obesity apply to the stratification of risk in this group of adults with CF

(continued on next page)

Table 2
(continued)

	Strengths	Considerations
	• Measuring abdominal circumference may be useful for identifying excess central adipose tissue in adults with high BMI and for monitoring the effect of interventions in individuals identified as suitable for weight loss	
Whole-body (air-displacement) plethysmography	Has been studied in CF	Not widely available; difficult to acquire and expensive

Adapted from Saxby N., Painter C., Kench A., King S., Crowder T., van der Haak N. and the Australian and New Zealand Cystic Fibrosis Nutrition Guideline Authorship Group (2017). Nutrition Guidelines for Cystic Fibrosis in Australia and New Zealand, ed. Scott C. Bell, Thoracic Society of Australia and New Zealand, Sydney; with permission.

hydration status[29]; SF require training to perform. Evidence for the predictive value of body composition assessment in PwCF remains moderate; longitudinal studies are needed to better understand the role of body composition in the assessment of nutrition status in CF.[27–30]

The Baby Observational and Nutrition Study (BONUS) also adds to our understanding of what nutrition can and cannot do.[31] This multicenter, longitudinal observational cohort study over the first 12 months of life in infants with CF enrolled 231 infants at 28 CF Foundation accredited Care Centers in the United States. The BONUS infants had lower birth weights than healthy newborns but recovered the weight in the first year of life, with weights at 12 months equivalent between BONUS infants and healthy infants. Birth lengths of BONUS infants were greater than those of healthy infants, but BONUS infants accrued length more slowly and were significantly shorter than healthy infants at 3, 6, and 12 months after birth. Head circumference was normal at birth and at 12 months. This study demonstrated that maintaining normal weight gain in infants with CF was not necessarily associated with achievement of normal length.

Obesity, Cardiovascular Risk, and Diet Quality

Nutrition outcomes, as measured by BMI, have continually improved in PwCF, likely for multiple reasons.[25] The median BMI percentile of individuals 2 to 19 years has increased from 46.4% in 2005 to 61.3% in 2020, and for adults aged 20 to 40 years, the median BMI increased from 21.2 in 2005 to 23.1 in 2020 (**Table 3**). There has been an increase in overweight (26.7%) and obese

(10.3%) in 2020 compared with 2000 when just 14.3% of adults with CF were overweight or obese. The causes of this trend are complex. Individuals who are pancreatic sufficient (PS) have, on average, a higher BMI than those who are pancreatic insufficient (PI).[32,33] However, the prevalence of overweight and obesity is also increasing in PwCF who are PI.[34] Increasing age, male sex, dietary habits, cultural effects, and improved therapy have all been associated with weight gain.[34] This trend toward overweight and obesity will be monitored closely, as more PwCF are surviving into adulthood, a time when cardiometabolic disease risk increases.

Alvarez and colleagues demonstrated that some individuals with CF had normal-weight obesity, a condition in which there is high body fat percentage despite normal BMI.[35] Normal-weight obesity was inversely correlated with lung function in these PwCF, suggesting BMI alone was not a good criterion for obesity in this disease.

With the aging of the CF population, and the prolonged lifespan that modulators may achieve, the long-term cardiovascular health of the CF population has become more important. Elevated triglycerides are common.[36,37] Cholesterol levels increase with age and with degree of obesity and are generally higher in PS than in PI individuals.[36–38] Coronary artery disease has been reported in CF, as has myocardial ischemia.[39] A recent study showed that older PwCF, with moderate to severe lung disease, had general arterial stiffness compared with controls. The investigators found increasing arterial stiffness with age, PI status, absence of hepatic cirrhosis, and colonization with *Pseudomonas aeruginosa*. PS patients had higher common carotid artery intima-media thickness compared with PI

Table 3
GI/nutrition subsection of the summary of the Cystic Fibrosis Foundation Patient Registry, 2005–2020

GI/Nutrition	2005	2010	2015	2019	2020
Body mass index (BMI) percentile in individuals 2–19 y (median)	46.4	50.9	54.7	58.3	61.3
Weight < 10th CDC percentile (%)	19.1	14.8	12.0	10.0	9.1
Height <5th CDC percentile (%)	14.1	11.7	10.2	9.5	9.5
BMI in individuals 20–40 y (median)	21.2	21.7	22.1	22.5	23.1
Pancreatic enzyme replacement therapy (%)	80.0	86.9	86.6	84.4	83.8
Supplemental feeding—tube (%)	9.5	10.3	11	10.2	9.0
Supplemental feeding—oral only (%)	36.0	38.3	42.3	44.3	39.4

Cystic fibrosis patients under care at CF Foundation–accredited care centers in the United States, who consented to have their data entered.

Abbreviation: GI, gastrointestinal.

Adapted from Cystic Fibrosis Foundation Patient Registry 2020 Annual Data Report, Bethesda, Maryland, ©2021 Cystic Fibrosis Foundation; with permission.

patients.[40] More information is needed to determine how we can modify CF diets to reduce risk of cardiac disease in this population.

The diet recommendations for PwCF have aimed for energy intake in 110% to 200% of non-CF individuals, with a high fat and high sodium intake to account for increased energy demands and sodium chloride losses in sweat[41,42]; this has become known as the legacy diet. There is a concern for age-related and metabolic conditions known to be associated with high fat, added sugar, high sodium diets, with low dietary quality.[41,43] High energy intake with excess saturated fat, trans-fats, and added sugars and low micronutrient intake in PwCF have been observed on 3 different continents—Australia,[44] Europe,[45,46] and North America.[43]

Sutherland and colleagues completed a cross-sectional study of 102 children with CF and controls in Australia, ages 2 to 18 years, evaluating nutrient dense (ND) and energy dense-nutrient poor (EDNP) intake.[44] ND foods are those that contain high amounts of essential nutrients, associated with prevention of diet-related chronic disease, but have lower calories, whereas EDNP foods are high in saturated fat and added sugars and contribute few dietary micronutrients. Children with CF consumed more energy from both EDNP and ND; EDNP contributed more total energy intake in children with CF than in controls. Children with CF consumed nearly twice as many sweetened drinks, confectionary, and packaged snacks. In Greece, children and adolescents with CF reported adequate fat and protein intake with suboptimal carbohydrate and fiber and excess saturated fat intake.[46] The average KIDMED score—a questionnaire that evaluates adherence to a Mediterranean

diet—was moderate, indicating mediocre diet quality and poor adherence to a Mediterranean diet. In a multicenter European study, Calvo-Lerma and colleagues showed that sugar and saturated fat contribute greater than 10% *each* to total calorie intake of children with CF.[45] The nutrient profiles of these European children were suboptimal—high saturated fat and sugar intake from meat, dairy, and processed foods, with low intake of fish, nuts, and legumes. Bellissimo and colleagues showed that adults with CF in Atlanta, Georgia, reported higher total energy intake compared with controls, meeting CF recommendations, while also consuming more trans-fatty acids and added sugars and less dietary fiber than controls.[43] PwCF had lower Healthy Eating Index-2015 scores compared with healthy controls and had significantly more visceral adipose tissue (VAT); added sugar and saturated fat were positively associated with VAT.

A systematic review by McDonald and colleagues concluded macronutrient distribution is not associated with nutrition-related outcomes in PwCF, leaving little evidence for an outcomes-related benefit of a higher fat diet.[41] In the non-CF population there is a relationship between suboptimal dietary intake, chronic disease, and mortality.[47] Although the legacy diet is not obsolete and should be used in those at risk of malnutrition to provide a high volume of calories in a low volume of food,[41,44] facilitated individualized nutrition interventions and counseling should promote nutrient dense diets; this is needed to reduce the risk of age-related metabolic diseases associated with overweight and obesity.[43]

Physical activity and its structured component, exercise, have become part of standard care for

PwCF in part because individuals with little physical activity have poorer pulmonary function, glycemic control, and BMD.[48,49] Van Biervliet and colleagues demonstrated that a 3-week supervised pulmonary, nutrition, and physical activity exercise intervention improved both BMI and FFM index in 34 PwCF ages 12 to 27 years.[50] FFM was measured by DXA. Prevotat and colleagues demonstrated similar improvement in FFM with an 8-week intervention in adults with CF.[51] In this case, the intervention was more structured, including aerobic exercise, muscle strengthening, and circuit training 3 times each week. In the 28 adults completing the program, BMI did not change, but FFM, measured by BIA, improved significantly as did a measure of physical fitness, the 6-minute walk test.

These pilot studies show that the use of different measurements for FFM may introduce difficulties in comparing studies and developing conclusions, as well as that the range of potential interventions in physical activity is large and may be confusing to patients or providers looking for the "best" intervention. The appropriate program for PwCF may vary from person to person and may involve more than one activity. Dietitians could be crucial to helping PwCF see the link between physical activity, improved strength, and pulmonary function and could team up with physical therapists when identifying an exercise recommendation.

Supplemental Feeding and New Products

Despite improvements in nutrition outcomes, the use of enteral tube feeding has remained steady over the years, with about 10% of PwCF reporting use of tube feedings and about 40% of people reporting use of oral nutrition supplements (see **Table 3**).[25] The CFF evidence-informed guidelines recommend enteral tube feeding to meet age-dependent growth parameters for those PwCF unable to consume adequate calories or protein to meet growth/maintenance needs.[52]

An updated Cochrane Review found no randomized controlled trials assessing effects of enteral tube feeding on nutrition outcomes in PwCF likely due to the ethical conflict of withholding a beneficial therapy from some.[53] However, the review identified that enteral tube feeding remains an accepted nutrition intervention, resulting in improvements in body weight, height, height velocity, BMI, nutritional status, and lung function, as well as being generally well tolerated.

New products made available may help improve nutrition in PwCF. See **Fig. 3**[54] for current oral enzymes available in the United States as well as helpful points when managing PERT.

Encala, an oral calorie supplement of a structured lipid matrix of lysophosphatidylcholine, monoglycerides, and essential fatty acids, demonstrated safety and tolerability in a double-blind placebo-controlled trial.[55] The product is water soluble and does not require lipase for digestion and so is helpful for those PwCF who have continued fat malabsorption despite optimization of PERT. It is easily mixed with food and fluids, providing additional calories without adding large volumes to meals/snacks.

RELiZORB is a Food and Drug Administration (FDA)-approved single-use, immobilized lipase, in-line cartridge to hydrolyze fats in enteral formula, as it passes through the cartridge.[56,57] Overall, the addition of RELiZORB provides a safe, tolerable alternative to oral PERT with enteral nutrition administration, improving fat absorption and gastrointestinal symptoms. It eliminates the need to awaken at night to take PERT during enteral infusions, reducing the burden for PwCF and their caretakers.

Digestive Care, Inc and Chiesi USA, Inc received FDA approval for updated labeling for gastrostomy tube administration of the 4000 USP lipase unit capsule of Pertzye.[58] This product contains microspheres that are ∼35% smaller than those in the higher dose capsules and may be helpful to some families who cannot obtain inline cartridges.

Borowitz and colleagues noted that the frequent feedings required of young infants led to total daily doses of PERT that often exceeded the 10,000 units of lipase/kg/d dosing recommendation limit.[59] It was suggested that, for the short period of early infancy, this dosing may be safe. However, there is no formal recommendation for this nor clear evidence supporting it. Schechter and colleagues found in a CFFPR study that infants with initial PERT doses greater than or equal to 1500 units lipase/kg/meal with their largest meal had better weight-related outcomes at 2 years of age measured as weight-for-age z-scores and weight-for-length percentile.[60] The BONUS study demonstrated no dose-response of PERT with weight at 12 months of age.[61] PERT doses in BONUS centers averaged about 1800 units of lipase/kg/meal over the first 12 months of life. There was no difference in weight-for-age z-scores or length-for-age z-scores in centers using higher or lower doses than the mean.

Relationship of Bone Health and Nutrition

In a systematic review of body composition and health outcomes of PwCF done by Calella and colleagues, there were 10 case-controlled studies that assessed BMD and bone mineral content (BMC).[62] Seven of these studies noted reduced BMD or

FDA Approved Enzyme Brands				Enzyme Dosing Guidelines
Product/Manufacturer/ Dosage Form/Strength	Lipase USP units	Amylase USP units	Protease USP units	**Based on units of lipase/kg/meal** ≥4y of age: Begin with 500 units lipase/kg/meal
Creon® (AbbVie Inc.) Pancrelipase				May increase up to 2,500 units lipase/kg/meal
3,000	3,000	15,000	9,500	or 10,000 lipase/kg/d
6,000	6,000	30,000	19,000	
12,000	12,000	60,000	38,000	**Based on units of lipase/grams of fat eaten**
24,000	24,000	120,000	76,000	Infant formula or Breast milk: 2,000–4,000 units
36,000	36,000	180,000	114,000	lipase/120mL Other solids and liquids: 500–4,000
Pancreaze® (Vivus, Inc.), Pancrelipase				units lipase/gm fat eaten
2,600 (MT2)	2,600	10,850	6,200	
4,200 (MT4)	4,200	24, 600	14,200	Mean of 1,800 units lipase/gm fat eaten/d in divided doses.
10,500 (MT10)	10,500	61,500	35,500	Use caution with >4,000 units lipase/gm fat eaten.
16,800 (MT16)	16,800	98,400	56,800	
21,000 (MT20)	21,000	83,900	54,700	**Factors that may Reduce Enzyme Efficacy**
37,000 (MT37)	37,000	149,900	97,300	▪ Expired or inappropriately stored enzymes
Zenpep® (Nestle) Pancrelipase				▪ Crushed or chewed enzyme beads
3,000	3,000	14,000	10,000	▪ Taking enzymes after eating or forgetting
5,000	5,000	24,000	17,000	▪ Acidic small intestine milieu **(see Acid Reducers)
10,000	10,000	42,000	32,000	▪ Prolonged exposure to alkaline foods
15,000	15,000	63,000	47,000	▪ Exposure to extreme temperatures
20,000	20,000	84,000	63,000	**Tests to Assess Exocrine Pancreatic Function (Qualitative)**
25,000	25,000	105,000	79,000	**Pancreatic (Fecal) Elastase:** Indirect test of exocrine pancreatic
40,000	40,000	168,000	126,000	function; Levels <100 µg/g = PI; 100–200µg/g borderline PI (repeat)
Viokace™ (Nestle) Tablet*, * not enteric-coated				Specimen requirements: ≥3 d FT infant; ≥2 wk PT infant; off TPN and near full feeds; no watery stools no ostomy output; on PERT OK
10,440	10,440	39,150	39,150	**Immunoreactive Trypsinogen (IRT):** Measures the amount of
20,880	20,880	78,300	78,300	trypsinogen in the blood. Levels may be high at birth, but generally
Pertzye® (Chiesi) Pancrelipase, Bicarb Buffered				will decrease with age. By the age of 8y low levels are
4,000	4,000	14,375	15,125	associated with PI. Levels are increased with acute pancreatitis.
8,000	8,000	30,250	28,750	**Other causes of malabsorptive symptoms**
16,000	16,000	60,500	57,500	Intestinal resection/short bowel syndrome, bacterial
24,000	24,000	90,750	86,250	overgrowth of the small intestine, Pseudomembranous
**Acid Reducers: PPI and H2 Blocker				enteritis, C. difficile enteritis, severe malnutrition, lactose
Decreased or absent bicarbonate secretion from the pancreas leads to an acidic intestinal environment, ineffective dissolution of enteric coating on enzymes, precipitation of bile salts, & subsequent maldigestion and malabsorption. Adding a PPI or H2-Blocker may reduce acid & promote the timely release of				malabsorption, Giardia or other parasites, hepatobiliary disease, inflammatory bowel disease, Celiac disease, fibrosing colonopathy, obstipation (leads to gassiness, can see "overflow incontinence")
Proton Pump Inhibitors (PPI)				**CF Mutations and Pancreatic Function (phenotype trumps genotype) * www.cftr2.org**
Generic name		Trade name		**Common Pancreatic-Sufficient Dominant Mutations:***
Omeprazole		Prilosec		G55 S 1 R334W T3381
Omeprazole/sodium bicarbonate		Zegerid		R352Q P574H R117H
Lansopraole		Prevacid		**Variable Pancreatic-Sufficient Mutations:***
Esomeprazole		Nexium		G85E A455E R347P 2789 5G → A
Pantoprazole		Protonix		3849 +10kb C →T *see above website for complete list
Rabeprazole		Aciphex		**Enzymes with TF**
H₂-receptor site Blocker				RELiZORB is a digestive enzyme cartridge that hydrolyzes
Generic name		Trade name		available fats in enteral formula immediately prior to ingestion. It
Cimetidine		Tagamet		connects directly to most tube feeding pump systems.
Famotidine		Pepcid		https://www.relizorb.com/docs/pdfs/Compatible-Formulas-and-
Nizatidine		Axid		Pumps.pdf for compatible pumps & formulas. See CF Nutr. 101
Ranitidine		Zantac		document for other methods of enzyme delivery with TF
72 Hour Fecal Fat Test (Quantitative). Measures the total stool fat content for 72 consecutive hours. Determines the Coefficient of Fat Absorption (%) and degree of steatorrhea					
☐ **Normal result:** Infants <6mo ≥ 85% coefficient of fat absorption; >6mo of age ≥93% CFA * ☐ **Abnormal result:** indicates steatorrhea and occurs when levels of lipase <5–10% of normal enzyme output. CF pts may not ever achieve normal CFA despite adequate enzyme dosing. **Test Procedure:** For accurate results, must eat high fat diet (Teens/Adults:>100 gm fat/d ; Infants/Children: >40% kcals from fat) for 3d prior to the start of the test and each day during the collection period. Meticulous diet records required to accurately calculate grams fat intake.					
***72H Fecal Fat Calculation:**	$\dfrac{\text{Grams Ingested fat} - \text{Grams fat in stool}}{\text{Grams Ingested fat}}$ X 100% = Coefficient of Fat Absorption				
To prevent diaper rash: Triple Paste Medicated Diaper Rash Ointment.1-800-533-7546 or: www.sumlab.com					

Fig. 3. Pancreatic enzyme replacement therapy (PERT) cheat sheet—available commercial formulations, dosing guidelines, management, and concomitant medications. (*Data from* CF Resource Library, Available at: (https://my.cff.org/cfx-docrep/document/detail/enzyme%20cheat%20sheet%208-2021.docx), accessed November 28, 2021.)

BMC, whereas 3 studies did not find any difference in BMD and BMC between PwCF compared with controls matched for age, sex, height, and LBM. PwCF often display one or more risk factors for low BMD, including suboptimal vitamin D status, delayed puberty, malnutrition, chronic inflammation, frequent glucocorticoid treatment, or physical inactivity.[63] Recently, it is understood CFTR protein is present in osteoclasts and osteoblasts,

suggesting dysfunctional CFTR might play a direct role in CF bone disease.[63]

Baker and colleagues conducted a longitudinal observational cohort study to assess associations between lean/fat mass and baseline and 2-year changes in BMD.[64] Sixty-three PwCF ages 18 to 57 years underwent DXA scanning of the posteroanterior spine, were asked about fracture history, had laboratory clinical assessments, and body fat composition estimated by tetrapolar BIA. Low BMD was observed in 52% of participants. These investigators suggest that lower LBM with greater adiposity are risk factors for BMD loss in PwCF; therefore, a focus on identifying and treating lean mass deficits are appropriate clinical targets to reduce risk of bone deficits in PwCF.

Putman and colleagues conducted a prospective observational multiple cohort study to evaluate the impact of ivacaftor on BMD, bone microarchitecture, and estimated bone strength. The clinical setting was children and adults with CF and the G551D mutation compared with age-, race-, and gender-matched PwCF not taking ivacaftor and similarly matched healthy controls.[65] Calcium, vitamin D intake, and physical activity were assessed by a registered bionutritionist. Serum 25-OH vitamin D was assessed, in addition to other serum samples. Over a 2-year period, this study noted improvements in cortical microarchitecture in the radius and tibia in PwCF treated with ivacaftor without significant differences in FEV1pp, number of CF exacerbations, oral glucocorticoid use, or bone turnover markers between the CF control and ivacaftor cohorts. There was a slight decrease in the BMD at femoral neck (3%) and total hip (2%) in the CF control cohort. The improvement in cortical microarchitecture is likely multifactorial, resulting from improved nutrition status and pulmonary function, among others. The most current recommendations for management of BMD in PwCF are summarized in **Box 1**.[63]

Nutrition considerations for abnormal glycemia in cystic fibrosis

Impaired glucose tolerance and CF-related diabetes (CFRD) continues to be a common comorbidity of CF and is associated with weight loss, lung function decline, and increased mortality.[66] The 2020 CFFPR annual report indicates 29.8% of those aged 18 years and older (18.6% of all) have CFRD.[25] The treatment of CFRD varies from chronic insulin treatment (71.4%) to dietary change (21.2%) to no treatment (13.3%). Although microvascular complications of diabetes are known to occur in those with CFRD,[67,68] the most common complication noted in 2020 were episodes of severe hypoglycemia (4.5% of all people with CFRD[25]).

Nutrition recommendations for glycemic abnormalities remain relatively unchanged since 2010 when the clinical care guidelines for CFRD were published.[69] Dietary recommendations are similar to general nutrition guidelines for PwCF with a few adjustments, namely limiting or eliminating sugary beverages and adjusting insulin dose based on carbohydrate intake to achieve glycemic control.[69,70]

Box 1
Biological measurements and nonpharmacological nutrition recommendations to optimize bone health in people with cystic fibrosis

Maintain normal BMI and aim for normal lean body mass

Engage in weight-bearing physical activity

Aim for adequate protein intake, PERT dosage, and physical activity

Vitamin D:

- Continue annual serum measurements of 25-hydroxyvitamin D, preferably at the end of winter
- Aim to maintain serum 25-hydroxyvitamin D > 30 ng/mL, supplementing accordingly

Calcium:

- Aim for a calcium-rich diet, which should be assessed at least annually in all PwCF
- Supplement accordingly for suboptimal calcium intake

Vitamin K:

- Supplement with vitamin K1 daily
- Consider evaluating PIVKA-II or carboxylated/undercarboxylated osteocalcin ratio, which is expensive but more sensitive than prothrombin time

Optimize lifestyle and nutrition goals before initiation of pharmacologic treatments, as well as during

Data from Putman MS, Anabtawi A, Le T, Tangpricha V, Sermet-Gaudelus I. Cystic fibrosis bone disease treatment: Current knowledge and future directions. J Cyst Fibros. 2019;18 Suppl 2:S56-S65.

A recent study compared quality of diet of 18 adults with CF living in Australia with the Australian Dietary Guidelines and compared glycemic index and glycemic load with glycemic response using continuous glucose monitoring.[71] Study participants consumed significantly more grains, protein, and saturated fat than dietary guideline recommendations, consistent with CF nutrition recommendations. Total energy, carbohydrate, sugar, and added sugar, as well as glycemic load, were significantly positively associated with mean amplitude glycemic excursions and standard deviation. Glycemic index was positively associated with more time spent in hyperglycemic range (>7.8 mmol/L; 140 mg/dL), and both glycemic index and glycemic load were negatively associated with percentage of time spent in euglycemic range. These investigators suggest glycemic index and glycemic load manipulation can have beneficial effects on glycemia. More evidence is needed, and future recommendations to manage glycemia in PwCF should become increasingly personalized.

Micronutrient Therapy: What Changes, What Is New

Despite widespread knowledge of fat-soluble vitamin deficiencies in CF, a recent study from Australia noted fat-soluble vitamin deficiencies in up to one-third of children with CF with EPI.[72] Possible reasons for persistent deficiencies include inconsistent use of supplement and/or PERT, liver disease, or short gut syndrome.[73] Dosing recommendations for vitamins in patients with CF are mostly based on expert consensus.[74] It is unclear if HEMT will significantly affect vitamin dosing recommendations in CF. Deficiencies of other micronutrients in CF are also recognized. Complete reviews of fat-soluble vitamins and other micronutrients in PwCF are available.[11,75] Some relevant considerations are discussed in the following section.

Vitamin A deficiency is usually limited to unsupplemented/undersupplemented patients with PI or patients with cholestatic liver disease. In 39 infants with CF diagnosed by newborn screening, 51% had low vitamin A levels that normalized at 1 year of age with supplementation.[76] Vitamin A may be toxic in excess dosing, or when administered with retinol-based supplements, in chronic kidney disease, and/or in individuals posttransplant (because of improved absorption).[77,78] Interpretation of vitamin A levels can be challenging due to effects of inflammation as well as reliance on retinol binding protein for transport. An individualized approach to vitamin A supplementation has been suggested.[79]

Deficient and insufficient levels of vitamin D in PwCF remain common. There are likely multiple causes such as decreased absorption, reduced sunlight exposure, decreased intake of vitamin D–rich foods and insufficient supplementation.[80] The current guidelines should be followed, with an understanding that modulator therapy may change recommendations in the future.

Obvious clinical symptoms of vitamin E deficiency are now uncommon in individuals treated with PERT and CF vitamins, and supplementation may not be needed for PS individuals.[10] Aggressive supplementation may lead to elevated serum α-tocopherol levels and/or suppression of γ-tocopherol levels.[81] A recent Polish study involving young children and adults with CF identified vitamin E deficiency in 8% and high levels in 11.4%.[82]

Assessment of vitamin K status is the least known of all fat-soluble vitamins in terms of type and amount of dosing and optimal methods for monitoring. Although it is commonly known for its importance in synthesizing proteins necessary for blood clotting, these proteins are also important for bone metabolism and cell growth regulation. Subclinical vitamin K deficiency may increase risk of osteoporosis and cancer.[83]

Outside of infancy, there are no specific recommendations for salt intake for individuals with CF, other than adding salt at meals and providing additional sources of salt when exercising and/or exposed to excessive heat.[74] Changes in sweat chloride levels are an outcome measure of modulator therapy. Although there is a significant decrease in sweat chloride levels on ivacaftor, the changes are variable and do not seem to be associated with improvements in lung function.[84] It is yet unknown if salt recommendations should be modified in individuals with CF after starting modulator therapy.

The Gut Microbiome and Nutrition

The gut microbiome has critical roles in nutrition, immunology, and hormone regulation. A recent review explores the importance of the gut microbiome in nutrition.[85,86] Ongoing research examining the microbiome in PwCF seeks to determine the impact of CF therapies on the gut microbiome, whether microbiome changes are associated with changes in gut health and nutrition, and whether manipulation of the gut microbiome is possible or effective.

The gut in PwCF is rapidly colonized in infancy, but the gut microbiome that develops differs from that of healthy controls.[87] The gut of children with CF demonstrates decreased species diversity with dysbiosis (as measured by fecal calprotectin). Hayden and colleagues showed that worsening fecal dysbiosis (decreased prevalence Bacteroidetes and increased prevalence Proteobacteria) was seen more commonly in infants with CF and was associated with delayed linear growth.[88] They highlight the important role of the gut microbiome on endocrine function and nutrient harvest.

Identifying a therapy to modify the gut microbiome in CF is a work in progress. Acid blockade does not affect the intestinal/respiratory microbiome.[89] Probiotics have been studied in CF in several studies involving varying methods, probiotic strain, length of treatment, and outcome measure. A Cochrane review of these data concluded that probiotic therapy generally reduced fecal calprotectin but had no effect on overall lung function,

SUMMARY

Nutrition affects many clinical aspects of CF. The relationship between current therapies, diet quality, body composition, and comorbid conditions needs further investigation (**Box 2**). Nutrition status of PwCF has improved dramatically, particularly in the postmodulator era. In this era of increasing weight, it is important to not only rely on anthropometric measures of BMI but to also consider incorporating body composition analysis; these can provide early markers of suboptimal nutrition status. Individualized nutrition recommendations are needed that take into account personal preferences, cultural traditions, and budgetary considerations,[9] promoting nutrient-dense foods that incorporate more unsaturated fats, fruits, vegetables, whole grains, and less added sugar. Although weights and BMI are trending up for many PwCF, the need for enteral or oral nutrition support remains for some and should start early. It should be noted that HEMT is not available for everyone with CF, underscoring the importance of individualized and targeted medical nutrition therapy so that every person with CF is well nourished.

Box 2
Nutrition-related research considerations for the future

1. How will highly effective CFTR modulators (HEMT) affect nutrition outcomes for people with CF? What are the mechanisms by which these changes occur?

2. Although overweight and obesity are increasing, are they having a negative impact on pulmonary, cardiovascular, and/or cardiometabolic outcomes?

3. What are modifiable dietary and physical activity behaviors that will result in the best overall health outcomes for people with CF?

4. Which methods of body composition assessment can be used regularly in clinical settings to identify those at risk of malnutrition and/or declining pulmonary function?

5. Will more regular body composition assessment affect body image?

6. Is there a "best" body fat to lean body mass ratio for people with CF to meet and maintain pulmonary health?

7. How can registered dietitians, or international equivalents, partner with physical therapists to promote physical activity regimens that are effective and sustainable for people with CF?

8. Are there specific dietary patterns that are preferred for people with CF in the era of HEMT? How can individualized, nutrient-dense dietary recommendations be transferred to those that will continue to require a high-fat, high-calorie, high-salt diet because they do not have access to CFTR modulators?

9. Which dietary strategies best manage glycemia for those PwCF with abnormal glycemia?

10. How will the gut microbiome change in response to HEMT, and how does this affect overall nutrition?

11. Will salt needs change in response to HEMT?

12. How will HEMT affect micronutrient supplementation in PwCF?

CLINICS CARE POINTS

- Regular nutrition assessment by a clinical dietitian, preferably with expertise in CF, remains essential, annually or more often as needed.

- Consider replacing the legacy diet with one with higher nutrient density and lower saturated and trans-fat.

- Body composition may be a useful clinical tool, particularly in those at higher risk, including those with declining pulmonary function.

- Consider if your patients with CF might benefit from Encala or RELiZORB.

- At present, there is no change in recommendations for salt supplementation.

- HEMT will continue to challenge us, as it changes the needs of PwCF; maintaining a close eye on the literature will be crucial in the coming years.

growth, hospitalization, and quality of life.[90] There are ongoing studies of the impact of modulators[24] on the gut microbiome. In summary, manipulation of the gut microbiome is a potential modifier of nutrition in PwCF, but much more research remains to be done.

DISCLOSURE

S.J. Schwarzenberg is a consultant for Abbvie, Mirium, Nestle, and UpToDate and has grant funding from the Cystic Fibrosis Foundation, the National Institutes of Health, and Gilead. T.

Schindler is on the speaker board for Chiesi and Abbvie. The remaining authors have nothing to disclose.

REFERENCES

1. Corey M, McLaughlin FJ, Williams M, et al. A comparison of survival, growth, and pulmonary function in patients with cystic fibrosis in Boston and Toronto. J Clin Epidemiol 1988;41(6):583–91.

2. Yen EH, Quinton H, Borowitz D. Better nutritional status in early childhood is associated with improved clinical outcomes and survival in patients with cystic fibrosis. J Pediatr 2013;162(3):530–535 e1.

3. Sanders DB, Fink A, Mayer-Hamblett N, et al. Early life growth trajectories in cystic fibrosis are associated with pulmonary function at age 6 years. J Pediatr 2015;167(5):1081–1088 e1.

4. Sanders DB, Slaven JE, Maguiness K, et al. Early-life height attainment in cystic fibrosis is associated with pulmonary function at age 6 years. Ann Am Thorac Soc 2021;18(8):1335–42.

5. Siuba M, Attaway A, Zein J, et al. Mortality in adults with cystic fibrosis requiring mechanical ventilation. cross-sectional analysis of nationwide events. Ann Am Thorac Soc 2019;16(8):1017–23.

6. Stephenson AL, Tom M, Berthiaume Y, et al. A contemporary survival analysis of individuals with cystic fibrosis: a cohort study. Eur Respir J 2015;45(3):670–9.

7. Borowitz D, Durie PR, Clarke LL, et al. Gastrointestinal outcomes and confounders in cystic fibrosis. J Pediatr Gastroenterol Nutr 2005;41(3):273–85.

8. Colombo C, Nobili RM, Alicandro G. Challenges with optimizing nutrition in cystic fibrosis. Expert Rev Respir Med 2019;13(6):533–44.

9. McDonald CM, Alvarez JA, Bailey J, et al. Academy of nutrition and dietetics: 2020 cystic fibrosis evidence analysis center evidence-based nutrition practice guideline. J Acad Nutr Diet 2021;121(8):1591–15636 e3.

10. Saxby N, Painter C, Kench A, King S, Crowder T, van der Haak N, et al. Nutrition guidelines for cystic fibrosis in Australia, 2017 Australia and New Zealand. Bell S, editor, Sydney: Thoracic Society of Australia and New Zealand; 2017. Available from: https://www.thoracic.org.au/journal- publishing/area?command=record&id=46.

11. Turck D, Braegger CP, Colombo C, et al. ESPEN-ESPGHAN-ECFS guidelines on nutrition care for infants, children, and adults with cystic fibrosis. Clin Nutr 2016;35(3):557–77.

12. Foundation CF. Age-specific guidelines. Available at: https://www.cff.org/medical-professionals/clinical-care-guidelines.

13. Davies JC, Cunningham S, Harris WT, et al. Safety, pharmacokinetics, and pharmacodynamics of ivacaftor in patients aged 2-5 years with cystic fibrosis and a CFTR gating mutation (KIWI): an open-label, single-arm study. Lancet Respir Med 2016;4(2):107–15.

14. Davies JC, Wainwright CE, Canny GJ, et al. Efficacy and safety of ivacaftor in patients aged 6 to 11 years with cystic fibrosis with a G551D mutation. Am J Respir Crit Care Med 2013;187(11):1219–25.

15. Ramsey BW, Davies J, McElvaney NG, et al. A CFTR potentiator in patients with cystic fibrosis and the G551D mutation. N Engl J Med 2011;365(18):1663–72.

16. Stalvey MS, Pace J, Niknian M, et al. Growth in prepubertal children with cystic fibrosis treated with ivacaftor. Pediatrics 2017;139(2).

17. Guimbellot JS, Taylor-Cousar JL. Combination CFTR modulator therapy in children and adults with cystic fibrosis. Lancet Respir Med 2021;9(7):677–9.

18. Borowitz D, Lubarsky B, Wilschanski M, et al. Nutritional status improved in cystic fibrosis patients with the G551D mutation after treatment with ivacaftor. Dig Dis Sci 2016;61(1):198–207.

19. Stallings VA, Sainath N, Oberle M, et al. Energy balance and mechanisms of weight gain with ivacaftor treatment of cystic fibrosis gating mutations. J Pediatr 2018;201:229–237 e4.

20. Gelfond D, Heltshe S, Ma C, et al. Impact of CFTR modulation on intestinal pH, motility, and clinical outcomes in patients with cystic fibrosis and the G551D mutation. Clin Transl Gastroenterol 2017;8(3):e81.

21. Rosenfeld M, Wainwright CE, Higgins M, et al. Ivacaftor treatment of cystic fibrosis in children aged 12 to <24 months and with a CFTR gating mutation (ARRIVAL): a phase 3 single-arm study. Lancet Respir Med 2018;6(7):545–53.

22. Griese M, Costa S, Linnemann RW, et al. Safety and efficacy of elexacaftor/tezacaftor/ivacaftor for 24 weeks or longer in people with cystic fibrosis and one or more f508del alleles: interim results of an open-label phase 3 clinical trial. Am J Respir Crit Care Med 2021;203(3):381–5.

23. Heijerman HGM, McKone EF, Downey DG, et al. Efficacy and safety of the elexacaftor plus tezacaftor plus ivacaftor combination regimen in people with cystic fibrosis homozygous for the F508del mutation: a double-blind, randomised, phase 3 trial. Lancet 2019;394(10212):1940–8.

24. Nichols DP, Paynter AC, Heltshe SL, et al. Clinical effectiveness of elexacaftor/tezacftor/ivacaftor in people with cystic fibrosis. Am J Respir Crit Care Med 2021;205(5):529–39.

25. Cystic Fibrosis Foundation .Cystic Fibrosis Foundation Patient Registry 2020 Annual Data Report Bethesda, Maryland ©2021 Cystic Fibrosis Foundation.

https://www.cff.org/medical-professionals/patient-registry.

26. van der Haak N, King SJ, Crowder T, et al. Highlights from the nutrition guidelines for cystic fibrosis in Australia and New Zealand. J Cyst Fibros 2020; 19(1):16–25.

27. King SJ, Nyulasi IB, Strauss BJ, et al. Fat-free mass depletion in cystic fibrosis: associated with lung disease severity but poorly detected by body mass index. Nutrition 2010;26(7–8):753–9.

28. Calella P, Valerio G, Thomas M, et al. Association between body composition and pulmonary function in children and young people with cystic fibrosis. Nutrition 2018;48:73–6.

29. Calella P, Valerio G, Brodlie M, et al. Tools and methods used for the assessment of body composition in patients with cystic fibrosis: a systematic review. Nutr Clin Pract 2019;34(5):701–14.

30. Gomes A, Hutcheon D, Ziegler J. Association between fat-free mass and pulmonary function in patients with cystic fibrosis: a narrative review. Nutr Clin Pract 2019;34(5):715–27.

31. Leung DH, Heltshe SL, Borowitz D, et al. Effects of diagnosis by newborn screening for cystic fibrosis on weight and length in the first year of life. JAMA Pediatr 2017;171(6):546–54.

32. Harindhanavudhi T, Wang Q, Dunitz J, et al. Prevalence and factors associated with overweight and obesity in adults with cystic fibrosis: a single-center analysis. J Cyst Fibros 2020;19(1):139–45.

33. Madde A, Okoniewski W, Sanders DB, et al. Nutritional status and lung function in children with pancreatic-sufficient cystic fibrosis. J Cyst Fibros 2021;S1569-1993(21):02173–81.

34. Kutney KA, Sandouk Z, Desimone M, et al. Obesity in cystic fibrosis. J Clin Transl Endocrinol 2021;26: 100276.

35. Alvarez JA, Ziegler TR, Millson EC, et al. Body composition and lung function in cystic fibrosis and their association with adiposity and normal-weight obesity. Nutrition 2016;32(4):447–52.

36. Figueroa V, Milla C, Parks EJ, et al. Abnormal lipid concentrations in cystic fibrosis. Am J Clin Nutr 2002;75(6):1005–11.

37. Rhodes B, Nash EF, Tullis E, et al. Prevalence of dyslipidemia in adults with cystic fibrosis. J Cyst Fibros 2010;9(1):24–8.

38. Coderre L, Fadainia C, Belson L, et al. LDL-cholesterol and insulin are independently associated with body mass index in adult cystic fibrosis patients. J Cyst Fibros 2012;11(5):393–7.

39. Poore TS, Taylor-Cousar JL, Zemanick ET. Cardiovascular complications in cystic fibrosis: a review of the literature. J Cyst Fibros 2021;21(1):18–25.

40. Nowak JK, Wykretowicz A, Madry E, et al. Preclinical atherosclerosis in cystic fibrosis: two distinct presentations are related to pancreatic status. J Cyst Fibros 2021;21(1):26–33.

41. McDonald CM, Bowser EK, Farnham K, et al. Dietary macronutrient distribution and nutrition outcomes in persons with cystic fibrosis: an evidence analysis center systematic review. J Acad Nutr Diet 2021; 121(8):1574–15790 e3.

42. Stallings VA, Stark LJ, Robinson KA, et al. Clinical Practice Guidelines on G, et al. Evidence-based practice recommendations for nutrition-related management of children and adults with cystic fibrosis and pancreatic insufficiency: results of a systematic review. J Am Diet Assoc 2008;108(5):832–9.

43. Bellissimo MP, Zhang I, Ivie EA, et al. Visceral adipose tissue is associated with poor diet quality and higher fasting glucose in adults with cystic fibrosis. J Cyst Fibros 2019;18(3):430–5.

44. Sutherland R, Katz T, Liu V, et al. Dietary intake of energy-dense, nutrient-poor and nutrient-dense food sources in children with cystic fibrosis. J Cyst Fibros 2018;17(6):804–10.

45. Calvo-Lerma J, Hulst J, Boon M, et al. The relative contribution of food groups to macronutrient intake in children with cystic fibrosis: a European multicenter assessment. J Acad Nutr Diet 2019;119(8): 1305–19.

46. Poulimeneas D, Grammatikopoulou MG, Devetzi P, et al. Adherence to dietary recommendations, nutrient intake adequacy and diet quality among pediatric cystic fibrosis patients: results from the greecf study. Nutrients 2020;12(10):3126.

47. Micha R, Penalvo JL, Cudhea F, et al. Association between dietary factors and mortality from heart disease, stroke, and type 2 diabetes in the United States. JAMA 2017;317(9):912–24.

48. Puppo H, Torres-Castro R, Vasconcello-Castillo L, et al. Physical activity in children and adolescents with cystic fibrosis: a systematic review and meta-analysis. Pediatr Pulmonol 2020;55(11):2863–76.

49. Shelley J, Boddy LM, Knowles ZR, et al. Physical activity and associations with clinical outcome measures in adults with cystic fibrosis; a systematic review. J Cyst Fibros 2019;18(5):590–601.

50. Van Biervliet S, Declercq D, Dereeper S, et al. The effect of an intensive residential rehabilitation program on body composition in patients with cystic fibrosis. Eur J Pediatr 2021;180(6):1981–5.

51. Prevotat A, Godin J, Bernard H, et al. Improvement in body composition following a supervised exercise-training program of adult patients with cystic fibrosis. Respir Med Res 2019;75:5–9.

52. Schwarzenberg SJ, Hempstead SE, McDonald CM, et al. Enteral tube feeding for individuals with cystic fibrosis: cystic Fibrosis Foundation evidence-informed guidelines. J Cyst Fibros 2016;15(6): 724–35.

53. Shimmin D, Lowdon J, Remmington T. Enteral tube feeding for cystic fibrosis. Cochrane Database Syst Rev 2019;7(7):CD001198.

54. Foundation CF. Enzyme cheat sheet. Available at: https://my.cff.org/cfx-docrep/document/detail/enzyme%20cheat%20sheet%208-2021.docx2021.

55. Lepage G, Yesair DW, Ronco N, et al. Effect of an organized lipid matrix on lipid absorption and clinical outcomes in patients with cystic fibrosis. J Pediatr 2002;141(2):178–85.

56. Freedman S, Orenstein D, Black P, et al. Increased fat absorption from enteral formula through an in-line digestive cartridge in patients with cystic fibrosis. J Pediatr Gastroenterol Nutr 2017;65(1): 97–101.

57. Stevens J, Wyatt C, Brown P, et al. Absorption and safety with sustained use of RELiZORB evaluation (ASSURE) study in patients with cystic fibrosis receiving enteral feeding. J Pediatr Gastroenterol Nutr 2018;67(4):527–32.

58. Inc. DC. Digestive Care, Inc. Announces FDA labeling revision approval for PERTZYE(R) (pancrelipase). Available at: https://www.globenewswire.com/news-release/2017/07/12/1180176/0/en/Digestive-Care-Inc-Announces-FDA-Labeling-Revision-Approval-for-PERTZYE-R-pancrelipase.html 2017.

59. Borowitz D, Gelfond D, Maguiness K, et al. Maximal daily dose of pancreatic enzyme replacement therapy in infants with cystic fibrosis: a reconsideration. J Cyst Fibros 2013;12(6):784–5.

60. Schechter MS, Michel S, Liu S, et al. Relationship of initial pancreatic enzyme replacement therapy dose with weight gain in infants with cystic fibrosis. J Pediatr Gastroenterol Nutr 2018;67(4): 520–6.

61. Gelfond D, Heltshe SL, Skalland M, et al. Pancreatic enzyme replacement therapy use in infants with cystic fibrosis diagnosed by newborn screening. J Pediatr Gastroenterol Nutr 2018;66(4):657–63.

62. Calella P, Valerio G, Brodlie M, et al. Cystic fibrosis, body composition, and health outcomes: a systematic review. Nutrition 2018;55-56:131–9.

63. Putman MS, Anabtawi A, Le T, et al. Cystic fibrosis bone disease treatment: current knowledge and future directions. J Cyst Fibros 2019;18(Suppl 2): S56–65.

64. Baker JF, Putman MS, Herlyn K, et al. Body composition, lung function, and prevalent and progressive bone deficits among adults with cystic fibrosis. Joint Bone Spine 2016;83(2):207–11.

65. Putman MS, Greenblatt LB, Bruce M, et al. The effects of ivacaftor on bone density and microarchitecture in children and adults with cystic fibrosis. J Clin Endocrinol Metab 2021;106(3):e1248–61.

66. Moran A, Becker D, Casella SJ, et al. Epidemiology, pathophysiology, and prognostic implications of cystic fibrosis-related diabetes: a technical review. Diabetes Care 2010;33(12):2677–83.

67. Lind-Ayres M, Thomas W, Holme B, et al. Microalbuminuria in patients with cystic fibrosis. Diabetes Care 2011;34(7):1526–8.

68. Schwarzenberg SJ, Thomas W, Olsen TW, et al. Microvascular complications in cystic fibrosis-related diabetes. Diabetes Care 2007;30(5): 1056–61.

69. Moran A, Brunzell C, Cohen RC, et al. Clinical care guidelines for cystic fibrosis-related diabetes: a position statement of the American Diabetes Association and a clinical practice guideline of the Cystic Fibrosis Foundation, endorsed by the Pediatric Endocrine Society. Diabetes Care 2010;33(12): 2697–708.

70. Kaminski BA, Goldsweig BK, Sidhaye A, et al. Cystic fibrosis related diabetes: nutrition and growth considerations. J Cyst Fibros 2019;18(Suppl 2):S32–7.

71. Armaghanian N, Atkinson F, Taylor N, et al. Dietary intake in cystic fibrosis and its role in glucose metabolism. Clin Nutr 2020;39(8):2495–500.

72. Rana M, Wong-See D, Katz T, et al. Fat-soluble vitamin deficiency in children and adolescents with cystic fibrosis. J Clin Pathol 2014;67(7):605–8.

73. Siwamogsatham O, Dong W, Binongo JN, et al. Relationship between fat-soluble vitamin supplementation and blood concentrations in adolescent and adult patients with cystic fibrosis. Nutr Clin Pract 2014;29(4):491–7.

74. Borowitz D, Baker RD, Stallings V. Consensus report on nutrition for pediatric patients with cystic fibrosis. J Pediatr Gastroenterol Nutr 2002;35(3):246–59.

75. Maqbool A, Stallings VA. Update on fat-soluble vitamins in cystic fibrosis. Curr Opin Pulm Med 2008; 14(6):574–81.

76. Bines JE, Truby HD, Armstrong DS, et al. Vitamin A and E deficiency and lung disease in infants with cystic fibrosis. J Paediatr Child Health 2005;41(12): 663–8.

77. Graham-Maar RC, Schall JI, Stettler N, et al. Elevated vitamin A intake and serum retinol in preadolescent children with cystic fibrosis. Am J Clin Nutr 2006;84(1):174–82.

78. Maqbool A, Graham-Maar RC, Schall JI, et al. Vitamin A intake and elevated serum retinol levels in children and young adults with cystic fibrosis. J Cyst Fibros 2008;7(2):137–41.

79. Brei C, Simon A, Krawinkel MB, et al. Individualized vitamin A supplementation for patients with cystic fibrosis. Clin Nutr 2013;32(5):805–10.

80. Tangpricha V, Kelly A, Stephenson A, et al. An update on the screening, diagnosis, management, and treatment of vitamin D deficiency in individuals with cystic fibrosis: evidence-based recommendations from the Cystic Fibrosis Foundation. J Clin Endocrinol Metab 2012;97(4):1082–93.

81. Wolf G. How an increased intake of alpha-tocopherol can suppress the bioavailability of gamma-tocopherol. Nutr Rev 2006;64(6):295–9.

82. Sapiejka E, Krzyzanowska-Jankowska P, Wenska-Chyzy E, et al. Vitamin E status and its determinants in patients with cystic fibrosis. Adv Med Sci 2018; 63(2):341–6.

83. Vermeer C. Vitamin K: the effect on health beyond coagulation - an overview. Food Nutr Res 2012;56: 1. https://doi.org/10.3402/fnr.v56i0.5329.

84. Heltshe SL, Mayer-Hamblett N, Rowe SM. Understanding the relationship between sweat chloride and lung function in cystic fibrosis. Chest 2013; 144(4):1418.

85. Mills S, Lane JA, Smith GJ, et al. Precision nutrition and the microbiome part II: potential opportunities and pathways to commercialisation. Nutrients 2019;11(7):1468.

86. Mills S, Stanton C, Lane JA, et al. Precision nutrition and the microbiome, part I: current state of the science. Nutrients 2019;11(4):923.

87. Coffey MJ, Nielsen S, Wemheuer B, et al. Gut microbiota in children with cystic fibrosis: a taxonomic and functional dysbiosis. Sci Rep 2019;9(1):18593.

88. Hayden HS, Eng A, Pope CE, et al. Fecal dysbiosis in infants with cystic fibrosis is associated with early linear growth failure. Nat Med 2020;26(2):215–21.

89. Khalaf RT, Furuta GT, Wagner BD, et al. Influence of acid blockade on the aerodigestive tract microbiome in children with cystic fibrosis. J Pediatr Gastroenterol Nutr 2021;72(4):520–7.

90. Coffey MJ, Garg M, Homaira N, et al. Probiotics for people with cystic fibrosis. Cochrane Database Syst Rev 2020;1(1):CD012949.

91. Castellani C, Duff AJA, Bell SC, et al. ECFS best practice guidelines: the 2018 revision. J Cyst Fibros 2018;17(2):153–78.

92. Lahiri T, Hempstead SE, Brady C, et al. Clinical practice guidelines from the cystic fibrosis foundation for preschoolers with cystic fibrosis. Pediatrics 2016; 137(4):e20151784.

93. Sermet-Gaudelus I, Mayell SJ, Southern KW, European Cystic Finrosis Society NSWG. Guidelines on the early management of infants diagnosed with cystic fibrosis following newborn screening. J Cyst Fibros 2010;9(5):323–9.

94. Cystic Fibrosis F, Borowitz D, Parad RB, et al. Cystic fibrosis foundation practice guidelines for the management of infants with cystic fibrosis transmembrane conductance regulator-related metabolic syndrome during the first two years of life and beyond. J Pediatr 2009;155(6 Suppl):S106–16.

95. Edenborough FP, Borgo G, Knoop C, et al. Guidelines for the management of pregnancy in women with cystic fibrosis. J Cyst Fibros 2008;7(Suppl 1): S2–32.

96. Yankaskas JR, Marshall BC, Sufian B, et al. Cystic fibrosis adult care: consensus conference report. Chest 2004;125(1 Suppl):1S–39S.

Update in Advancing the Gastrointestinal Frontier in Cystic Fibrosis

Christopher Vélez, MD[a], Steven D. Freedman, MD, PhD[b],
David N. Assis, MD[c],*

KEYWORDS

- Cystic fibrosis • GERD • Dysmotility • SIBO • Pancreatic insufficiency • Liver involvement
- Constipation

KEY POINTS

- Gastrointestinal (GI) and hepatobiliary complications in persons with cystic fibrosis (pwCF) will assume a significantly greater relevance as this population lives longer and as more patients are diagnosed in adulthood with GI-predominant manifestations.
- GERD is very common in pwCF and should be treated primarily with PPI therapy.
- Empiric treatment of SIBO in pwCF should use rifaximin as the first-line agent.
- Liver biopsy to distinguish cirrhotic versus non cirrhotic causes of portal hypertension may be valuable in pwCF.
- Early colon cancer screening in all adults with CF should begin at age 40.

INTRODUCTION

Gastrointestinal (GI) manifestations were among the first complications observed with cystic fibrosis (CF).[1] (**Fig. 1**). Yet, with pulmonary disease being the major driver of morbidity and mortality in persons with CF (pwCF), the impact of CF on the GI tract and the hepatobiliary system historically has not been given the same attention. Additionally, most pwCF have their care directed principally by pulmonology providers, who may have completed training before the advent of new medications for constipation that have been developed relatively recently. Furthermore, the definition and scope of liver involvement in pwCF have not been clear, impairing the clinical characterization and management of hepatic complications in these individuals. The advent of highly effective modulator therapy (HEMT) (see Chapter 8) provides pwCF the best chance of the longest life span ever possible and this development builds on decades of incremental improvement in longevity through attention to nutrition and multidisciplinary care models. Undoubtedly, GI and hepatobiliary symptoms will assume a significantly greater clinical priority as this population ages and also as many new patients are diagnosed in adulthood due to improved clinical diagnosis and testing for genetic variants in pwCF who may have missed detection as children as a result of pancreatic sufficiency. Fortunately, emerging advances occurring in CF more broadly and in persons with CF-related gastrointestinal disease (CFGD) specifically will likely reduce symptom burden in the coming years.

PwCFGD can have disturbances from both the luminal and extra-luminal tract. When dividing the luminal GI tract into regions of embryologic origin (fore-, mid-, and hindgut), pathology attributable to CF is found in each region. In the foregut, comprising

[a] Division of Gastroenterology, Department of Medicine, Center for Neurointestinal Health, Massachusetts General Hospital, Harvard Medical School, 15 Parkman Street Suite 535, Boston, MA 0211, USA; [b] Beth Israel Medical Center, Harvard Medical School, 330 Brookline Avenue, Boston, MA 02215, USA; [c] Section of Digestive Diseases, Yale School of Medicine, 333 Cedar Street, 1080 LMP, New Haven, CT 06510, USA
* Corresponding author.
E-mail address: david.assis@yale.edu

Clin Chest Med 43 (2022) 743–755
https://doi.org/10.1016/j.ccm.2022.07.001
0272-5231/22/© 2022 Elsevier Inc. All rights reserved.

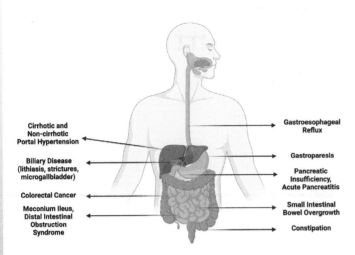

Fig. 1. Luminal and hepatobiliary manifestations of cystic fibrosis.

Cirrhotic and Non-cirrhotic Portal Hypertension

Biliary Disease (lithiasis, strictures, microgallbladder)

Colorectal Cancer

Meconium Ileus, Distal Intestinal Obstruction Syndrome

Gastroesophageal Reflux

Gastroparesis

Pancreatic Insufficiency, Acute Pancreatitis

Small Intestinal Bowel Overgrowth

Constipation

the esophagus and stomach, it is known that gastroesophageal reflux (GER) is burdensome in pwCF. In the mid-gut, consisting predominantly of the small intestine, there are issues with dysmotility and distal intestinal obstruction syndrome (DIOS) as well as perturbations in gut microbiome communities that can result in small intestinal bacterial overgrowth (SIBO). Finally, the hindgut consisting predominantly of the colon is impacted by constipation and increased risk for colorectal cancer malignancy. Similarly, the extra-luminal GI tract (consisting of the liver, biliary tree, and pancreas) experiences the consequences of dysfunction of the CF transmembrane conductance regulator (CFTR) protein, including the development of cirrhotic and noncirrhotic portal hypertension, sclerosing cholangitis, and both exocrine and endocrine pancreatic insufficiency (PI).

CFGD burden is substantial, as shown by the recent multicenter study of patient-reported GI symptoms in pwCF (GALAXY) study (NCT03801993).[2] GALAXY, an observational study investigating GI symptoms in more than 400 pwCFGD, found that 20.3% of patients with CF strained to pass bowel movements, 18.3% experienced fullness, 16.4% experienced bloating, and 5.2% and 7.5% had upper and lower abdominal pain, respectively.[2] Patient-reported outcome measures (PROMs) like the "Patient Assessment of Gastrointestinal Disorders – Symptom Severity" (PAGI-SYM), the "Patient Assessment of Constipation Symptoms" (PAC-SYM) and the "Patient Assessment of Constipation Quality of Life" (PAC-QoL) indices are well-validated questionnaires that detail GI symptom burden[3–5] that have been deployed systematically for the first time in pwCF. Here, we will review CFGD and

highlight recent advances or future research avenues that may be explored.

GASTROINTESTINAL MANIFESTATIONS OF CYSTIC FIBROSIS
Gastroesophageal Reflux

Gastroesophageal reflux is a normal physiologic event that occurs when gastric contents move in retrograde fashion into the esophagus, surpassing the barrier called the esophagogastric junction (EGJ) which consists of the gastric cardia, the diaphragm, as well as the lower esophageal sphincter. It is particularly common in infancy, ultimately resolving for the vast majority of children. Manifestations vary by age, and GER may be associated with difficulty with feeding and regurgitation in children and in adults may be either esophageal in nature (heartburn and regurgitation) or extra-esophageal (like cough).[6,7]

Gastroesophageal reflux becomes pathologic (ie, gastro-esophageal reflux disease (GERD)) either based on symptom patterns or after ambulatory reflux monitoring confirms an elevated exposure time (**Table 1**). PwCF can have reasons for developing this pathology that is similar to the population at large.[8] For example, impairment of appropriate EGJ function such as from transient lower esophageal reflux relaxations (TLESRs), decreased resting lower esophageal sphincter, and hiatal hernias can result in GERD in both pwCF and those without CF. When gastric emptying delays are present, the retention of contents can result in increased troublesome reflux. There are also CF-related factors that are thought to contribute to GERD in pwCF.[9] Gastric emptying delays can be provoked by lung transplantation as

Table 1 Reflux/heartburn in infants versus older children and adults	
Infants	**Older Children/ Adults**
• Refusal of feedings • Recurrent vomiting • Poor weight gain • Irritability • Sleep disturbance • Respiratory symptoms	• Abdominal pain/ heartburn • Recurrent vomiting • Dysphagia • Asthma • Recurrent pneumonia • Extra-esophageal symptoms (chronic cough, hoarse voice)

Adapted from Lightdale JR, Gremse DA; Section on Gastroenterology, Hepatology, and Nutrition. Gastroesophageal reflux: management guidance for the pediatrician. Pediatrics. 2013 May;131(5):e1684-95.

well as in those with CF-related diabetes. High-fat diets that historically have been recommended for pwCF also can provoke GERD symptoms.[10] Additionally, lung hyperinflation from obstructive lung disease and positional changes related to lung physical therapy are thought to contribute to GER development in pwCF.[8] It has been known since 1975 that pwCF have GER-related complaints. Determining GER prevalence is problematic due to the heterogeneity of definitions that have been used: symptom reporting or use of ambulatory-based reflux testing (described later in discussion).[9] As such, the reported prevalence has ranged from 35% to 81%.[11,12]

The principal diagnostic tools in the evaluation of GER include endoscopy, esophagram, high-resolution manometry, and ambulatory reflux monitoring.[13] Various algorithms[13,14] have been proposed recently for the diagnostic work-up and management of GER and GERD, and in the absence of data tailored specifically to pwCF, population-wide guidance should be offered by CF-focused clinicians. Reasonable recommendations include[1]: starting proton pump inhibitors (PPIs) empirically with typical esophageal reflux symptoms such as heartburn and regurgitation[2]; attempting the discontinuation of PPIs with responsive symptoms[3]; diagnostic endoscopy in patients not responsive to PPI[4]; ambulatory reflux testing in patients with typical symptoms; and[5] avoidance of using barium swallow as the sole proof of resource. There is greater variability in both pwCF and patients without CF in terms of the application of additional diagnostic testing such as high-resolution esophageal manometry

(HRM) and ambulatory reflux monitoring. In general, these tests are considered when there is a concern for esophageal motor abnormalities that may contribute to GER, when evaluating for dysphagia with a negative endoscopic examination when there are atypical GER symptoms (particularly relevant for pwCF with chronic cough), or to guide decision making regarding long-term PPI usage. Further information regarding when to apply the various modalities of esophageal testing can be found in **Table 2**.

The mainstay for pharmacologic GERD treatment remains PPIs, although various other agents can be used (**Table 3**). Care must be made to ensure that patients with CF also include lifestyle modification to reduce the need for PPI therapy (such as reduction in weight if obese in the context of pancreatic sufficiency or use of CFTR modulators), dietitian counseling to reduce insults from GERD-provoking foods, and avoidance of meals within 2 to 3 hours of bedtime.[13] The use of PPIs has proven controversial not only in the wider patient community but also in pwCF. There also have been reported concerns of risks like intestinal infections, bone density-related considerations, and electrolyte disturbances.[15] There have been conflicting considerations about PPIs in pwCF. Use of PPIs is common in patients taking pancreatic enzyme replacement therapy (PERT) to improve their efficacy.[16] Some evidence points to GER in CF contributing to respiratory exacerbations, which likely is part of the reason why more than half of patients treated in the United States are given PPIs.[8] Yet, other work associates PPI usage with increased pulmonary exacerbations in CF.[17] One must caution that the findings of adverse PPI events are based on flawed and often poorly generated data that lack plausible, pathophysiologic mechanisms; thus, ultimately the benefits of PPIs are likely greater than the risks.[15]

However, further prospective study is needed (and preferentially in conjunction with objective GER assessments with ambulatory reflux monitoring) to target which pwCF would benefit most from PPI therapy. Beyond PPI therapy, as there are limited data regarding the efficacy of antireflux procedures in pwCF (although published data do suggest a potential benefit[18]), it is unclear how aggressively antireflux procedures should be made available to pwCF. This question is particularly relevant given the increased adoption of endoluminal antireflux techniques such as transoral incisionless fundoplication (TIF) which offers a less invasive alternative to more invasive surgical approaches but whose long-term efficacy compared with traditional laparoscopic fundoplication remains unproven.[19]

Table 2
Routine diagnostic testing for heartburn and reflux

Diagnostic Testing Modality	Considerations and Recommendations
Endoscopy	• Exclude erosive esophagitis • Indicated when there are alarm signs (weight loss, dysphagia, melena, anemia) • May miss some anatomic abnormalities (large hiatal hernia, stricture/stenosis) • Consider with PPI-refractory symptoms • Used to place wireless pH monitoring
Esophagram and/or upper GI series	• Can comment on major abnormalities of esophageal motor function (esophagram) and, at times, on reflux (esophagram/upper GI series is <u>not</u> a recommended way to diagnose gastro-esophageal reflux) • Can highlight hernias, strictures/stenoses
High resolution manometry	• Identifies esophageal motor abnormalities (peristalsis and lower esophageal sphincter relaxation) that may be associated with pathologic GER • Used to identify lower esophageal sphincter and guide catheter-based ambulatory reflux and impedance monitoring • Indicated before lung

(continued on next page)

Table 2
(continued)

Diagnostic Testing Modality	Considerations and Recommendations
	transplantation or anti-reflux procedures
Catheter-based ambulatory reflux/impedance monitoring	• Two types: pH testing and pH multichannel intraluminal impedance (pH-MII) testing • pH-MII identifies both acidic reflux and weakly acid reflux (both can provoke worsening lung function in any pulmonary condition including CF) • Uses parameters like symptom index • Requires tolerance of nasal probe for 24 h • Diagnoses reflux hypersensitivity or functional heartburn, both conditions usually responding to neuromodulation with agents like tricyclic antidepressants, selective serotonin reuptake inhibitors, serotonin-norepinephrine reuptake inhibitors, trazodone
Wireless-based ambulatory reflux monitoring	• Only provides information on elevated acid exposure time and association of acidic reflux with symptoms • Provides 48–96 h of data • Can be associated with chest pain; rarely requires endoscopy to remove with snare

(continued on next page)

Table 2 *(continued)*	
Diagnostic Testing Modality	**Considerations and Recommendations**
	• Requires endoscopic placement; capsule can become dislodged particularly during placement and require bronchoscopy to remove • Will detach spontaneously and pass

Gastrointestinal Dysmotility in Persons with Cystic Fibrosis

Gastrointestinal dysmotility in pwCF is an important yet troublesome complication of the disease with difficult-to-manage symptoms that can consist of nausea, vomiting, abdominal pain, and bloating.[20] The provoking factor, as in the airway, is a cycle of impaired luminal flow due to highly viscous mucus that is associated with inflammation, infection, and dysbiosis and dysmotility. Dysmotility in pwCF can impact the entire gut, although lower GI motility considerations will be addressed subsequently in the setting of meconium ileus, DIOS, and chronic constipation is given particular considerations regarding the management and diagnoses of these diseases.

Motility disturbances of the GI tract refer to diseases arising from perturbed transit, either hastened or slowed through a variety of mechanisms such as iatrogenic injury or nerve dysfunction. A canonical motility disorder is gastroparesis. Gastroparesis has been recognized as a disease entity since the early 1900s, with the pioneering work of Boas and Ferroir demonstrating that gastric retention could be found in patients with diabetes in the setting of chronic weaker motor responses with slow contractions that fail to propagate correctly.[21–23] Traditionally, the management of gastroparesis has focused on the motor aspects of the disease. However, there is increasing recognition that there is likely a sensory component to patients' complaints which should also be addressed in patients deemed to be refractory before pursuing surgical intervention in the form of pyloroplasty or gastric electrical stimulation as this may better reflect a diagnosis of functional dyspepsia versus gastroparesis.[24] It is thought that gastroparesis is common in pwCF, although true prevalence is hindered by the heterogeneity of studies.[25]

Diabetes, a recognized risk factor for GI dysmotility, can result in acute changes in GI sensorimotor function due to temporary fluctuations in glycemic control and progressive autonomic neuropathy from long-term damage[26] and presumably this is a mechanism of dysmotility that is also present in persons with CF-related diabetes (pwCFRD). While studies cite different GI symptom prevalence depending on the sampled cohort, at least 70% of patients with diabetes in non-CF populations have such complaints.[26] It is estimated that upwards of 50% of diabetes in patients without CF (ie, type 1 diabetes and type 2 diabetes – T1D and T2D) is associated with delays in gastric emptying.[27] Acute hyperglycemia is associated with changes in GI motor function/motility including delays in stomach emptying and intestinal transit.[28–30] While both diabetes and CF independently impact the GI tract, it is not yet known if CFRD can compound CFGD.

In pwCF, symptoms of GI dysmotility such as nausea and vomiting can overlap both with other causes of GI illness (both CF-related and independent of CF) and a broad differential should be considered before settling on a diagnosis of GI dysmotility as a cause of a patient's complaints (**Box 1**). Evaluation to distinguish between these potential diagnoses before settling on GI dysmotility as an explanation begins first with the patient history to ensure both patients and clinicians are using the same word to describe the same complaint. For example, nausea is a sensation, vomiting is used exclusively to describe forceful emesis, and regurgitation which at times is described as "vomiting," but differs in that it is passive and effortless. Time course is also crucial, as the etiology of acute nausea, vomiting, and/or abdominal discomfort differs substantially from chronic causes. Beyond the history, evaluation includes tests familiar to any clinician, such as computerized tomography, abdominal x-ray, endoscopy, ultrasound, and gastric emptying scan (4-h with solid phase emptying preferred). Other modalities can be used including upper GI series[31] and wireless motility capsule.[32]

Management of GI dysmotility in pwCF can be as challenging as in those without CF and can include prokinetic therapy in the form of metoclopramide, erythromycin for patients with sluggish transit (in particular gastroparesis).[33] In pwCF in whom pain and discomfort are predominant symptoms, use of "neuromodulation" or medications like low dose antidepressants may be as critical as the use of prokinetic therapy given the overlap map between disorders of dysmotility like gastroparesis and disordered gut–brain interaction like functional dyspepsia.[24] Pyloric-

Table 3
Selected medical management for gastro-esophageal reflux symptoms

Agent	Recommendations/Considerations
Calcium carbonate	• Can be used for mild or breakthrough symptoms • Over-the-counter dosing depends on the product
Famotidine	• Histamine-2 antagonism can be used as needed for symptoms • Ranitidine no longer used due to potential carcinogenic risk • Potential for tachyphylaxis • Generally start famotidine 20 mg as needed, 1–2 times daily
Omeprazole/esomeprazole/pantoprazole/lansoprazole/dexlansoprazole/rabeprazole	• Proton pump inhibitors are the mainstay of heartburn/reflux symptom management • Must be given approximately 30-min before a meal; incorrect timing is a common mechanism of refractory symptoms • Each PPI has different dosing recommendations, follow accordingly • If typical GER symptoms (heartburn/regurgitation), generally purse ambulatory pH/pH-MII testing ON PPI to determine reflux hypersensitivity or esophageal hypersensitivity • If atypical GER symptoms (coughing, hoarseness), generally pursue ambulatory pH/PH-MII testing OFF PPI to determine if they truly have GERD • Given to pancreatic insufficient CF patients to assist in efficacy of pancreatic enzyme replacement • Long-term use may be problematic from CF perspective (may cause pulmonary exacerbations) and non-CF perspective (increased risk of enteric infections, decreased bone density)
Sucralfate	• At times given as an adjunctive agent for PPI-refractory symptoms • For PPI-refractory symptoms, should generally perform EGD and ambulatory reflux monitoring before resorting to sucralfate • Can inhibit the absorption of other medications, so must be timed far apart from other medications

directed therapy, in particular, pyloroplasty (surgical vs per-oral approaches) have not been studied in gastroparesis in pwCF, and its use somewhat limited.[34]

Small Intestinal Bacterial Overgrowth in Persons with Cystic Fibrosis

SIBO, defined as an abnormal increase in small intestinal bacterial burden beyond 10 colony-forming units per mL of intestinal fluid, is associated with CF.[20] Indeed, several studies have indicated a frequency of SIBO in up to 40%[35] in pwCF with symptoms including bloating, flatulence, abdominal pain, and diarrhea. If untreated, malabsorption of relevant nutrients (ie, fat-soluble vitamins, vitamin B12, and iron) can also occur. The frequency of these symptoms in pwCF and the predisposition to nutritional deficiency raise the need for an elevated suspicion of SIBO and early treatment in this population. One challenge, however, that is specific to pwCF is the difficulty in ascertaining a diagnosis of SIBO. This challenge occurs due to[1]: difficulty in the interpretation of breath tests in CF due to delayed intestinal transit, confounding by gas retention in the lungs from mucus plugs, and frequent exposure to antibiotics; and[2] a highly adherent mucus layer in the intestine of pwCF which makes adequate aspiration of small bowel fluid during endoscopy suboptimal.

Due to these limitations in diagnostic testing, pwCF with symptoms concerning SIBO in whom infectious pathogens (ie, *Clostridium difficile*) and suboptimal treatment of PI are ruled out can be given empirical treatment. In these patients, improvement in symptoms following empiric treatment is helpful to confirm the clinical diagnosis. First-line treatment options include rifaximin and metronidazole. A recent randomized, case-control clinical trial specifically evaluating SIBO in pwCF studied the efficacy of rifaximin, dosed at 1200 mg/d for 14 days versus observation.[36] Although the study was modest in size (13 patients received rifaximin and 10 received no treatments), the authors reported a clear difference among the groups with the eradication of symptoms in 90% of those who received rifaximin versus 33.3% of the observation group (*P* < .05). Patients who do not respond to rifaximin can be treated with alternative, second-line antibiotics including metronidazole, trimethoprim-sulfamethoxazole, doxycycline and amoxicillin/clavulanate, although overall the number and quality of studies on antibiotic therapy for SIBO is limited.[37] Failure to respond to more than one empiric trial of SIBO in pwCF should lead to a search for alternative explanations for the symptoms.

Pancreatic Insufficiency and Acute Pancreatitis

Pancreatic insufficiency was the first reported manifestation of what came to be known as CF,[1] and remains a seminal characteristic of CF in many patients with classes I, II, and III CFTR mutations.[38] Classic clinical manifestations can present soon after birth and include steatorrhea, failure to thrive, bloating and flatulence. Advanced PI is easily recognized on cross-sectional imaging with atrophy and fatty replacement of the pancreas. Left untreated, patients are at risk of progressive nutritional impairment, mineral bone deficiency, and growth delay. Early recognition and treatment of PI are one of the key factors responsible for the improved nutritional health and survival in pwCF over the past several decades.

A diagnosis of PI in pwCF can be made through a formal 72-hour fecal fat study in which more than 7 g of fat quantified over a 24 hour period is diagnostic.[39] However, this mode of testing is an impractical burden in routine clinical care, and a semiquantitative "spot" fecal fat test is not recommended due to lack of specificity. Therefore, the fecal elastase-1 test, using a monoclonal ELISA, is the preferred method for quantifying the degree of insufficiency and can be measured over time. This test has the additional advantage that it can be performed while patients are taking PERT. Fecal elastase was found to have an area under the receiver operating curve of 0.861 for the diagnosis of PI,[40] and a concentration of less than 84 ug/g had the best cutoff with a positive and negative predictive value of 66.7% and 93.9%, respectively. Conversely, a fecal elastase level greater than 100 ug/g is associated with a 99% negative predictive value.[41] All pwCF should be tested for PI with a fecal elastase measurement, and patients with class I, II, or III mutations and a low baseline fecal elastase level should receive PERT. In pwCF found to be pancreatic sufficient but who harbor the above class mutations, serial measurement is advised as the decline in pancreatic function can occur over time.[42]

Management of PI in pwCF includes the measurement of fat-soluble vitamins (ie, A,E,D,K) on a yearly basis with repletion under the input from CF-experienced nutritionists. Initiation of PERT should be started as soon as possible after the diagnosis of PI and maintained indefinitely. A typical starting dose may be 500 lipase units per kilogram per meal, with a maximum of 2500 lipase units per kilogram of body weight at meals, with half doses used for snacks. A Cochrane review of available studies comparing enteric versus non-enteric coated microsphere-based PERT found low quality of evidence and heterogeneity making formal comparisons difficult.[43] Recently, studies have evaluated the administration of PERT in pwCF who rely on enteral feedings. RELiZORB is an in-line digestive enzyme cartridge designed for patients receiving enteral feeding and has been found to be safe and well tolerated in pwCF with significant improvement in fat absorption.[44]

PwCF who are pancreatic sufficient may be at risk of acute pancreatitis, typically in the setting of milder CFTR mutations (those that confer some degree of CFTR function/chloride transport), milder lung disease, and a CF diagnosis in adolescence or adulthood.[45] In addition, there is a recognition that pwCF who develop acute pancreatitis often have a "second hit" such as alcohol, tobacco, drugs/metabolites, hypertriglyceridemia or ductal abnormalities (ie, pancreas divisum) as a key contributor, and thus the existence of additional triggers should be evaluated.[39] Recurrent acute pancreatitis in pwCF raises the risk of chronic pancreatitis with parenchymal damage and eventual insufficiency. Therefore, individuals

Box 1
A focused differential diagnosis for the CF
patient complaining of nausea and vomiting

Nausea and vomiting in CF patients

CF-related causes

- Gastroparesis
- Distal intestinal obstruction syndrome (DIOS)
- Chronic constipation
- Pancreatitis
- Gallstone disease

Non–CF-related acute causes

- Infection (including appendicitis)
- Mechanical obstruction
- Mesenteric ischemia
- Intoxication
- Non-GI causes (migraine, diabetic ketoacidosis, pregnancy, myocardial infarction, and so forth)

Miscellaneous chronic nausea and vomiting

- Functional nausea/vomiting disorders (such as cyclic vomiting syndrome)

with these complications should have monitoring for PI with fecal elastase levels over time.

Hepatobiliary Involvement in Persons with Cystic Fibrosis

The hepatobiliary system is commonly involved in pwCF and can affect patients with any of the CFTR mutation classes.[46,47] The CFTR protein is highly expressed in the gallbladder and entire biliary tree.[48] Dysfunctional expression may manifest clinically in the form of biliary strictures, microgallbladder, and hepatic lithiasis. Despite the absence of CFTR on hepatocytes, parenchymal liver damage is common in CF and manifestations include steatosis, focal biliary cirrhosis, cholestasis, and advanced liver disease with cirrhosis. One of the limitations which historically hindered the understanding of hepatic manifestations of CF is a lack of clear definitions and clinical characterization. The term cystic fibrosis liver disease (CFLD) is imprecise and can refer to a variety of liver abnormalities. Various criteria have been proposed (ie, Colombo,[49] Debray,[50] Flass/Narkewicz,[51] Koh[52]) which differ regarding the reliance on physical examination and the use of noninvasive markers of fibrosis such as transient elastography. A consensus on terminology and clear distinctions between mild liver involvement in CF (ie, elevation of AST and ALT, GGT, simple steatosis) versus advanced liver disease (biliary cirrhosis, portal hypertension) will allow for better delineation of disease phenotypes.

PwCF of all ages can demonstrate liver involvement, such as mild hepatomegaly, steatosis, elevated liver enzymes, and biliary abnormalities. A smaller minority of patients develop advanced liver disease, frequently in adolescence and early adulthood.[46] Given that clinical symptoms of liver disease are often absent until late stages, there may be a benefit for proactive screening for liver involvement in all pwCF although such screening is not yet standardized. It also is likely that physical examination for hepatosplenomegaly in combination with laboratory liver tests can be beneficial to detect advanced liver involvement. Liver ultrasound imaging can demonstrate the presence of heterogeneous parenchyma and may be useful to distinguish between those at risk of subsequent liver disease over time.[53] For those diagnosed with liver manifestations of CF, determining the extent of disease and particularly fibrosis is important for monitoring and prognostication. Calculated scores based on laboratory tests (ie, aspartate-to-platelet ratio or APRI; FIB-4) may help with the early identification of pwCF and advanced liver disease including portal hypertension.[52,54] In addition, recent studies have demonstrated a benefit of noninvasive measurements of fibrosis from transient elastography.[55] Indeed, a baseline assessment of fibrosis should be performed in patients with documented liver involvement to distinguish between minimal fibrosis (stage 0–1) and advanced liver fibrosis (stage 3–4), since this information carries prognostic significance.

PwCF and advanced liver disease who have clinical manifestations of portal hypertension are at higher risk of needing liver transplantation.[46] Traditionally, the assumption has been that patients with morphologic changes suggestive of cirrhosis (ie, nodularity on imaging) with portal hypertension findings (ie, varices, ascites) have well-established cirrhosis. However, a recent series of studies reported a surprisingly frequent occurrence of noncirrhotic portal hypertension in the explants of patients who underwent liver transplantation.[56–58] The pathophysiology of noncirrhotic portal hypertension in pwCF is not well understood, but histologic findings include obliterative portal venopathy causing nodular regenerative hyperplasia, possibly resulting from inflammatory or coagulable changes in the context of CF. Importantly, the absence of synthetic dysfunction in noncirrhotic portal hypertension may allow for nontransplant management strategies. Therefore, consideration should be given to

Table 4
Management options for chronic constipation in pwCF

Agent	Typical Indications	Dosing Recommendations/ Considerations
Laxative therapy		
Polyethylene glycol (Miralax, GoLytely)	• As-needed or baseline bowel regimen	• Generally benign regimen with ability to uptitrate and downtitrate • Start 0.5 capful daily for 1 wk, can increase to 1 capful daily as baseline regimen • Can use as frequently as twice or 3 times daily • Can use heavier dose preparations (ie, 119 g in 40 oz of water or 235 g in 80 oz of water) if symptoms acutely worsening • Same active ingredient as many large volume preps like GoLytely, follow dosing instructions
Sennosides/bisacodyl	• As-needed or baseline bowel regimen	• Can be associated with abdominal pain • Start Senna 2 tablets (17.2 mg) once daily, can uptitrate to 5 tablets twice daily • Start bisacodyl 5 mg daily, can be increased to 5 mg three times daily
Magnesium citrate	• As-needed or baseline bowel regimen	• Try to use mainly as rescue therapy given potential electrolyte disturbance • 300 mL given at once or divided over the course of the day
Pro-secretory or pro-kinetic therapy		
Linaclotide	• Laxative-refractory constipation	• Secretagogue • Mechanism is via CFTR • Start 72 mcg daily, can increase eventually to 290 mcg daily • Can be associated with diarrhea, abdominal pain
Lubiprostone	• Laxative-refractory constipation	• Secretagogue • Start lubiprostone 8 mcg daily, can increase to 25 mcg twice daily • Can be associated with headache, abdominal pain, and diarrhea
Plecanatide	• Laxative-refractory constipation	• Secretagogue • 3 mg once daily
Prucalopride	• Laxative-refractory constipation	• Prokinetic • 2 mg daily • Can be considered if there is underlying gastroparesis

a liver biopsy to rule in or out histologic cirrhosis in pwCF found to have portal hypertension. Ultimately, patients with portal hypertension and signs of decompensated liver disease with ascites, synthetic dysfunction, or variceal bleeding should be considered for transplant evaluation.

PwCF who develop acute cholangitis should be evaluated with MRI/MRCP imaging to evaluate for sclerosing cholangitis features with large duct biliary strictures.[59] Another manifestation of CF that can lead to biliary obstruction and cholangitis is intrahepatic lithiasis, also best evaluated with MRI imaging. Patients found to have large duct abnormalities and/or stones should receive therapeutic endoscopic retrograde cholangiopancreatography (ERCP) for removal of stones and/or treatment of strictures with balloon dilation or stenting.

Cystic Fibrosis and the Lower Gastrointestinal Tract

PwCF can develop several classic diagnoses related to CFGD of the lower GI tract: meconium ileus of the neonate and DIOS. Symptoms in part overlap with disorders of CF dysmotility, but, alterations in bowel habits (in particular, frequency, consistency, and association with pain) can be distinct. Meconium ileus management remains relatively unchanged from the historical standard of care with the prioritization of medical management over surgical approaches whenever possible.[60] It is increasingly recognized that chronic constipation begets DIOS, with DIOS first described as being a "meconium ileus equivalent" (61). The prevention and management of DIOS are analogous to that of meconium ileus with the following goals[1]: primary and secondary prevention through adequate hydration, optimized use of PERT in the setting of PI, and treatment of constipation[2]; treatment through noninvasive means with agents such as gastrografin enemas; and[3] avoidance of surgical intervention if possible.

As with more proximal GI dysmotility, history is key. Patients will use the terms "constipation" and "diarrhea" in ways that providers would not necessarily use (eg, mistaken belief that failure to have a bowel movement daily constitutes constipation). It is important to ask clarifying questions such as stool consistency, straining, bloating/pain, need for manual disimpaction to maneuvers. Potential iatrogenic causes of altered bowel habits need to be explored. Once history is clarified, diagnostic testing can include colonoscopy, stool testing, serologic assessment for the systemic illness that can result in a change in bowel habits (such hypo- or hyper-thyroid states). Anorectal manometry can be used to identify pelvic dyssynergia as a cause of constipation for which patients may benefit from pelvic floor therapy. Likewise, the differential of diarrhea is broad in pwCF and may be related to PI that is not treated or is undertreated with PERT, "overflow" diarrhea associated with chronic constipation, antibiotic-related diarrhea, C difficile-related diarrhea, or other pathologies.

Management of chronic constipation in pwCF generally follows options available to the patient population at large given the lack of robust trials studying treatment efficacy, particularly of a whole host of new agents available over the past 10 years (**Table 4**). Mainstays of constipation treatment include osmotic laxatives, stimulant laxatives, and fiber. Despite the lack of evidence demonstrating efficacy in patients with CF, linaclotide, lubiprostone, plecanatide, and prucalopride can be used (and can be considered if older medications fail to control constipation). When pain is a predominant feature (vs frequency and consistency of bowel habits), as in GI dysmotility, neuromodulation may be used, again based on provider preference given the lack of evidence.

As the majority of patients with CF are now adults, the risk of colorectal cancer development is an area of lower GI health in pwCF of increasing relevance. There is a concern that CF can almost be considered a hereditary cancer syndrome, with risk factors including chronic inflammation in the setting of constipation, and in patients with lung transplant, the risk factor is the use of immunosuppressants.[61] Guidelines from the Cystic Fibrosis Colorectal Screening Task Force[62] recommend that[1]: colonoscopy should be favored over noninvasive modalities[2]; screening should begin at age 40 be repeated every 5-year if no adenomatous lesions are observed– within 3-year if adenomatous lesions are found; and[3] should include adults over 30 years within 2 years of solid organ transplant. These recommendations include aggressive intervals driven by concern that colon cancer incidence is several folds higher in pwCF than in the rest of the population: more research is needed to justify this degree of intervention (62).

SUMMARY

The wide spectrum of GI and hepatobiliary manifestations of CF makes it imperative for the clinician to maintain an open-minded approach to patient symptoms and an updated skill set for evaluation and management of these complications in pwCF. As the CF population continues to live longer and benefit from HEMT for pulmonary complications, there will be a need to focus on luminal and hepatobiliary disease which will account for an increasing share of the disease burden for pwCF. Scientific and clinical innovations that can improve diagnostic and management strategies are necessary and should be prioritized through coordinated approaches by multiple stakeholders.

CLINICS CARE POINTS

- GERD is common in pwCF, may be exacerbated by lung hyperinflation due to CF itself, and should be treated with PPI as the mainstay of therapy.
- pwCF with GI dysmotility who have pain and discomfort as predominant symptoms may benefit from neuromodulation or low-dose antidepressants as much as prokinetic therapy.
- Empirical treatment of suspected SIBO in pwCF should use rifaximin as the first-line agent.
- All pwCF should be tested for PI with a fecal elastase measurement, and those with CFTR class I, II, and III mutations found to be sufficient should have serial measurement over time to monitor for a decline in function.
- pwCF found to have portal hypertension may have noncirrhotic causes such as nodular regenerative hyperplasia, and a liver biopsy to distinguish between cirrhosis and noncirrhotic histology can be considered.
- Treatment of constipation in pwCF can include laxatives as well as newer nonlaxative agents such as linaclotide and lubiprostone.
- The increased risk of colorectal cancer in CF requires early screening with colonoscopy beginning at age 40 for all adults with CF, and at age 30 in those who are at least 2 years postsolid organ transplant.

DISCLOSURE

C. Velez – Cystic Fibrosis Foundation (CFF) funding for research in the gastrointestinal manifestations of cystic fibrosis, CFF DIGEST faculty award, CFF Data Safety Monitoring Board. S.D. Freedman – CFF funding for research in the gastrointestinal manifestations of cystic fibrosis, CFF DIGEST faculty. D.N. Assis – Prior CFF DIGEST faculty award, CFF research funding.

REFERENCES

1. Andersen DH. Cystic fibrosis of the pancreas and its relation to celiac disease: a clinical and pathologic study. Am J Dis Child 1938;56:344–99.
2. Moshiree B., Freeman A.J., Vu P., et al., Multicenter prospective study of gastrointestinal symptom prevalence and severity in CF: GALASY results, Pediatr Pulmonol, 55 (S2), 2020, 127 (Abstract 227).
3. Revicki DA, Rentz AM, Tack J, et al. Responsiveness and interpretation of a symptom severity index specific to upper gastrointestinal disorders. Clin Gastroenterol Hepatol 2004;2:769–77.
4. Slappendel R, Simpson K, Dubois D, et al. Validation of the PAC-SYM questionnaire for opioid-induced constipation in patients with chronic low back pain. Eur J Pain 2006;10:209–17.
5. Marquis P, De La Loge C, Dubois D, et al. Development and validation of the patient Assessment of constipation quality of life questionnaire. Scand J Gastroenterol 2005;40:540–51.
6. Maqbool A, Pauwels A. Cystic Fibrosis and gastroesophageal reflux disease. J Cyst Fibros 2017; 16(Suppl 2):S2–13.
7. Lightdale JR, Gremse DA, Section on Gastroenterology, Hepatology, and Nutrition. Gastroesophageal reflux: management guidance for the pediatrician. Pediatrics 2013;131:e1684–95.
8. Robinson NB, DiMango E. Prevalence of gastroesophageal reflux in cystic fibrosis and implications for lung disease. Ann Am Thorac Soc 2014;11:964–8.
9. Pauwels A, Blondeau K, Dupont LJ, et al. Mechanisms of increased gastroesophageal reflux in patients with cystic fibrosis. Am J Gastroenterol 2012; 107:1346–53.
10. Omari T. Gastro-oesophagel reflux disease and children: new insights, developments and old chestnuts. J Pediatr Gastroenterol Nutr 2005;41(Suppl 1):S21–3.
11. Button BM, Roberts S, Kotsimbos TC, et al. Gastroesophageal reflux (symptomatic and silent): a potentially significant problem in patients with cystic fibrosis before and after lung transplantation. J Heart Lung Transpl 2005;24:1522–9.
12. Ledson MJ, Tran J, Walshaw MJ. Prevalence and mechanisms of gastro-oesophageal reflux in adult cystic fibrosis patients. J R Soc Med 1998;91:7–9.
13. Katz PO, Dunbar KB, Schnoll-Sussman FH, et al. ACG clinical guideline for the diagnosis and management of gastroesophageal reflux disease. Am J Gastroenterol 2022;117:27–56.
14. Gyawali CP, Carlson DA, Chen JW, et al. ACG clinical guidelines: clinical use of esophageal physiologic testing. Am J Gastroenterol 2020;115:1412–28.
15. Freedberg DE, Kim LS, Yang YX. The risks and benefits of long-term use of proton pump inhibitors:

expert review and best practice advice from the American Gastroenterological Association. Gastroenterology 2017;152:706–15.

16. Lindkvist B. Diagnosis and treatment of pancreatic exocrine insufficiency. World J Gastroenterol 2013; 19:7258–66.

17. Ayoub F, Lascano J, Morelli G. Proton pump inhibitor use is associated with an increased frequency of hospitalization in patients with cystic fibrosis. Gastroenterol Res 2017;10:288–93.

18. Ng J, Friedmacher F, Pao C, et al. Gastroesophageal reflux disease and need for antireflux surgery in children with cystic fibrosis: a systematic review on incidence, surgical complications, and postoperative outcomes. Eur J Pediatr Surg 2021;31:106–14.

19. Richter JE, Kumar A, Lipka S, et al. Efficacy of laparoscopic nissen fundoplication vs transoral incisionless fundoplication or proton pump inhibitors in patients with gastroesophageal reflux disease: a systematic review and network meta-analysis. Gastroenterology 2018;154:1298–1308 e7.

20. Dorsey J, Gonska T. Bacterial overgrowth, dysbiosis, inflammation, and dysmotility in the Cystic Fibrosis intestine. J Cyst Fibros 2017;16(Suppl 2): S14–23.

21. Saltzman MB, McCallum RW. Diabetes and the stomach. Yale J Biol Med 1983;56:179–87.

22. Navas CM, Patel NK, Lacy BE. Gastroparesis: medical and therapeutic advances. Dig Dis Sci 2017;62: 2231–40.

23. Sullivan A, Temperley L, Ruban A. Pathophysiology, aetiology and treatment of gastroparesis. Dig Dis Sci 2020;65:1615–31.

24. Pasricha PJ, Grover M, Yates KP, et al. Functional dyspepsia and gastroparesis in tertiary care are interchangeable syndromes with common clinical and pathologic features. Gastroenterology 2021; 160:2006–17.

25. Corral JE, Dye CW, Mascarenhas MR, et al. Is Gastroparesis found more frequently in patients with cystic fibrosis? a systematic review. Scientifica (Cairo) 2016;2016:2918139.

26. Du YT, Rayner CK, Jones KL, et al. Gastrointestinal symptoms in diabetes: prevalence, assessment, pathogenesis, and management. Diabetes Care 2018;41:627–37.

27. Bharucha AE, Kudva YC, Prichard DO. Diabetic gastroparesis. Endocr Rev 2019;40:1318–52.

28. de Boer SY, Masclee AA, Lamers CB. Effect of hyperglycemia on gastrointestinal and gallbladder motility. Scand J Gastroenterol Suppl 1992;194: 13–8.

29. Keshavarzian A, Iber FL. Gastrointestinal involvement in insulin-requiring diabetes mellitus. J Clin Gastroenterol 1987;9:685–92.

30. Rayner CK, Samsom M, Jones KL, et al. Relationships of upper gastrointestinal motor and sensory function with glycemic control. Diabetes Care 2001;24:371–81.

31. Szarka LA, Camilleri M. Methods for the assessment of small-bowel and colonic transit. Semin Nucl Med 2012;42:113–23.

32. Saad RJ, Hasler WL. A technical review and clinical assessment of the wireless motility capsule. Gastroenterol Hepatol (N Y) 2011;7:795–804.

33. Camilleri M, Parkman HP, Shafi MA, et al. Clinical guideline: management of gastroparesis. Am J Gastroenterol 2013;108:18–37 [quiz: 38].

34. Lebares C, Swanstrom LL. Per-oral pyloromyotomy (POP): an emerging application of submucosal tunneling for the treatment of refractory gastroparesis. Gastrointest Endosc Clin N Am 2016;26: 257–70.

35. Lewindon PJ, Robb TA, Moore DJ, et al. Bowel dysfunction in cystic fibrsis: importance of breath testing. J Paediatr Child Health 1998;34:79–82.

36. Furnari M, De Alessandri A, Cresta F, et al. The role of small intestinal bacterial overgrowth in cystic fibrosis: a randomized case-controlled clinical trial with rifaximin. J Gastroenterol 2019;54:261–70.

37. Shah SC, Day LW, Somsouk M, et al. Meta-analysis: antibiotic therapy for small intestinal bacterial overgrowth. Aliment Pharmacol Ther 2013;38:925–34.

38. Ahmed N, Corey M, Forstner G, et al. Molecular consequences of cystic fibrosis transmembrane regulator (CFTR) gene mutations in the exocrine pancreas. Gut 2003;52:1159–64.

39. Assis DN, Freedman SD. Gastrointestinal disorders in cystic fibrosis. Clin Chest Med 2016;37:109–18.

40. Gonzalez-Sanchez V, Amrani R, Gonzalez V, et al. Diagnosis of exocrine pancreatic insufficiency in chronic pancreatitis: 13C-mixed triglyceride breath test versus fecal elastase. Pancreatology 2017;17: 580–5.

41. Beharry S, Ellis L, Corey M, et al. How useful is fecal pancreatic elastase 1 as a marker of exocrine pancreatic disease? J Pediatr 2002;141:84–90.

42. Walkowiak J, Nousia-Arvanitakis S, Agguridaki C, et al. Longitudinal follow-up of exocrine pancreatic function in pancreatic sufficient cystic fibrosis patgients using the fecal elastase-1 test. J Pediatr Gastroenterol Nutr 2003;36:474–8.

43. Somaraju URR, Solis-Moya A. Pancreatic enzyme replacement therapy for people with cystic fibrosis. Cochrane Database Syst Rev 2020;5:CD008227.

44. Stevens J, Wyatt C, Brown P, et al. Absorption and safety with sustained use of RELiZORB Evaluation (ASSURE) study in patients with cystic fibrosis receiving enteral feeding. J Pediatr Gastroenterol Nutr 2018;67:527–32.

45. Durno C, Corey M, Zielinski J, et al. Genotype and phenotype correlations in patients with cystic fibrosis and pancreatitis. Gastroenterology 2002; 123:1857–64.

46. Leung DH, Narkewicz MR. Cystic fibrosis-related cirrhosis. J Cyst Fibros 2017;(Supppl 2):S50–61.

47. Assis DN, Debray D. Gallbladder and bile duct disease in Cystic Fibrosis. J Cyst Fibros 2017;(Suppl 2):S62–9.

48. Cohn JA, Strong TV, Picciotto MR, et al. Locatlization of the cystic fibrosis transmembrane conductance regulator in human bile duct epithelial cells. Gastroenterology 1993;106:1857–64.

49. Colombo C, Battezzati PM, Crosignani A, et al. Liver disease in cystic fibrosis: a prospective study on incidence, risk factors, and outcome. Hepatology 2002;36:1374–82.

50. Debray D. Cystic fibrosis associated with liver disease. Arch Pediatr 2012;(Suppl 1):S23–6.

51. Flass T, Narkewicz MR. Cirrhosis and other liver disease in cystic fibrosis. J Cyst Fibros 2013;12:116–24.

52. Koh C, Sakiani S, Surana P, et al. Adult-onset cystic fibrosis liver disease: diagnosis and characterization of an underappreciated entity. Hepatology 2017;66:591–601.

53. Siegel MJ, Freeman AJ, Ye W, et al. Heterogeneous liver on research ultrasound identifies children with cystic fibrosis at high risk of advanced liver disease: interim results of a prospective observational case-controlled study. J Pediatr 2020;219:62–9.

54. Klotter V, Gunchick C, Siemers E, et al. Assessment of pathologic increase in liver stiffness enables earlier diagnosis of CFLD: results from a prospective longitudinal cohort study. PLoS One 2017;12:e0178784.

55. Lewindon PJ, Puertolas-Lopez MV, Ramm LE, et al. Accuracy of transient elastography data combined with APRI in detection and staging of liver disease in pediatric patients with cystic fibrosis. Clin Gastroenterol Hepatol 2019;17:2561–9.

56. Wu H, Vu M, Dhingra S, et al. Obliterative portal venopahty without cirrhosis is prevalent in pediatric cystic fibrosis liver disease with portal hypertension. Clin Gastroenterol Hepatol 2019;17:2134–6.

57. Witters P, Libbrecht L, Roskams T, et al. Liver disease in cystic fibrosis presents as non-cirrhotic portal hypertension. J Cyst Fibros 2017;16:e11–3.

58. Hillaire S, Cazals-Hatem D, Bruno O, et al. Liver transplantation in adult cystic fibrosis: clinical, imaging, and pathological evidence of obliterative portal venopathy. Liver Transpl 2017;23:1342–7.

59. Durieu I, Pellet O, Simonot L, et al. Sclerosing cholangitis in adults with cystic fibrosis: a magnetic resonance cholangiographic prospective study. J Hepatol 1999;30:1052–6.

60. Sathe M, Houwen R. Meconium ileus in cystic fibrosis. J Cyst Fibros 2017;16(Suppl 2):S32–9.

61. Abraham J, Taylor C. Cystic Fibrosis & disorders of the large intestine: DIOS, constipation, and colorectal cancer. J cystic fibrosis 2017;16.

62. Hadjiliadis D, Khoruts A, Zauber AG, et al. Cystic Fibrosis colorectal cancer screening consensus recommendations. Gastroenterology 2018;154:736–45.

Transitions of Care in Cystic Fibrosis

Eunice M.M. DeFilippo, MD[a], Jaideep S. Talwalkar, MD[a,b], Zachary M. Harris, MD[b],
Jennifer Butcher, PhD[c], Samya Z. Nasr, MD[d,*]

KEYWORDS

- Cystic fibrosis • Health care transition • CF rise • Transition readiness evaluation
- Self-management • Quality improvement • Adolescents

KEY POINTS

- What should transition look like in chronic diseases?
- There are barriers and challenges associated with cystic fibrosis (CF) transition.
- Several models of transition have been described to create an appropriate transition landscape.
- Establishment of formal, standardized programs and models of care is important in the transition process.
- There are recommended mechanisms to enhance training and establishment of programs for transition.

INTRODUCTION

Health care transition (HCT) is defined as the process of transitioning and transferring adolescents and young adults from a pediatric/family-centered model of care to an adult/patient-centered one.[1–3] Medical advances related to the care of people with cystic fibrosis (pwCF) have been improving since the creation of the Cystic Fibrosis Foundation (CFF) in 1955.[4,5] Today, more than 50% of pwCF are adults who manage complex medication regimens.[6] Accordingly, the best practice for HCT requires the utilization of a systematic and planned process involving careful attention to the skills necessary for pwCF to make a safe and stable transition to the adult health care system that is tailored to their needs.[2,4,7]

Ideally, at the end of the transition process, pwCF should be prepared with pertinent disease-related knowledge and skills in self-management, and the independence to implement these skills. To optimize their integration into the adult care model, pwCF should be equipped with the appropriate care coordination, insurance coverage, social services, behavioral health support, and family support.[7–10]

Despite the progress made in CF management, as pwCF emerge into adulthood, they continue to face many challenges.[5] These challenges often stem from developmental changes leading to more risk-taking behaviors, difficulty with disease self-management and autonomy, health care system changes between pediatrics and adult medicine, and disease-related comorbidities that cooccur with the transition to adulthood.[9] Standardized transition programs for pwCF can address these challenges.

Due to the growing calls for the structured transition to comprehensive adult care for pwCF, in 2000, the CFF mandated the development of adult CF programs for centers with over 40 adults. This

All authors have nothing to disclose.
[a] Internal Medicine and Pediatrics, Yale School of Medicine, New Haven, CT, USA; [b] Yale Adult Cystic Fibrosis Program, Section of Pulmonary, Critical Care, and Sleep Medicine, Yale School of Medicine, New Haven, CT, USA; [c] Department of Pediatrics, Division of Pediatric Psychology, Mott Children's Hospital, University of Michigan Health, Ann Arbor, MI, USA; [d] Department of Pediatrics, Division of Pediatric Pulmonology, Mott Children's Hospital, University of Michigan Health, 1500 E. Medical Center Dr., Ann Arbor, MI 48109-5212, USA
* Corresponding author.
E-mail address: snasr@umich.edu

Clin Chest Med 43 (2022) 757–771
https://doi.org/10.1016/j.ccm.2022.06.016
0272-5231/22/© 2022 Elsevier Inc. All rights reserved.

chestmed.theclinics.com

mandate led to the swift emergence of diverse models of adult CF care centers nationwide, and the development of a variety of protocols, tools, and frameworks to support transition and transfer for pwCF.[11] However, HCT among CF care centers was inconsistent and generally lacking in timely transfer, readiness assessments, and other metrics for the optimal transition. For centers that were most successful with transition efforts, broad dissemination of best practices across centers was lacking.[12] The development of formal transition models emerged to combat this variability in care, including CF RISE (CF: responsibility, independence, self-care, and education) which provided a standardized and modular transition program including knowledge assessments, self-management checklists, and milestones for pwCF and their families, with successful broad implementation.[12,13] Despite these interventions, recent outcomes continue to suggest that the approach to the transition period remains suboptimal.

Problems Associated with Transition

Adolescents transitioning to adulthood often face an overall decline in health (**Fig. 1**) and are associated with lower rates of health care system utilization, difficulties navigating the adult health care system, poor medical regimen adherence, and gaps in insurance coverage.[2,9,14] A retrospective analysis using the Nationwide Inpatient Sample showed that among pwCF hospitalized with CF between 2002 and 2017, young adults had more comorbidities, hospitalizations, and in-hospital mortality compared to children hospitalized with CF. Also, opioid use, alcohol use, depression, and weight loss increased among adults compared with children with CF.[9] In 2019, Dunbar

and colleagues[15] showed that compared to people hospitalized with type 1 diabetes, sickle cell disease, spina bifida, and inflammatory bowel disease, hospitalized pwCF had the highest increase in readmission rates between adolescence and adulthood.

In addition, using data from the CFF registry, Sawicki and colleagues[16] showed that for pwCF transferring to an adult program between 2007 and 2013, there was an average gap in outpatient care of 183 days, with 13% of pwCF having a gap in the care of over 1 year. These gaps occurred despite recommendations for quarterly follow-up. Furthermore, around the time of the standard age of transition, pwCF tend to develop new complications such as CF-related diabetes (CFRD), multidrug-resistant-infection, or , considerations for transplant in those with advanced disease.[17–19]

What Should Transition Look Like in Chronic Diseases?

The purpose of structured HCT is to intervene in the preventable aspects of these barriers.[20] According to a 2017 systematic review, a structured HCT intervention can decrease ED utilization, and improve medical regimen adherence, health literacy, and patient and family satisfaction.[20] It can also decrease anxiety, increase perceived readiness, and improve autonomy, disease self-management, and satisfaction posttransition.[21] Follow-up rates may improve when pwCF and providers agree on the timing of transfer.[22]

Best practices for transfer include having a joint visit with the pediatric and adult provider, a medical summary of disease course with a treatment plan, and proper care coordination to facilitate transfer.[3,7,23] The process of transition, however,

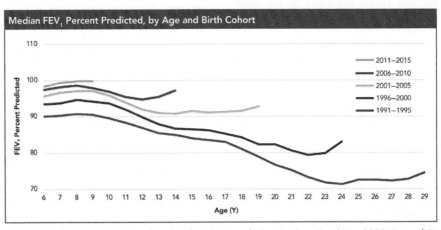

Fig. 1. Deterioration of FEV1 over time. (Cystic Fibrosis Foundation Patient Registry, 2020 Annual Data Report, Bethesda, Maryland, ©2021 Cystic Fibrosis Foundation.)

is not one-size-fits-all and must be adjusted based on disease burden and the needs or preferences of pwCF and their families.[3]

The challenges of implementing structured HCT programs are not unique to CF. In 2015, as part of the *Healthy People 2030 adolescent health objective to improve HCT,* the Maternal and Child Health Bureau began tracking the percent of children who received HCT services as part of their 2015–2017 block grant cycle. A subsequent analysis noted that only about 70% of respondents reported that a health care provider worked with them to gain self-care skills or to understand changes in health care that occur at age 18, a measure that is fundamental to optimal HCT.[24,25] Across specialists, primary care pediatricians, and adult providers, less than 20% of children reported receiving the recommended transition support.[24,26]

BARRIERS AND CHALLENGES ASSOCIATED WITH CYSTIC FIBROSIS TRANSITION
Medical Complexity

While there are adult CF care guidelines, the HCT-related recommendations have not been updated since 2004 and were based on consensus statements (**Tables 1** and **2**).[27] Medical treatment of CF is complex, requiring significant time, knowledge, and health literacy,[28,29] and has advanced considerably since the 2004 guidelines (eg, advances in pancreatic enzyme replacement, CFRD management, and therapies directed at the basic CF defect, CF transmembrane conductance regulator [CFTR] modulation).[30,31] Often, technology assistance (TA) is indicated in CF care, defined as an indwelling medical device required to maintain health status.[3,18] TA signals that pwCF may require further specialized care during the transition to adulthood. The intense work involved in CF medical care can create a substantial treatment burden on pwCF and their families,[32] with ongoing research dedicated to simplifying medical regimens in CF.[33] Treatment complexity may increase with age. In a large, multi-site study, complexity was highest for adults compared with children and adolescents and increased over a 3-year period for all 3 groups.[34] As one example, during puberty, there is a 25–30% decrease in insulin sensitivity, consistent with that seen in pregnancy.[35] Many pwCF with CFRD are started on insulin during early adulthood. However, reassessment of the need for insulin when sensitivity may have improved is infrequent. Discontinuation of insulin therapy in early adulthood is an area of active investigation.[36] Therefore, providers should be cognizant of physiologic changes associated

with HCT. Given these factors, many adult-focused primary care providers are not comfortable managing pwCF,[37] and thus, the high degree of complexity associated with CF care is an important consideration during HCT.

There are specific considerations related to transition timing for pwCF with Advanced CF Lung Disease (ACFLD). ACFLD is defined as forced expiratory volume in one-second percent predicted (ppFEV1) less than 40. In spite of recent therapeutic advances, because 20% of pwCF over 30 years have ACFLD,[38] CF care centers should be prepared to refer for transplant, optimize palliative care, and defer transition to adult care if there is unstable disease.[38] Palliative care services can alleviate suffering and disease-related burden for pwCF; however, literature on palliative care and HCT is limited.[39] In 2021, consensus guidelines were developed for palliative care in CF, suggesting that it occur alongside routine care and be individualized according to the goals, hopes, and values of pwCF.[39]

Challenges Associated with Adolescence

Medication adherence often decreases as adolescents take more responsibility for their own care. Adolescents can be concerned about how their peers view their disease and may hide their need to take medications.[40] Consequently, poor adherence to CF treatment plans is known to adversely affect the quality of life and lead to worse outcomes.[40] Pediatric providers should plan effective interventions to prevent these complications from occurring.[41]

CFF emphasizes the importance of pwCF planning for life events and milestones that seemed out of reach a generation ago.[42] Adolescents with CF should be encouraged to plan for life after high school.[43] As of 2019, nearly 70% of pwCF 18 years and older attended college, and rates of college graduation have quadrupled in the past 20 years. Similarly, nearly 70% of adults with CF were actively working or attending school in 2019.[44] Success in school or work requires knowledge about accommodations that may be necessary (eg, private bathroom, access to private space for treatments) and available scholarship opportunities. Care teams should offer anticipatory guidance about time management, treatment adherence, maintenance of exercise routines, and adequate caloric intake.[42]

Conversations during adolescence should focus on sexual and reproductive health. While the American Academy of Pediatrics and Society for Adolescent Health and Medicine have clear recommendations on what should be included in

Table 1
Barriers and challenges associated with cf transition

Patient-related Barriers	Health care Utilization	• Lower rates of health care system utilization • Difficulties navigating the health care system • Increased gaps in CF care during transition
	Medical Complexity	• Increased burden for pwCF and caregivers due to complex treatment regimens • Increased technology assistance • Increasing disease complexity with age (eg, CFRD, ACFLD)
	Adolescence and Emerging Adulthood	• Increased risk-taking behavior • Poor medication adherence • Difficulty with executive function, eg, time management, memory, planning • Inconsistency with meeting caloric needs • Family planning and the challenges of pregnancy for PwCF • Worsening depression and anxiety
	Transition Readiness	• Lack of CF-related knowledge • Lack of self-management skills • Neurocognitive deficits and developmental limitations
	Family and Caregivers	• Fears associated with leaving pediatric care • Reluctance to provide independence/autonomy with CF care
Provider-related Barriers	Patient-Centered Care Education	• Lack of time alone with pwCF during visits • Inadequate education and counseling regarding CF care
	Structured Transition	• Delayed initiation of transition services • Inconsistent methods of transition across providers • Inconsistent skill-building to support transition • Inappropriate timing of transfer
System-related Barriers	Access to Care	• Lack of primary care providers comfortable with the complexity of CF care • Gaps in insurance coverage during transition
	Guidelines	• Lack of updated CF care guidelines related to transition
	Research Limitations	• Paucity of standardized assessment tools to gauge the efficacy of transfer • Lack of prospective studies evaluating the long-term impact of transition strategies

such discussions, studies reveal much room for improvement in meeting these guidelines,[45,46] especially as CFF registry data indicate that almost half of adults with CF are married or living with an intimate partner, and pregnancy numbers are steadily climbing over time.[44] As they consider intimate relationships, pwCF must wrestle with a multitude of complexities including disclosure of health status, and the impact on the health of pregnancy and raising children. (See Lauren N. Meiss and colleagues' article, "Family Planning and Reproductive Health in Cystic Fibrosis," in this issue.) The CFF offers resources for pwCF to navigate sexual and reproductive health issues with active decision-making.[42]

Transition Readiness

Successful planning and implementation of a transition program rely on the evaluation of transition readiness, defined as "the degree to which adolescents and young adults and supportive partners (eg, parents) are able and willing to initiate and progress through the transition process."[47] Measurement of transition readiness is considered best practice for transition programs.[48] Several measures of readiness assessment have been developed.

A recent systematic review concluded that best practices in readiness assessment are measures that are grounded in theory, can be used

Table 2
Best practices for optimizing CF transition

Patient-Focused	Health care Utilization and Self-Management	• Develop skills in health care navigation: Making appointments, communicating with providers, maintaining insurance • Develop skills in self-management: Treatment adherence, equipment use, adequate caloric intake, exercise
	Medical Complexity	• Simplify medication regimens • Ensure early referral to transplant for ACFLD and optimize palliative care • Defer transition if disease is unstable
	Adolescence and Emerging Adulthood	• Assess neurodevelopmental ability • Counsel PwCF regarding time management and keeping a schedule • Provide anticipatory guidance regarding smoking, substance use, peer pressure influence, and reproductive health • Provide mental health screening and support services
Provider-Focused	Patient-Centered Care	• Improve communication skills (listening, empathy, honesty); Increase telehealth utilization • Devote a portion of scheduled visits to time alone with pwCF • Provide targeted family and caregiver support and education, eg, support groups
	Structured Transition	• Initiate transition services when developmentally ready; use shared decision-making regarding the timing of transfer • Provide developmentally appropriate education about CF and rationale for treatments • Measure transition readiness using validated tools, eg, TRAQ survey • Create a medical summary, treatment plan, and emergency care plan for pwCF • Assess social complexity and provide social work support • Schedule the first adult visit; consider a joint visit between pediatric and adult care teams • Monitor for the successful transition, including changes in lung function
	Access to Care	• Establish relationships with local primary care providers who are willing to care for pwCF • Ensure maintenance of insurance coverage prior to transition
System-Focused	Guidelines	• Update CF care guidelines to include optimal transition strategies
	Next Steps in Research	• Define outcomes of successful transition and standardize assessment tools in CF transition • Utilize registry data (including patient-reported quality-of-life outcomes) in CF transition research • Integrate registry date with patient-reported quality-of-life outcomes • Increase QI initiatives between pediatric and adult CF care teams

longitudinally, are validated for a wide age range, measure multiple stakeholders' perspectives, and have strong psychometrics.[49] Another systematic review identified 19 transition readiness tools.[49] The majority originated in the United States (13/19) and about half were disease-neutral (9/19).[50] Of the 8 psychometrically sound measures, the Transition Readiness Assessment Questionnaire (TRAQ) and Self-Management and Transition to Adulthood with the Rx = Treatment (STARx)[51] included pwCF in their development.[51–54] The TRAQ[52,53] includes a 20-item scale with 5 subscales that are skill-based (managing medications, appointment keeping, tracking health issues, talking with providers, and managing daily activities) rated on a 5-point Likert scale. The STARx[51] includes a 13-item scale rated on a 5-point Likert scale with 3 factors identified (disease knowledge, self-management, and provider communication).[54] The authors concluded that the TRAQ was the gold standard at that time.[52]

Individual factors, such as transition readiness,[48] are central to models of HCT as they are some of the best predictors of successful transition.[55] One way to conceptualize individual factors is to divide them into those that are amenable to change through intervention, such as knowledge, and those that are considered stable, such as culture.[56] Other nonmodifiable factors include socio-demographic influences, access to medical care, insurance coverage, medical health, and neurocognitive factors.[56]

A meta-analysis of transition studies in chronic illness found that the most consistent associations between socio-demographic factors and transition readiness were age, female gender, higher median household income, living in a two-parent household, having private insurance, having higher health literacy scores, and better academic performance, although not all studies found these associations.[48] Further, a combination of factors conceptualized as "social complexity" (overall health, family factors, mental/behavioral health, and education) has been found to predict hospitalization[57] and decline in lung function[58] after transfer to adult care in CF, even when controlling for treatment complexity.

Among the factors that were hypothesized as amenable to change, self-efficacy has shown the most consistent relationship for individuals with chronic illnesses,[48] including CF.[8] Other relationships in chronic illness have been found between transition readiness and illness-related knowledge, disease management responsibility, parental involvement, and perceived barriers to self-management, but these are less well studied.[48] In a study that included pwCF and other chronic illnesses, a model including age, self-reported health care responsibility, barriers to self-management, and academic performance was found to predict a significant variation in self-reported transition readiness.[59] Further, transition readiness has been positively related to adolescents' beliefs about being able to manage their own care in a survey that included pwCF.[60]

Age is one of the static factors that has most consistently demonstrated a relationship with transition readiness. As pwCF moves from early to late adolescence, transition readiness skills improve.[26] However, recent evidence demonstrates the importance of separating chronological age from developmental maturity and ensuring that transition is patient-centered and tailored to the individual.[61] In these models, care responsibility is shifted to the adolescent based on developmental maturity, and not chronological age.[62]

Although psychological functioning is thought to play a role in transition readiness,[47,56] few direct links have been found. One recent study in epilepsy found a negative relationship between adolescent inattention and readiness to transition, but not between internalizing (depression, anxiety) and externalizing (disruptive behaviors) symptoms and transition readiness.[63] Other studies have found no relationship between psychological functioning/distress and transition readiness,[64] satisfaction,[65] or changes in psychological well-being pre and posttransition.[66] Some research has shown that being anxious about aspects of transition decreases transition readiness.[67]

There is evidence that psychological functioning can negatively influence illness self-management,[68,69] which is an integral component of transition readiness[47,56]; therefore, the links may be indirect. This finding is important because pwCF have an increased psychological burden[70] demonstrated by reporting elevated depression and anxiety symptoms at 2–3 times those of community samples.[71] Although rates of externalizing behaviors have not been found to be elevated among pwCF,[72] illness self-management may be problematic for those who do demonstrate elevations.[73]

Physician/Provider-Related Barriers and Timing of Health Care Transition

A 2017 survey of pwCF assessing needs and strategies for improving communication between pwCF and their providers recommended a focus on listening, empathy, honesty, personalized education, detailed medical explanations, and different communication options as best practices.[74] Participants stated that childhood and adolescence is a crucial time to have incremental education and counseling about the different components of CF care.[74]

To prepare for transfer to the adult health care system, there should be a discussion between pwCF, their family, and their CF team about the appropriate time for the transfer. It could be the following graduation from high school or after starting college, as this is a significant milestone. Preparation for transfer can occur by setting goals for each visit, providing educational materials, and assessing their skills and demonstrating of equipment use.[74]

Loss or change in insurance coverage can present a significant barrier to care for young adults with CF. Using a national database, a study demonstrated a 7.7-fold increase in lack of insurance over a 7-year period during which adolescents with special health care needs to be aged into adulthood.[75] The study was performed prior to the Affordable Care Act which extended dependent coverage through age 26 and liberalized income eligibility for Medicaid, thereby decreasing the number of uninsured children and young adults.[76] However, the substantial portion of pwCF who rely on Medicaid[44] still face more stringent qualifying medical and financial criteria when they shift to adult status by their state Medicaid programs.[77] Care teams must offer specific attention to the maintenance of adequate health insurance.

MODELS OF TRANSITION/LANDSCAPE OF TRANSITION
Education, Health-Literacy, Transition Self-Readiness

The goal of a planned transition is to reduce the interruption of care, maximize well-being, and improve quality of life.[78] Unfortunately, this typically occurs when pwCF are struggling with biological, emotional, and psychological changes that accompany adolescence, which can be more stressful for those with chronic illness.[79–81] A structured transition program can optimize health and continuity of care, and improve adherence, satisfaction, perceived health status, and independence.[81]

Best Practices of Transition and Implementation

It is important to focus on educating adolescents about their disease. Education should include the rationale for therapies, assessment of the adolescent's ability to independently manage them, and navigation of the health care system in general.[82] The challenges of adolescence can adversely affect the health of individuals with chronic illness.[83] PwCF who participate in shared decision-making in health care are likely to be more informed, feel more prepared, and experience less anxiety about the unknown.[82] Skov, and colleagues implemented changes to their CF clinic including staff training on communication, a youth-friendly feel to the outpatient clinic, the introduction of youth consultations partly alone with the adolescent, and a parents' evening focused on CF in adolescence. The adolescents were assessed at baseline and 12 months after the implementation of the program.[83] The transition readiness checklist score increased significantly over the study period which indicates increased readiness to transfer and improved self-management skills.[84] Health care professionals and parents must recognize that pwCF can develop an increasing ability to manage the complex decisions involving their care and therefore must support them in a developmentally appropriate incremental way.[85] A study reported that pwCF (as well as their parents) preferred age of transition to be 16–18 years,[86] and that older age at a final pediatric visit was significantly associated with successful transfer.[87] In another analysis, pwCF preferred that transition occur between 14 and 19 years of age.[88]

CFF and other professional societies recommend an early start to the transition process, involving pwCF (who usually lack knowledge about their disease in early childhood), parents, and families, to improve the knowledge base for pwCF and their families.[89,90] Education should include the rationale for therapies, assessment of independence in care management, and navigation of the health care system in general.[82] In addition, work, relationships, reproductive health issues, and family planning are important issues to address during the transition period and at the time of transfer.[11] Haarbauer-Krupa and colleagues examined perceptions of transition readiness and health-care satisfaction across chronic disease groups to better understand what factors may be universally important to consider when caring for adolescents with chronic illness. Greater adolescents' satisfaction with their care was related to gender and fewer perceived barriers to medication adherence.[59] These findings suggest that behavioral interventions targeting improving self-management and reducing barriers to adherence may be universally helpful to adolescents with chronic illness.[59]

In addition, scheduling an adult clinic visit after the last pediatric visit, touring the adult clinic before the first visit, organizing a formal departure/reception time, identifying indicators to evaluate the process periodically, and making adjustments to the process as needed should also be part of the institutional and center protocol for HCT and transfer.[91]

ESTABLISHMENT OF FORMAL, STANDARDIZED PROGRAMS, AND MODELS OF CARE
Cystic Fibrosis Responsibility, Independence, Self-Care, and Education Transition Readiness Program

CF RISE is a comprehensive program designed to address the needs of pwCF in preparation for transitioning toward independence (**Fig. 2**).[85] It provides CF centers with tools to prepare pwCF for taking responsibility for their care. CF RISE offers a comprehensive package focused on issues specifically pertaining to CF. Gilead Sciences, Inc. funded the development and ongoing maintenance of the CF RISE program, but the program is unbranded.[12,13] As of January 1st, 2022, the ownership of the program was being transferred to CFF.

CF RISE includes CF Knowledge Assessments and Responsibilities Checklist. The Knowledge Assessments' objective is to assess knowledge of various aspects of CF care. It includes 12 modules for 16–25 years of age: Lung Health & Airway Clearance, Pancreatic Insufficiency & Nutrition, CF Liver Disease, CFRD, General CF Health, Screening and Prevention, Equipment Maintenance & Infection Control, Sexual Health, Lifestyle, Insurance and Finance, College and Work, and CF and Your Body. The Responsibilities Checklist's objective is to assess and support pwCF's current level of responsibility for care. It helps them to develop age-appropriate self-care skills by working with the CF care team to transfer responsibility from caregivers. A progress report for each individual is provided to track results and record transition goals over time. In addition, the program includes an educational resource guide to remediate knowledge gaps identified through the CF RISE toolset. It contains links to resources from CFF and other CF publications. All material is available on a digital portal and as a hard copy. The digital format provides timesaving, automated scoring, a process for remediation, and a longitudinal tracking of results over time. This program is HIPAA compliant.[80] CF RISE is flexible in implementation, can complement existing transition programs, and has recently been extended to children aged 10–15 (**Fig. 3**).

There is great flexibility in implementing CF RISE which can vary from full implementation to partial implementation.[86] Outcome's data support the CF RISE program. For example, Riekert and colleagues[92] identified knowledge gaps that might hinder transition and CF RISE was able to address these gaps.

Additional Programs and Models

A number of other transition programs for pwCF have been described.[21,93,94] Good2Go is a transition readiness program developed in France, Got Transition is a federally funded resource center in the US, and a more exhaustive list of resources can be found within a multispecialty clinical report.[95]

MECHANISMS TO ENHANCE THE TRAINING AND ESTABLISHMENT OF PROGRAMS FOR TRANSITION

There are a growing number of initiatives to enhance training and help develop adult programs to care for pwCF. The CFF Program for Adult Care Excellence (PACE) award provides three years' salary support to train physicians in the care of adults with CF,[96] which has included transition-specific initiatives.[80] The CFF Learning and Leadership Collaborative (LLC) is a structured program for interprofessional CF care teams to utilize longitudinal coaching to develop quality improvement (QI) solutions to local challenges. Over 90% of CFF accredited care centers have participated,[97] and centers have used the LLC framework to improve processes and outcomes related to transition.[80,98] In addition, CFF sponsors other

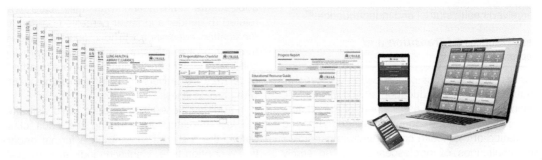

Fig. 2. Component of CF RISE. (*From* Cystic Fibrosis Foundation CF R.I.S.E. Bethesda, Maryland, © 2021 Cystic Fibrosis Foundation.)

CF Milestones At A Glance

Legend:
- ○ Parent/Support Person Completely Responsible
- ◔ Parent/Support Person Primarily Responsible
- ◑ Parent/Support Person and Person with CF Share Responsibility
- ◕ Person with CF Primarily Responsible
- ● Person with CF Completely Responsible

MILESTONE	Early School Age (6–9)	Late Elementary & Middle School (10–12)	Early High School (13–15)	Late High School (16–18)	Early Adulthood (18–25)
MANAGING CF CARE					
Leads all aspects of clinic visit—asks/answers questions about health status, treatment changes, insurance, etc	◔	◑	◕	◕	●
Proactively identifies and reports changes in health/symptoms and alerts parent or care team	◔	◑	◕	●	●
Keeps track of FEV$_1$ and BMI and implements recommended nutrition/treatment changes, as needed	○	◔	◑	◕	●
Monitors and maintains appropriate sleep schedule	○	◔	◑	◕	●
Creates and maintains proper diet and nutrition plan	○	◔	◑	◕	●
Prepares for hospital visits (packing, alerting school/work, etc)	○	◔	◑	◕	◕
Coordinates care with healthcare providers outside the CF center (primary care, psychologist, OB/GYN)	○	◔	◔	◑	◕
Person with CF is open to and ready for transfer to adult center	○	◔	◔	◑	◕
Schedules appointments and tracks all doctor's appointments/clinic visits	○	○	◔	◑	◕
Manages all insurance and financial aspects of CF care (ordering new treatments, coordinating refills, co-pays, etc)	○	○	◔	◑	◕
Arranges transportation to all doctor's appointments/clinic visits	○	○	○	◑	●
TAKING CF TREATMENTS & THERAPIES	(6–9)	(10–12)	(13–15)	(16–18)	(18–25)
Sets up all equipment and treatments	◑	◕	◕	●	●
Remembers to take and carry pills and enzymes	◔	◑	◕	◕	●
Remembers and takes medicines and treatments as prescribed by doctor	◔	◑	◕	◕	●
Cleans and disinfects equipment	◔	◑	◕	◕	●
Sorts and tracks medications, identifies need for refills, and informs care team/pharmacy if running low	◔	◑	◕	◕	●
Stores medication properly	◔	◑	◕	◕	●
Has a plan or system for taking medicines and treatments when on the road (on vacation, at school, at work)	◔	◑	◕	◕	●
LIVING WITH CF	(6–9)	(10–12)	(13–15)	(16–18)	(18–25)
Pictures and openly talks about a future for the person with CF	◑	◑	◕	◕	●
Able to identify warning signs and apply strategies for managing anxiety and depression	◔	◔	◑	◕	◕
Maintains and monitors exercise plan	○	◔	◑	◕	●
Educates school, family, friends, and coaches about CF	○	◔	◑	◕	●
Able to speak up/advocate for the person with CF in the medical system, school, or other social settings	○	◔	◑	◕	●
Makes healthy lifestyle choices (drinking, drugs, infection control, etc)	○	◔	◑	◕	●
Understands the importance of—and utilizes—a support system of peers with CF	◔	◑	◕	◕	●

NOTE to reader: This chart begins at early school age (age 6). This chart will be updated to include milestones for newly diagnosed through age 5 in the future.

Fig. 3. CF milestones at A Glance. (Recommended Cystic Fibrosis (CF) Milestones by Age & Stage, CF Milestones At A Glance. https://cfrise.com/Content/pdfs/Milestones/Milestones%20At%20a%20Glance.pdf, 2021. Accessed Jun. 15, 2022. Cystic Fibrosis Foundation CF R.I.S.E. Bethesda, Maryland, ©2021 Cystic Fibrosis Foundation.)

programs to promote the career development of specialists caring for the needs of pwCF across the lifespan. Examples include career development awards for endocrinologists, gastroenterologists, and mental health professionals.[99]

Health Care Transition Quality Improvement Outcomes

Critical to CF HCT research is defining outcomes of the successful transition. First, outcomes need to be evaluated across a long period of time because the downstream effects of transition may persist for several years after the completion of transfer.[4] Second, outcomes must be defined broadly and should not be produced solely based on the discrete markers of disease severity and outcome. A recent

Delphi process[100] determined that CF HCT outcomes should merge individual patient-/family-reported outcomes (eg, quality of life), health-services outcomes (eg, cost of care), social functioning outcomes, and key clinical and biometric measurements. PwCF and their families should be involved in developing research questions for HCT.[4]

Role of Comparative Effectiveness Research, Registry Data, and Quality Improvement in Transforming Cystic Fibrosis Health Care Transition

While prospective trials are necessary to evaluate the long-term impact of HCT strategies, these trials take considerable time to achieve results and are vulnerable to issues with follow-up for pwCF.

Utilization of registry data is critical; however, studies incorporating these data require data sharing and may lack details of organization practices that influence outcomes.[4] CER examines different strategies for the prevention and/or therapy for a specific disease or disease outcomes for the purpose of evidence-based decision-making regarding human health. CER that evaluates and compares health outcomes, as well as risks and benefits associated with medical treatments, services, and/or protocols, is predicted to be an important component of HCT research in CF moving forward.[4]

Measures of quality of life and patient/family experience of quality of care are included with clinical (eg, forced expiratory volume in 1 second [FEV1]), biometric (eg, body mass index [BMI]), and process-oriented (eg, attendance at quarterly clinic visits, hospitalizations) measures in the CFF registry data.[101] Thus, studies using CFF registry data to examine pwCF and their families as they are preparing for transition (ie, 13–18 years old) and during transfer (ie, 18–21 years old) could integrate clinical, biometric, and process-oriented data with measures of quality of life and experiences to deliver a more comprehensive picture of how the transfer experience impacts both pwCF and their families.[11]

In 2002, the CFF launched a multifaceted QI program to accelerate improvement in CF care.[102] There is substantial evidence that QI initiatives improve key process measures in CF, such as more consistent outpatient follow-up.[102] QI initiatives are integral to improving HCT in CF. Engagement of both the pediatric and adult care teams in the transition process is likely to improve the experience for pwCF and their families during this pivotal time,[81,103] and QI programs provide the opportunity for both teams to collaborate on system-wide initiatives. When QI efforts are aligned between the 2 teams, HCT may improve as an ancillary benefit.[104] In a single-center QI initiative, recognition of deficiency in nutritional assessment and infection control practices were identified as barriers to transition. Development of a standardized approach to these issues ameliorated the consistency of the center's message, thus improving outcomes.[105]

To summarize, clinical and biometric outcomes, patient-/family-reported outcomes, health services outcomes, and social functioning outcomes are key metrics in research on CF HCT. Development and standardization of assessment tools to gauge the efficacy of transfer from pediatric to adult care is a high research priority. Such tools should incorporate both clinical and patient-centered outcomes to provide a comprehensive picture of the progress and deficiencies of the HCT process. CER is an important research paradigm that could evaluate interventions in the transition process and their effect on patient-centered outcomes. In keeping with a pragmatic, patient-centered approach, studies utilizing registries containing patient-/family-reported outcomes as well as QI research that facilitate the rapid translation of results into practice have the potential to positively influence practice patterns for CF HCT.

TRANSITION IN POST–COVID-19 ERA/FUTURE DIRECTIONS

CF care significantly improved following the introduction of the CF modulators. The improved health status has been redefining how adolescents perceive their sense of self, seeing possibilities for the future beyond being defined by CF.[106] Another change in CF care occurred with the COVID-19 pandemic which has made telehealth a necessity in health care delivery.[107] Even though telehealth has been part of CF care for over a decade, it's use has been limited.[108] However, the COVID-19 pandemic rapidly accelerated the use of telehealth delivery across CF care centers. In 2020 there was a 5-fold increase in telehealth visits across CFF care centers, in addition to the delivery of more than 17,000 home spirometers to pwCF.[6] Targeted visits following interventions can be scheduled more easily; height, weight, and pulmonary function can be measured; and direct observation in the home environment can be helpful.[109] Additional potential benefits could be relevant to HCT. Telehealth visits could offer improved efficiency for meeting future caregivers. Telemedicine has significant benefits for transition, as studies have shown that virtual visits can improve patient-centered aspects of care, decrease barriers to engagement, and improve satisfaction.[110–112] In addition, for pwCF, telemedicine can improve the connection between subspecialists and primary care providers.[113–115]

SUMMARY

CF transition research has led the way for other chronic diseases and has been an example for the implementation of HCT to achieve optimal high-quality care.[116] In addition, the work of the CFF and CF care centers to improve the HCT landscape by investing in multidisciplinary care has been a pillar of successful transition strategy for national and international HCT programs.[41] CF clinicians should utilize structured transition programs such as CF RISE, researchers must work toward standardizing assessment tools to gauge the efficacy of transfer from pediatric to adult care, and such programs and tools should incorporate both clinical and patient-centered outcomes to provide a comprehensive picture of progress and deficiencies of the HCT process.

CLINICS CARE POINTS

- Transition of care from pediatrics to adult for people with chronic illnesses is challenging.
- CF transition has been more organized than that of other chronic diseases.
- A structured transition program should be established and followed by the medical team taking care of people with chronic diseases.

REFERENCES

1. Rosen DS, Blum RW, Britto M, et al. Transition to adult health care for adolescents and young adults with chronic conditions: position paper of the Society for Adolescent Medicine. J Adolesc Health 2003;33(4):309–11.
2. National Research Council. Investing in the health and well-being of young adults. Washington, DC: The National Academies Press; 2015.
3. White P, Schmidt A, Shore J, et al. Six core elements of health care transition 3.0. The national alliance to advance adolescent health. Available at: https://www.gottransition.org/6ce/?leaving-full-package. Accessed October 21, 2021.
4. Lanzkron S, Sawicki GS, Hassell KL, et al. Transition to adulthood and adult health care for patients with sickle cell disease or cystic fibrosis: current practices and research priorities. J Clin Transl Sci 2018;2(5):334–42.
5. Mahan JD, Betz CL, Okumura MJ, et al. Self-management and transition to adult health care in adolescents and young adults: a team process. Pediatr Rev 2017;38(7):305–19.
6. Cystic Fibrosis Foundation. 2020 Annual report. Available at: https://www.cff.org/about-us/annual-report. Accessed November 26, 2021.
7. White P, Cooley W. Supporting the health care transition from adolescence to adulthood in the medical home. Article Pediatr 2018;142(5). no pagination.
8. Torun T, Cavusoglu H, Dogru D, et al. The effect of self-efficacy, social support and quality of life on readiness for transition to adult care among adolescents with cystic fibrosis in Turkey. J Pediatr Nurs 2021;57:e79–84.
9. Ramsey ML, Lara LF, Gariepy CE, et al. National trends of hospitalizations in cystic fibrosis highlight a need for pediatric to adult transition clinics. Pancreas 2021;50(5):704–9.
10. Collins R, Singh B, Payne DN, et al. Effect of transfer from a pediatric to adult cystic fibrosis center on clinical status and hospital attendance. Pediatr Pulmonology 2021;56(7):2029–35.
11. Okumura MJ, Kleinhenz ME. Cystic fibrosis transitions of care: lessons learned and future directions for cystic fibrosis. Clin Chest Med Mar 2016;37(1):119–26.
12. Baker AM, Riekert KA, Sawicki GS, et al. CF RISE: implementing a clinic-based transition program. Pediatr Allergy Immunol Pulmonology 2015;28(4):250–4.
13. Are. Education. Gilead Sciences Inc.. Available at: https://www.cfrise.com/. Accessed December 4, 2021.
14. Sibanda D, Singleton R, Clark J, et al. Adult outcomes of childhood bronchiectasis. Int J Circumpolar Health 2020;79(1):1731059.
15. Dunbar P, Hall M, Gay JC, et al. Hospital readmission of adolescents and young adults with complex chronic disease. JAMA Netw Open 2019;2(7):e197613.
16. Sawicki GS, Ostrenga J, Petren K, et al. Risk factors for gaps in care during transfer from pediatric to adult cystic fibrosis programs in the United States. Ann Am Thorac Soc 2018;15(2):234–40.
17. Dickinson KM, Collaco JM. Cystic fibrosis. Pediatr Rev 2021;42(2):55–65.
18. Hoppe JE, Guimbellot J, Martiniano SL, et al. Highlights from the 2019 North American cystic fibrosis conference. Pediatr Pulmonol 2020;55(9):2225–32.
19. Cystic Fibrosis Foundation Patient Registry. 2020 annual data report. 2021. Available at: https://www.cff.org/medical-professionals/patient-registry. Accessed December 15, 2021.
20. Gabriel P, McManus M, Rogers K, et al. Outcome evidence for structured pediatric to adult health care transition interventions: a systematic review. J Pediatr 2017;188:263–9.e15.
21. Middour-Oxler B, Bergman S, Blair S, et al. Formal vs. informal transition in adolescents with cystic fibrosis: a retrospective comparison of outcomes. J Pediatr Nurs 2021;62:177–83.
22. Lal RA, Maahs DM, Dosiou C, et al. The guided transfer of care improves adult clinic show rate. Endocr Pract 2020;26(5):508–13.
23. Zupanc ML. Models of transition. Semin Pediatr Neurol 2020;36:100853.
24. Lebrun-Harris LA, McManus MA, Ilango SM, et al. Transition planning among US youth with and without special health care needs. Pediatrics 2018;142(4):e20180194.
25. Health Research Services Administration. National performance measures. U.S. Department of health

and human services. Available at: https://mchb.
tvisdata.hrsa.gov/PrioritiesAndMeasures/National
PerformanceMeasures. Accessed December 2,
2021.

26. Yassaee A, Hale D, Armitage A, et al. The impact of
age of transfer on outcomes in the transition from
pediatric to adult health systems: a systematic review of reviews. Review. J Adolesc Health 2019;
64(6):709–20.

27. Keyt H, Yankaskas J. Adult care clinical care
guidelines. Cystic Fibrosis Foundation; 2019.
Available at: https://www.cff.org/node/1406#future-
directions-and-unanswered-questions. Accessed
December 3, 2021.

28. Mogayzel PJ, Naureckas ET, Robinson KA, et al.
Cystic fibrosis pulmonary guidelines. Chronic medications for maintenance of lung health. Am J Respir Crit Care Med 2013;187(7):680–9.

29. Flume PA, Robinson KA, O'Sullivan BP, et al. Cystic
fibrosis pulmonary guidelines: airway clearance
therapies. Respir Care 2009;54(4):522–37.

30. Kayani K, Mohammed R, Mohiaddin H. Cystic
fibrosis-related diabetes. Front Endocrinol (Lausanne) 2018;9:20.

31. Boggs EF, Foster C, Shah P, et al. Trends in technology assistance among patients with childhood
onset chronic conditions. Hosp Pediatr 2021;
11(7):711–9.

32. Sawicki GS, Sellers DE, Robinson WM. High treatment burden in adults with cystic fibrosis: challenges to disease self-management. J Cyst Fibros
2009;8(2):91–6.

33. Rowbotham NJ, Smith S, Leighton PA, et al. The top
10 research priorities in cystic fibrosis developed by
a partnership between people with CF and health-
care providers. Thorax 2018;73(4):388–90.

34. Sawicki GS, Ren CL, Konstan MW, et al. Treatment
complexity in cystic fibrosis: trends over time and
associations with site-specific outcomes. J Cyst Fibros 2013;12(5):461–7.

35. Kelsey MM, Zeitler PS. Insulin resistance of puberty. Curr Diab Rep 2016;16(7):64.

36. Ogbolu C, Arregui-Fresneda I, Daniels T, et al.
Some young adults with cystic fibrosis-related diabetes may safely stop insulin without any adverse
clinical sequelae. Diabet Med 2020;37(7):1205–8.

37. Okumura MJ, Heisler M, Davis MM, et al. Comfort
of general internists and general pediatricians in
providing care for young adults with chronic illnesses of childhood. J Gen Intern Med 2008;
23(10):1621–7.

38. Kapnadak SG, Ramos KJ, Dellon EP. Enhancing
care for individuals with advanced cystic fibrosis
lung disease. Rev Pediatr Pulmonology 2021;
56(S1):S69–78.

39. Kavalieratos D, Georgiopoulos AM, Dhingra L,
et al. Models of palliative care delivery for

individuals with cystic fibrosis: cystic fibrosis foundation evidence-informed consensus guidelines.
J Palliat Med 2021;24(1):18–30.

40. Dziuban EJ, Saab-Abazeed L, Chaudhry SR, et al.
Identifying barriers to treatment adherence and
related attitudinal patterns in adolescents with
cystic fibrosis. Pediatr Pulmonol 2010;45(5):450–8.

41. West NE, Mogayzel PJ. Transitions in health care:
what can we learn from our experience with cystic
fibrosis. review. Pediatr Clin North Am 2016;63(5):
887–97.

42. Cystic Fibrosis Foundation. Life with CF: transitions. Available at: https://www.cff.org/Life-With-
CF/Transitions/. Accessed October 26, 2021.

43. Smith M. Salt in my soul: an unfinished life. New
York City, NY: Random House; 2019.

44. Cystic Fibrosis Foundation Patient Registry. 2019
annual data report. Available at: https://www.cff.
org/Research/Researcher-Resources/Patient-
Registry/2019-Patient-Registry-Annual-Data-
Report.pdf. Accessed October 26, 2021.

45. Marcell AV, Burstein GR. Sexual and reproductive
health care services in the pediatric setting. Pediatrics 2017;140(5):e20172858.

46. Kazmerski TM, Borrero S, Tuchman LK, et al. Provider and patient attitudes regarding sexual health
in young women with cystic fibrosis. Pediatrics
2016;137(6):e20154452.

47. Devine K, Monaghan M, Schwartz L. Transition in
pediatric psychology: adolescents and young
adults. In: Roberts MC, Steele RG, editors. Hand-
book of pediatric psychology. New York City, NY:
The Guilford Press; 2017. p. 620–31.

48. Varty M, Popejoy LL. A systematic review of transition readiness in youth with chronic disease. West J
Nurs Res 2020;42(7):554–66.

49. Walton H, Hudson E, Simpson A, et al. Defining coordinated care for people with rare conditions: a
scoping review. Int J Integr Care 2020;20(2):14.

50. Cohen LL, La Greca AM, Blount RL, et al. Introduction to special issue: evidence-based assessment
in pediatric psychology. J Pediatr Psychol 2008;
33(9):911–5.

51. Ferris M, Cohen S, Haberman C, et al. Self-management and transition readiness assessment:
development, reliability, and factor structure of
the STARx questionnaire. J Pediatr Nurs 2015;
30(5):691–9.

52. Sawicki GS, Lukens-Bull K, Yin X, et al. Measuring
the transition readiness of youth with special
healthcare needs: validation of the TRAQ–Transition Readiness Assessment Questionnaire.
J Pediatr Psychol 2011;36(2):160–71.

53. Wood DL, Sawicki GS, Miller MD, et al. The transition readiness assessment questionnaire (TRAQ):
its factor structure, reliability, and validity. Acad Pediatr 2014;14(4):415–22.

54. Nazareth M, Hart L, Ferris M, et al. A parental report of youth transition readiness: the parent STARx questionnaire (STARx-P) and re-evaluation of the STARx child report. J Pediatr Nurs 2018;38:122–6.

55. Blum R, Hirsch D, Kastner T, et al. A consensus statement on health care transitions for young adults with special health care needs. Pediatrics 2002;110(6 Pt 2):1304–6.

56. Schwartz LA, Tuchman LK, Hobbie WL, et al. A social-ecological model of readiness for transition to adult-oriented care for adolescents and young adults with chronic health conditions. Child Care Health Dev 2011;37(6):883–95.

57. Crowley EM, Bosslet GT, Khan B, et al. Impact of social complexity on outcomes in cystic fibrosis after transfer to adult care. Pediatr Pulmonology. June 2018;53(6):735–40.

58. Crowley EM, Bosslet GT, Khan B, et al. Social complexity negatively influences lung function in cystic fibrosis after transfer to adult care. Pediatr Pulmonol 2020;55(1):24–6.

59. Haarbauer-Krupa J, Alexander NM, Mee L, et al. Readiness for transition and health-care satisfaction in adolescents with complex medical conditions. Child Care Health Dev 2019;45(3):463–71.

60. Sawicki GS, Kelemen S, Weitzman ER. Ready, set, stop: mismatch between self-care beliefs, transition readiness skills, and transition planning among adolescents, young adults, and parents. Clin Pediatr 2014;53(11):1062–8.

61. Towns S, Jayasuriya G, et al. Transition to adult care in cystic fibrosis: the challenges and the structure. Review. Paediatr Respir Rev 2022;41:23–9.

62. Willis LD. Transition from pediatric to adult care for young adults with chronic respiratory disease. Respir Care 2020;65(12):1916–22.

63. Smith AW, Gutierrez-Colina AM, Roemisch E, et al. Modifiable factors related to transition readiness in adolescents and young adults with epilepsy. Epilepsy Behav 2021;115:107718.

64. Gutierrez-Colina AM, Corathers S, Beal S, et al. Young adults with type 1 diabetes preparing to transition to adult care: psychosocial functioning and associations with self-management and health outcomes. Diabetes Spectr 2020;33(3):255–63.

65. Van Laar M, Glaser A, Phillips RS, et al. The impact of a managed transition of care upon psychosocial characteristics and patient satisfaction in a cohort of adult survivors of childhood cancer. Psycho-oncology 2013;22(9):2039–45.

66. While AE, Heery E, Sheehan AM, et al. Health-related quality of life of young people with long-term illnesses before and after transfer from child to adult healthcare. Child Care Health Dev 2017; 43(1):144–51.

67. Gray WN, Schaefer MR, Resmini-Rawlinson A, et al. Barriers to transition from pediatric to adult care: a systematic review. J Pediatr Psychol 2018;43(5):488–502.

68. Zheng K, Abraham C, Bruzzese JM, et al. Longitudinal relationships between depression and chronic illness in adolescents: an integrative review. J Pediatr Health Care 2020;34(4):333–45.

69. Hilliard ME, Eakin MN, Borrelli B, et al. Medication beliefs mediate between depressive symptoms and medication adherence in cystic fibrosis. Health Psychol 2015;34(5):496–504.

70. Quittner AL, Saez-Flores E, Barton JD. The psychological burden of cystic fibrosis. Curr Opin Pulm Med 2016;22(2):187–91.

71. Quittner AL, Goldbeck L, Abbott J, et al. Prevalence of depression and anxiety in patients with cystic fibrosis and parent caregivers: results of the International Depression Epidemiological Study across nine countries. Thorax 2014;69(12):1090–7.

72. Sheehan J, Massie J, Hay M, et al. The natural history and predictors of persistent problem behaviours in cystic fibrosis: a multicentre, prospective study. Arch Dis Child 2012;97(7):625–31.

73. Modi AC, Quittner AL. Barriers to treatment adherence for children with cystic fibrosis and asthma: what gets in the way? J Pediatr Psychol 2006; 31(8):846–58.

74. Cooley L, Hudson J, Potter E, et al. Clinical communication preferences in cystic fibrosis and strategies to optimize care. Pediatr Pulmonology 2020; 55(4):948–58.

75. Okumura MJ, Hersh AO, Hilton JF, et al. Change in health status and access to care in young adults with special health care needs: results from the 2007 national survey of adult transition and health. J Adolesc Health 2013;52(4):413–8.

76. Talwalkar JS, Fenick AM, eds. Yale primary care pediatrics curriculum, 15th edition. 2021. Available at: https://medicine.yale.edu/pediatrics/pcpc/.

77. Bogursky S. Acne vulgaris. In: Talwalkar JS, Fenick AM, editors. Yale primary care pediatrics curriculum, 15th edition. 2021. Available at: https://medicine.yale.edu/pediatrics/pcpc/.

78. Cooley WC, Sagerman PJ. Supporting the health care transition from adolescence to adulthood in the medical home. Pediatrics 2011;128(1):182–200.

79. Nasr SZ, Campbell C, Howatt W. Transition program from pediatric to adult care for cystic fibrosis patients. J Adolesc Health 1992;13(8):682–5.

80. Goralski JL, Nasr SZ, Uluer A. Overcoming barriers to a successful transition from pediatric to adult care. Rev Pediatr Pulmonology 2017; 52(Supplement 48):S52–60.

81. Chaudhry SR, Keaton M, Nasr SZ. Evaluation of a cystic fibrosis transition program from pediatric to adult care. Pediatr Pulmonol 2013;48(7):658–65.

82. Malone H, Biggar S, Javadpour S, et al. Interventions for promoting participation in shared

decisionmaking for children and adolescents with cystic fibrosis. Cochrane Database Syst Rev 2019;2019(5):Cd012578.

83. Skov M, Teilmann G, Damgaard IN, et al. Initiating transitional care for adolescents with cystic fibrosis at the age of 12 is both feasible and promising. Acta Paediatr 2018;107(11):1977–82.

84. Cronly J, Savage E. Developing agency in the transition to self-management of cystic fibrosis in young people. J Adolesc 2019;75:130–7.

85. Yankaskas JR, Marshall BC, Sufian B, et al. Cystic fibrosis adult care: consensus conference report. Chest 2004;125(1 Suppl):1s–39s.

86. Merz J, Enochs C, Nasr SZ. Expanding Our Transition Process. Conference Abstract presented at: North American CF Conference (NACF); November 1–4, 2017 2017; Indianapolis, IN. Session S 47.

87. Doug M, Adi Y, Williams J, et al. Transition to adult services for children and young people with palliative care needs: a systematic review. Arch Dis Child 2011;96(1):78–84.

88. Hallowell SC. Setting the stage for development of a program for adolescent heart transplant recipients to transition to adult providers: an integrative review of the literature. J Spec Pediatr Nurs 2014; 19 4(4):285–95.

89. Sawicki GS, Sellers DE, McGuffie K, et al. Adults with cystic fibrosis report important and unmet needs for disease information. J Cyst Fibros 2007;6(6):411–6.

90. Kerem E, Conway S, Elborn S, et al. Standards of care for patients with cystic fibrosis: a European consensus. J Cyst Fibros 2005;4(1):7–26.

91. Vion Genovese V, Perceval M, Buscarlet-Jardine L, et al. Quality criteria for the transition to adult care in French CF centers - results from the SAFETIM APP study? Criteres de qualite pour la transition dans la mucoviscidose en France (suivi des adolescents, des familles et des equipes, pour une transition ideale en mucoviscidose - analyse des pratiques professionnelles). Revue des Maladies Respiratoires 2019;36(5):565–77.

92. Riekert K, Bryson E, Capece C, et al. Identifying Knowledge Gaps That May Hinder Transitions: The CF R.I.S.E. Transition Program Knowledge Assessment Modules. Conference Abstract presented at: North American CF Conference (NACF); November 1–4, 2017 2017; Indianapolis, IN. Session S 47.

93. Available at: https://publications.aap.org/pediatrics/article/128/1/182/30310/Supporting-the-Health-Care-Transition-From.

94. Welsner M, Sutharsan S, Taube C, et al. Changes in clinical markers during a short-term transfer program of adult cystic fibrosis patients from pediatric to adult care. Open Respir Med J 2019;13(1):11–8.

95. Mellerio H, Jacquin P, Trelles N, et al. Validation of the "Good2Go": the first French-language transition readiness questionnaire. Eur J Pediatr 2020; 179(1):61–71.

96. Cystic Fibrosis Foundation. Program for adult care excellence. 2021. Available at: https://www.cff.org/Care/Clinician-Resources/Clinician-Awards/Clinician-Career-Development-Awards/Program-for-Adult-Care-Excellence/. Accessed November 5, 2021.

97. Godfrey MM, Oliver BJ. Accelerating the rate of improvement in cystic fibrosis care: contributions and insights of the learning and leadership collaborative. BMJ Qual Saf 2014;23(Suppl 1):i23–32.

98. Prunty L, Heritage R, Pamer C. Post-transition quarterly phone calls and emails increase contact with young adults with CF and address concerns between clinic visits. Conference Abstract 2021; Session S2.

99. Cystic Fibrosis Foundation. Clinician career development awards. 2021. Available at: https://www.cff.org/Care/Clinician-Resources/Clinician-Awards/Clinician-Career-Development-Awards/. Accessed November 5, 2021.

100. Fair C, Cuttance J, Sharma N, et al. International and interdisciplinary identification of health care transition outcomes. JAMA Pediatr 2016;170(3):205–11.

101. Quittner AL, Sawicki GS, McMullen A, et al. Psychometric evaluation of the cystic fibrosis questionnaire-revised in a national sample. Qual Life Res 2012;21(7):1267–78.

102. Marshall BC, Nelson EC. Accelerating implementation of biomedical research advances: critical elements of a successful 10 year Cystic Fibrosis Foundation healthcare delivery improvement initiative. BMJ Qual Saf 2014;23(Suppl 1):i95–103.

103. Steinkamp G, Ullrich G, Muller C, et al. Transition of adult patients with cystic fibrosis from paediatric to adult care–the patients' perspective before and after start-up of an adult clinic. Eur J Med Res 2001; 6(2):85–92.

104. Wildman MJ, Hoo ZH. Moving cystic fibrosis care from rescue to prevention by embedding adherence measurement in routine care. Paediatr Respir Rev 2014;15(Suppl 1):16–8.

105. Okumura MJ, Ong T, Dawson D, et al. Improving transition from paediatric to adult cystic fibrosis care: programme implementation and evaluation. BMJ Qual Saf 2014;23(Suppl 1):i64–72.

106. Page A, Goldenberg A, Matthews A. Lived experiences of individuals with cystic fibrosis on CFTR. BMC Pulm Med 2022;22:42. https://doi.org/10.1186/s12890-022-01825-2.

107. Baggio S, Vernaz N, Spechbach H, et al. Vulnerable patients forgo health care during the first wave of the Covid-19 pandemic. Prev Med 2021; 150:106696.

108. Cox NS, Alison JA, Rasekaba T, et al. Telehealth in cystic fibrosis: a systematic review. J Telemed Telecare 2012;18(2):72–8.

109. Dixon E, Dick K, Ollosson S. Telemedicine and cystic fibrosis: do we still need face-to-face clinics? Paediatr Respir Rev 2022;42:23–8.

110. Barney A, Buckelew S, Mesheriakova V, et al. The COVID-19 pandemic and rapid implementation of adolescent and young adult telemedicine: challenges and opportunities for innovation. J Adolesc Health 2020;67(2):164–71.

111. Nowicki M, Bazan-Socha S, Kłopotowski M, et al. Considerations for home-based treatment of fabry disease in Poland during the COVID-19 pandemic and beyond. Int J Environ Res Public Health 2021;18(16):8242.

112. Chang JE, Lai AY, Gupta A, et al. Rapid Transition to telehealth and the digital divide: implications for primary care access and equity in a Post-COVID era. Milbank Q 2021;99(2):340–68.

113. Kulkarni R. Use of telehealth in the delivery of comprehensive care for patients with haemophilia and other inherited bleeding disorders. Haemophilia 2018;24(1):33–42.

114. Nicholas J, Bell IH, Thompson A, et al. Implementation lessons from the transition to telehealth during COVID-19: a survey of clinicians and young people from youth mental health services. Psychiatry Res 2021;299:113848.

115. North S. Telemedicine in the time of COVID and beyond. J Adolesc Health 2020;67(2):145–6.

116. Onofri A, Broomfield A, Tan HL. Transition to adult care in children on long-term ventilation. Review. Front Pediatr 2020;8(no pagination):548839.

Endocrine Complications of Cystic Fibrosis

Andrea Kelly, MD, MSCE[a], Brynn E. Marks, MD, MSHPEd[b], Michael S. Stalvey, MD[c,d],*

KEYWORDS

- Cystic fibrosis-related diabetes • Cystic fibrosis bone disease • Diabetes management
- Diabetes technologies • Dual X- ray absorptiometry • Bone accrual • Body composition • Growth

KEY POINTS

- Progressive insulin secretion defects underlie abnormal glucose tolerance in cystic fibrosis (CF).
- Leveraging diabetes technologies and type 2 diabetes therapeutics may advance care in youth and adults with CF-related abnormal glucose tolerance.
- Advances in care and the introduction of highly effective modulator therapies may challenge the traditional paradigms that focus on the nutritional compromise that accompanies insulin secretion defects in CF.

INTRODUCTION

With advances in cystic fibrosis (CF) care, endocrine comorbidities, including diabetes (CFRD) and bone disease (CFBD), have become increasingly important medical considerations in people with CF. Although the underlying pathophysiology remains elusive, the medical community is leveraging novel technologies and therapeutics to manage these conditions while addressing patient-reported concerns. Previously recognized conditions in CF such as pubertal delay and short stature have been tempered whereas others such as hypogonadism are increasingly recognized. Enter the success of highly effective modulator therapies (HEMT) for many patients, and the established phenotypes for several of these conditions are now less clearly defined. Given the rapidly changing landscape, this review will discuss the more recent literature surrounding endocrine comorbidities and introduce non–CF-specific innovations that are being extended to address these co-occurring conditions in CF.

CYSTIC FIBROSIS-RELATED DIABETES
Introduction

The relevance of diabetes in CF cannot be understated. CFRD is common, traditionally associated with worse CF outcomes, adds additional patient burden,[1] and, like other forms of diabetes, associates with microvascular sequelae.

Cystic Fibrosis-Related Diabetes Screening Guidelines

As CFRD does not generally present with classic diabetes symptoms (polyuria, polydipsia) but can negatively impact pulmonary function and nutritional status despite its generally "indolent" nature, the Cystic Fibrosis Foundation (CFF) recommends

[a] Division of Endocrinology & Diabetes, University of Pennsylvania Perelman School of Medicine, Children's Hospital of Philadelphia, Room 14363, Roberts Building for Pediatric Research, 2716 South Street, Philadelphia, PA 19146, USA; [b] Division of Endocrinology & Diabetes, Department of Pediatrics, University of Pennsylvania Perelman School of Medicine, Children's Hospital of Philadelphia, Room 7547, The Hub for Clinical Collaboration, 3501 Civic Center Blvd, Philadelphia, PA 19104, USA; [c] Department of Pediatrics, UAB Gregory Fleming James Cystic Fibrosis Research Center, University of Alabama at Birmingham, Children's of Alabama, CPPII M30, 1600 7th Avenue South, Birmingham, AL 35233-1711, USA; [d] Department of Medicine, UAB Gregory Fleming James Cystic Fibrosis Research Center, University of Alabama at Birmingham, Children's of Alabama, CPPII M30, 1600 7th Avenue South, Birmingham, AL 35233-1711, USA
* Corresponding author. Children's of Alabama, CPPII M30, 1600 7th Avenue South, Birmingham, AL 35233-1711.
E-mail address: mstalvey@uabmc.edu

Clin Chest Med 43 (2022) 773–789
https://doi.org/10.1016/j.ccm.2022.06.013

annual screening with oral glucose tolerance testing (OGTT) starting by age 10 years,[2] **Table 1**. Unlike in type 2 diabetes (T2D) in which fasting glucose and hemoglobin A1c (HbA1c) are useful screening tools, fasting hyperglycemia (glucose >125 mg/dL) tends to be a late finding in CF although HbA1C is frequently normal (HbA1c <6.5%).

Cystic Fibrosis-Related Diabetes Screening Research

Recent clinical research has also attempted to find alternatives to OGTT for screening for CFRD. This work was recently briefly reviewed by Chan.[3] Lowering of the HbA1C threshold from the traditional threshold of 6.5% to 5.8% does not overcome the issue of lack of sensitivity of HbA1c, and further lowering renders the test completely nonspecific.[4,5] Clinically, HbA1c is frequently obtained in patients with CF because (1) an elevated HbA1c is consistent with CFRD and (2) high-normal values heighten awareness that CFRD or abnormal glucose tolerance (AGT) may be operative. Indeed, HbA1c has been proposed as a prescreen to identify the subset of individuals requiring OGTT for formal CFRD screening; patients with HbA1c greater than or equal to 6.5% do not require OGTT as they meet the diagnostic criteria and those with HbA1c less than 5.5% have a low likelihood of having CFRD and might delay OGTT.[6] This approach has not been rigorously tested beyond the cited study and is not a currently recommended approach for CFRD screening. Similarly, the nonfasting, single sample, 50-g glucose challenge test has been proposed as a prescreen to identify the subset of individuals

who should undergo OGTT, but the limited number of patients with CFRD in that group of 27 adolescents and young adults with pancreatic insufficient CF (PI-CF) made drawing conclusions surrounding sensitivity challenging.[7] Continuous glucose monitoring (CGM) has received increasing attention as a potential screening tool for CFRD, and although CGM identifies glycemic variability and frequent hyperglycemia under free-living conditions, its agreement with the OGTT diagnosis of CFRD is inconsistent.[8–12] Investigators and clinicians are now focusing on the CGM thresholds that associate with worse outcomes even among those with normal glucose tolerance[8,13–15] and at which treatment imparts improvements.

Mechanisms of Cystic Fibrosis-Related Diabetes Pathogenesis

CFRD shares features with but is distinct from type 1 diabetes (T1D) and T2D, and arises largely from insulin secretion defects (**Fig. 1**) with a contribution of reduced insulin sensitivity that has been best characterized in adults.[16] As a pancreatogenic form of diabetes, pancreatic exocrine inflammation extending to pancreatic islet tissue where fatty infiltration and fibrosis contribute to reductions in islet mass has traditionally been considered responsible for impaired insulin secretion. Indeed, pancreatic islets from individuals with CFRD also show disrupted architecture, abnormal aggregation, and variable encasement in fatty or fibrotic tissue as well as immune cell infiltration.[17] More recently, however, a 50% relative reduction in beta-cell number per islet, smaller insulin-positive area, and lower markers of beta-cell

---

Table 1
Definitions of glucose tolerance

| | Plasma Glucose (PG) Mg/dL | | |
| | | OGTT | |
	Fasting	1-h	2-h
Normal	<100	<140	<140
Impaired fasting glucose	100–125		
Fasting hyperglycemia	≥126		
Early Glucose Intolerance[a]		≥155 and < 200	<140
Indeterminate Glucose Intolerance (IND)		≥200	<140
Impaired glucose tolerance (IGT)			140–199
CFRD without fasting hyperglycemia	<126		≥200
CFRD	Random glucose ≥200 mg/dL with classic symptoms (polyuria, polydipsia) HbA1c ≥ 6.5%		

[a] Not included in 2010 CFF guidelines.

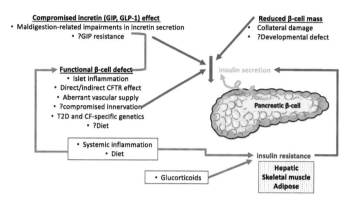

Fig. 1. Pathogenesis of CFRD arises largely from insulin secretion defects.

proliferation and ductal cells were found in pancreata from children with CF aged <4 years; these reductions were independent of the extent of pancreatic exocrine damage.[18] These data suggest beta-cell loss is not simply a by-product of exocrine tissue damage extending to islets but may reflect reduced survival of beta-cell progenitors, reduced beta-cell proliferation, or given the relative abundance of other islet cells, reduced beta-cell fate specification of progenitors.[18] Interestingly, neonatal CF transmembrane regulator (CFTR) knockout ferret islets also demonstrate 30% to 50% reductions in insulin content but upregulate insulin secretion.[19]

Research into Mechanisms of Cystic Fibrosis-Related Diabetes Pathogenesis

With the goal of delineating the mechanisms underlying insulin secretion defects in CF to develop interventions that delay, prevent, and treat CFRD, much attention has focused on the endocrine pancreas and its pancreatic exocrine neighborhood.

A primary role for defective beta-cell function in the insulin secretion defects of CF is receiving increasing attention. Insulin secretion defects in the pig model, in which islet mass is generally preserved, are unlikely fully explained by the modest reductions in overall insulin content of the pancreas.[20] Also suggesting that the islet "neighborhood" may be relevant, insulin secretion studies of islets isolated from pancreata of individuals with CFRD documented preserved insulin and glucagon secretion.[17] CF pigs demonstrate intact islet vasculature but reduction in neural fibers[20]; the contribution of aberrant innervation to islet function is not yet known albeit actively being studied. Supporting a role for inflammation in islet dysfunction are (1) immune cell infiltration of islets from people with CFRD,[17] (2) increased secretion of interleukin-6 by CFTR knockout ferret islets,

and (3) the recapitulation of the neonatal CFTR knockout ferret model's reduced insulin content but upregulation of insulin secretion following interleukin-6 application to the wild-type ferret.[19] Further highlighting the inflammatory milieu's potential negative impact upon beta-cell insulin secretion, increased interleukin-1 beta accompanied relatively preserved beta-cell area and higher alpha-cell area in pancreata from patients with CF with and without CFRD including in youth.[21]

The direct role of CFTR in islet-cell function has been debated. CFTR RNA expression is very low in beta cells,[17,22–24] and in extensive studies by Hart and colleagues, immunocytochemistry did not identify CFTR protein coexpression with insulin-positive, glucagon-positive, or somatostatin-positive cells in human islets whereas CFTR modulators and inhibitors did not appear to impact in vitro insulin secretion even at high glucose concentrations.[17] These studies contrast with other in vitro murine and human islet studies identifying impaired GLP-1-augmented and forskolin-augmented glucose-potentiated insulin secretion with CFTR inhibition—findings that were attributed to interfere with cyclic AMP-mediated exocytosis of insulin secretory granules.[25] By way of explanation, CFTR inhibition similarly reduced insulin secretion from isolated human, wild-type ferret, and CF ferret islets[19]—findings that suggest these CFTR inhibitors may be operating nonspecifically.

These questions surrounding the role of CFTR in islet cell function are not arcane. Case reports and series documenting improvements in insulin secretion and glucose excursion/tolerance with CFTR modulator therapy with ivacaftor[26,27] and the trend toward lower CFRD rates in the US and UK registries over the 4 to 5 years following ivacaftor treatment[28] underscore their relevance. Unfortunately, these data are unable to differentiate direct potentiation of insulin secretion by beta-cell CFTR modulation from indirect enhancements in insulin secretion related to improvements in systemic or peri-islet inflammation. In a multi-center French study of OGTT in individuals aged 12 years or older with IGT ($n = 31$) or CFRD ($n = 9$) at baseline, glucose tolerance improved following 1 year of lumacaftor/ivacaftor[29]; the enthusiasm was tempered with the reminder of the well-recognized variability in OGTT.[30] In contrast, the overall lack of improvement in glucose tolerance and insulin secretion in the US-based *PROSPECT* with lumacaftor/ivacaftor was disheartening but not unexpected given the modest impact of the modulator upon CF outcomes.[31] More recent CGM data from people with CFRD identified improvements in glucose excursion with elexacaftor/tezacaftor/ivacaftor (ETI).[32] The CFF-funded *PROMISE* endocrine substudy was organized to test the impact of 24 to 30 months of ETI on various aspects of glucose excursion as well as islet hormone and incretin secretion using multisample oral glucose tolerance tests performed at baseline, 12 to 18, and 24 to 30 months.[33] *PROMISE* would be unable to discern the direct and indirect impacts of ETI on beta-cell function, but analyses of the relationships of changes in OGTT outcomes to changes in BMI, body composition, pulmonary function, and, potentially, systemic inflammation, liver stiffness, and gastrointestinal health are planned. Worthy of consideration, aging and the emergence of overweight/obesity may unmask the residual compromised beta-cell function.

Enrichment in genome-wide associated (GWAS) T2D insulin secretion-affecting variants confers increased CFRD risk.[34] Candidate gene-based studies identified increased CFRD risk, specifically with T2D-related variants in *TCF7L2,* CDKAL1, CDKN2A/B, and IGF2BP2[35]. Variants in the gene encoding SLC26A9, a widely expressed anion transporter that has not been documented to associate with T2D, are associated with CFRD onset[34,35] and with meconium ileus in CF.[36] Providing further compelling evidence for a modifying role of SLC26A9, this protein has recently been demonstrated to be coexpressed with CFTR in a subset of pancreatic ductal cells where low-risk variants confer enhanced SLC26A9 expression.[22] A second CFRD-specific variant on chromosome 2 near PTMA, encoding prothymosin-α, has also been identified,[34] but its role remains undefined. Based upon these variants, a personalized CFRD risk assessment tool based on genetic and clinical measures at birth is now available online.[37]

Additional patient-oriented studies are attempting to distill the mechanisms underlying progressive insulin secretion defects and development of CFRD. Loss of early-phase insulin secretion (secretion within first 30 minutes of meal or glucose consumption) is one of the earliest markers of insulin secretion defects in CF, is accompanied by augmented second-phase insulin secretion that occurs 60 to 90 minutes after ingestion, and manifests clinically as an isolated OGTT 1-hour glucose equal to or greater than 155 mg/dL,[38,39] a threshold that is increasingly being recognized as abnormal in adults who will later advance to T2D,[40,41] **Fig. 2**. Insulin secretion is likely abnormal even prior to this "early glucose intolerance" (EGI) threshold as individuals with PI-CF and 1-hour glucose less than 155 mg/dL (1) have glucose concentrations that are higher at 1 hour than in otherwise healthy individuals without CF and (2) demonstrate augmented second-phase insulin secretion.[38] The mechanisms underlying the gradual loss of early-phase insulin secretion, worsening of glucose tolerance, loss of second-phase insulin secretion as glucose tolerance worsens,[38] and, in a subset of patients, emergence of fasting hyperglycemia are not known. The animal models described above will hopefully provide clarity on some of these questions.

Insulin resistance is recognized but has not been considered a major contributor to CFRD. Basing glucose tolerance strictly on OGTT 2-hour glucose in adults with pancreatic exocrine sufficient (PS) and pancreatic exocrine insufficient (PI) CF, Boudreau and colleagues identified baseline differences in OGTT insulin area under the curve (AUC) from 0 to 30 min and 30 to 120 min in the stable, improved, and worsened glucose tolerance status groups over approximately 21 months.[42] Worsening of these insulin AUC phases was not apparent in the group whose glucose tolerance worsened. Instead, lower insulin sensitivity was found.[42] Increasing rates of overweight and obesity in CF may propel a greater role for insulin resistance in CFRD development. At the University of Minnesota (2015–2017), overweight was present in approximately 25%, obesity in 6.6%, and underweight in only 5.2% of adults with CF.[43] In 2012, the University of Pittsburgh reported 15% overweight and 8% obesity in youth aged 2 to 18 years with CF.[44] With increasing use of highly effective modulator therapy and improvements in body mass index (BMI) that accompany that therapy,[45] undernutrition may become even less common.

Treatment of Cystic Fibrosis-Related Diabetes

Current CFRD clinical care guidelines recommend insulin therapy as the mainstay of CFRD treatment[2,46] These guidelines are based on

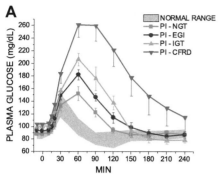
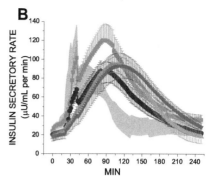

Fig. 2. Plasma glucose (*A*) and insulin secretory rates (*B*) in response to the mixed-meal tolerance test (MMTT) in subjects with pancreatic insufficient CF (PI-CF). Individuals were categorized based on a preceding oral glucose tolerance test (NGT, normal glucose tolerance; EGI, early glucose intolerance (plasma glucose at 1 hour > 155 mg/dL and plasma glucose at 2 hours < 140 mg/dL; IGT, impaired glucose tolerance; CFRD, CF-related diabetes). Significant decline in beta-cell secretory capacity is evident in PI-EGI. Reprinted under STM Permissions Guidelines from "Beta-cell secretory defects are present in pancreatic insufficient cystic fibrosis with 1-h oral glucose tolerance test glucose >/ = 155 mg/dL". (*From* Nyirjesy SC, Sheikh S, Hadjiliadis D, De Leon DD, Peleckis AJ, Eiel JN, Kubrak C, Stefanovski D, Rubenstein RC, Rickels MR, Kelly A. β-Cell secretory defects are present in pancreatic insufficient cystic fibrosis with 1-hour oral glucose tolerance test glucose ≥155 mg/dL. Pediatr Diabetes. 2018 Nov;19(7):1173-1182.)

associations of CFRD with worsening nutritional status and pulmonary function[47,48] that have been ascribed to reduced insulin secretion[49]; the former improved with a 12-month intervention with rapid-acting insulin. Many insulin formulations are available and the approach to CFRD management is highly individualized to meet the lifestyle and nutritional needs of patients. Current guidelines do not differentiate the management of CFRD among those with insulin deficiency versus insulin resistance; however, research exploring the use of T2D agents is ongoing. Compromised early-phase insulin secretion (robust insulin secretion occurring within the first 30 minutes following a meal) leads to early hyperglycemia and a compensatory, albeit delayed, insulin secretion. This excessive insulin secretion with a potential contribution of inadequate glucagon response appear to contribute to postprandial hypoglycemia in CF.[50,51] No studies have systematically addressed interventions to mitigate hypoglycemia development, but clinically (1) avoidance of quick acting sugars, (2) pairing quick-acting sugars with complex carbohydrates, proteins, and fats, (3) administering rapid-acting insulin 15 to 20 minutes before meals, and (4) switching premeal rapid-acting insulin to ultrafast-acting insulin are all trialed. The emerging technologies presented below may also help combat this nuisance.

Emerging Technologies

Rapid advances in diabetes technologies over the last decade have improved the care of people with CFRD. CGM monitors are wearable technologies that measure and report interstitial glucose values every 5 to 15 minutes with optional alerts for both hypoglycemia and hyperglycemia.[52] Since its development in 1999, CGM has become increasingly user friendly such that devices are factory calibrated, do not require calibration, and allow for diabetes treatment decisions to be made without a confirmatory fingerstick glucose value. Differences between the gold-standard Yellow Springs Instrument measurements of plasma glucose concentrations and CGM measurements are less than 10% among commercially available systems. The accuracy of CGM among people with CF is comparable to that among individuals without CF.[53] Most CGM sensors are worn for 7 to 14 consecutive days before being changed at home by the user with simple applicator devices. Glucose values may be sent to the user's smartphone or to a dedicated receiver that can display the glucose values (see example in **Fig. 3**).

CGM-defined glycemic targets have not yet been established for individuals with CFRD. However, International Consensus Guidelines for most individuals with T1D and T2D recommend targeting at least 70% of sensor glucose values between 70 to 180 mg/dL (time in range) and no more than 5% of time below 70 mg/dL (time below range).[54] These targets are derived from data demonstrating a strong correlation between 70% time in range and HbA1c less than 7%.[55] Given the HbA1c goal of less than or equal to 7% in CFRD, applying these targets for individuals with CFRD seems reasonable. Rates of CGM use in routine

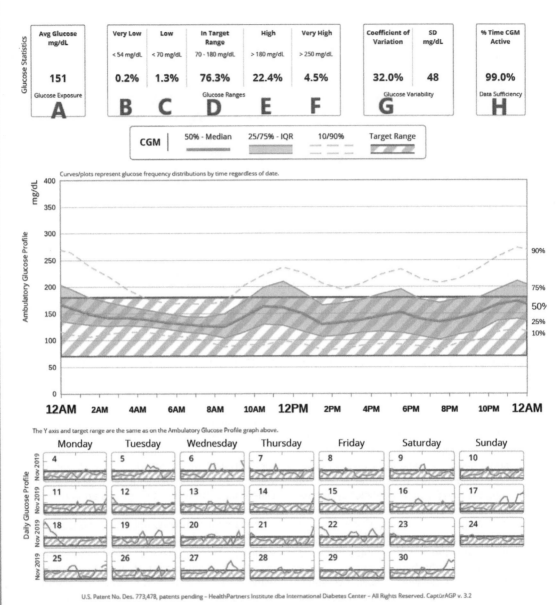

Fig. 3. Example of continuous glucose monitoring (CGM) usage. (*From* Marks BE, Wolfsdorf JI. Monitoring of Pediatric Type 1 Diabetes. Front Endocrinol (Lausanne). 2020 Mar 17;11:128.)

clinical care were 75% among a selected group of individuals with CFRD.[56] Despite positive perceptions of this technology among the CF community, including those with and without CFRD, and many perceived benefits of CGM use, 19% discontinued CGM mostly commonly due to cost and increased worry about glycemia. Greater evidence to support the benefits of CGM use among people with CFRD and better insurance coverage of this technology coupled with improved education about CGM may increase uptake and sustained use of this technology.

The last decade has also witnessed tremendous advances in insulin delivery systems. Insulin

pumps provide a continuous subcutaneous infusion of rapid-acting insulin that allows for greater customization of insulin delivery than with injection-based therapy. Data in this area are extremely limited, but continuous insulin infusion may optimize glycemic control for those with common gastrointestinal comorbidities of CF including exocrine pancreatic insufficiency, gastroparesis with alterations in intestinal transit, and periods of insulin resistance during illness. Improvements in lean body mass and glycemic control with insulin pump therapy have been demonstrated in CFRD.[57] Despite its potential benefits, insulin pump use is not sustained among a subset of people with CFRD and is less highly regarded than CGM among the CF community.[56]

Automated insulin delivery (AID), which uses CGM glucose data to guide pump delivery of insulin, is the most promising development in diabetes technology to date. AID systems increase insulin delivery in response to hyperglycemia and can also decrease or suspend insulin delivery in response to predicated or impending hypoglycemia. Among individuals with T1D, AID use improved glycemic control while simultaneously decreasing patient burden.[58,59] A pilot study ($n = 3$) of a dual hormone AID system employing insulin and glucagon showed nonsignificant improvements in mean CGM sensor glucose and patient reported outcomes with decreased treatment burden.[60] However, AID systems and insulin delivery algorithms were developed to meet the needs of individuals with T1D, who in contrast to people with CFRD, have near complete insulin deficiency. Further studies of AID efficacy and patient-reported outcomes in individuals with the unique physiology of CFRD are needed.

Research into Therapeutic Approaches for Cystic Fibrosis-Related Diabetes

Associations of early glucose abnormalities with worse CF outcomes have prompted interventions with insulin in the prediabetes state.[61–65] Results of various insulin regimens (long-acting, rapid) in prediabetes have been variable and may be more effective with worse baseline health.[65] Many of the recent clinical studies in CF report fairly preserved nutritional status in people with CFRD (average body mass index z-score (BMIZ): −0.6 to −0.8),[66] adults with abnormal glucose tolerance (average BMIZ: −0.05)[50] or abnormal glucose tolerance/CFRD without fasting hyperglycemia (FH),[67] and youth (NGT: −0.18; AGT: 0.14, CFRD: −0.65).[39] As a result, the focus of management may shift from nutritional status (and perhaps pulmonary function) to traditional diabetes-related microvascular outcomes, though less likely in CFRD than in T1D and T2D.

With the changing CF landscape and the goal of less encumbered CFRD care, several case series and acute, short-term, and longer-term trials are examining the role of T2D interventions in people with CF and abnormal glucose tolerance. Following 12 weeks of combined aerobic and resistance exercise program in 8 sedentary adults with abnormal glucose tolerance, glucose excursion improved while remaining unchanged in the control group.[68] Similarly, a randomized trial examining the impact of aerobic interval training upon glucose tolerance is planned for youth with CF.[69]

T2D incretin-based therapies are predicated on the ability of the gut derived hormones, glucagon-like peptide-1 (GLP-1) and glucose-dependent insulinotropic polypeptide (GIP), to augment insulin secretion in response to a meal or oral glucose load. In T2D, GLP-1 agonist treatment has the added advantage of weight loss, whereas dipeptidyl peptidase 4 inhibitors (DPP-4) like sitagliptin interfere with incretin catabolism but tend to be weight neutral. Incretin-based therapies are attractive in CF because data demonstrate improved meal-related incretin secretion and glucose excursion with pancreatic enzyme replacement in individuals with pancreatic insufficient CF.[70,71] Moreover, in the CF ferret, hyperglycemia is accompanied by dampened insulin, GLP-1, and GIP responses.[72] In a randomized, cross-over study of a single dose of either the short-acting GLP-1 agonist, exenatide, or placebo in 6 individuals aged 11 to 24 years with IGT, exenatide was associated with lower glucose and insulin following a high carbohydrate (50 g) meal (**Table 2**).[73] In a 6-month, randomized, placebo-controlled study, the oral DDP-4 inhibitor, sitagliptin, was well tolerated, associated with increased GLP-1 and GIP and improved early-phase insulin (first 30 minutes) secretion in response to a meal, but no improvement in glucose tolerance/excursion in adults with pancreatic insufficient CF and abnormal glucose tolerance; BMI remained unchanged.[67] A case series of 3 patients with CFRD treated with sitagliptin showed short-term improvements in glucose excursion as defined by CGM and continued CFRD control beyond 5 years in 2 in whom BMI was maintained or improved; the third participant had worsening obesity (BMI 32–30 kg/m²) and required insulin therapy beyond the 5 years.[74] These preliminary data suggest incretin-based therapies may have a role in a subset of people with CFRD in whom under-nutrition is not a concern. A 6-week, cross-over, proof-of-concept study will test the impact of weekly dulaglutide on early phase insulin secretion during a meal and will collect important data on gastrointestinal side effects and BMI (NCT04731272).

Ballmann and colleagues completed a 24-month, multicenter study of 3 times per day, premeal, oral repaglinide ($n = 34$; 14 of whom discontinued before 24 months) to 3 times per day, premeal, regular insulin ($n = 41$; 16 of whom discontinued before 24 months) in individuals aged 10 years or older with newly diagnosed CFRD. No between-group differences in HbA1c, FEV1%-predicted, or BMI were found at 24 months.[66] An additional ongoing study in people with CFRD is the cross-over *MIRE* study of 3-

Table 2
Trials of type 2 diabetes medications in CFRD

Authors. Year	Study Design	Sample Size	Inclusion Criteria	Treatment	Outcomes
Geyer, et al,[74] 2018	Double-blinded, Randomized, placebo-controlled, cross-over	N = 6	Ages 11–24 IGT	Single-dose Exenatide 2.5 mg vs Placebo	During MMTT, AUC over 240 min for blood glucose, insulin, and GLP-1 was lower with exenatide
Kelly, et al,[68] 2021	Randomized, placebo-controlled	N = 26	Adults AGT (1 h >155 and 2h <140), IGT, or CFRD	6-mo double-blind Sitagliptin 100 mg daily vs Placebo	During MMTT GLP-1, GIP insulin secretion rates improved while glucagon suppression increased without changes in postprandial glycemia
Olatunbosun,[75] 2021	Case series	N = 3	CFRD (44yo M, 38yo M, 19yo F)	5–10 y of Sitagliptin 100 mg daily	Improved BMI, HbA1c <6%; insulin required after 7 and 10 y in 2 patients
Ballmann, et al,[30] 2017	Open-label, randomized	N = 67	>10 y Newly diagnosed CFRD	24 mo Repaglinide vs Insulin	No significant difference in HbA1c over time between the two groups

month of preprandial aspart insulin versus postprandial faster-acting aspart insulin which will compare time in range by CGM (NCT04381429).

With individuals with CF overall healthier, a number of the traditional paradigms are being challenged. On a cautionary note, this recent literature many not be generalizable to the subsets of individuals around the world with limited access to care and highly effective modulator therapies, with *CFTR* mutations that are not amenable to highly effective modulator therapies or who do not tolerate highly effective modulator therapy, or with such profound insulin secretion defects that the prospect of using T2D therapies is unlikely to impact hyperglycemia.

CYSTIC FIBROSIS-RELATED BONE DISEASE
Introduction

Cystic fibrosis-related bone disease (CFBD) was first described by Mischler and colleagues in

1979, as an association of low bone density in CF. In their study, they found that 44% of CF individuals had reduced bone mineral content (BMC).[75] An interesting bit of foreshadowing for future research studies, they noted that these findings were confounded by short stature, delayed bone age and low body weight. In the past 40 years since that first report, numerous studies have documented bone disease in CF. These studies demonstrated the multitude of factors that contribute to bone disease. Probably the greatest presentation of bone disease in CF is found in the individuals referred for lung transplant, in whom 57% had osteoporosis,[76] translating to a 100-fold greater risk of vertebral compression fractures (a potential disqualifier for transplantation). In contrast, lower bone density and content does not necessarily translate to an increase fracture risk in youth. Rovner and colleagues, in a study of 186 CF children and young adults with mild to moderate lung disease, reported fracture rates that were comparable to those of healthy children.[77] Underscoring the potential implications of bone fragility in youth are case reports of significant fracture, including the spontaneous sternal fracture in a 16-year-old woman that caused severe respiratory distress.[78]

Screening Guidelines

The 2019 Cystic Fibrosis Foundation Patient Registry (CFFPR) reports a history fracture, osteopenia, and osteoporosis as 0.2%, 1.1%, and 0.3% (respectively) for children less than 18 years and 0.2%, 17.9%, and 7.0% (respectively) for adults older than 18 years.[79] In much need of revision, the CF guidelines for bone health screening in CF currently recommend baseline dual-energy x-ray absorptiometry (DXA) for all individuals aged 18 years or older, and for children aged 8 years or older with risk factors.[80] The guidelines also recommend DXA results guide timing of subsequent DXA. The CFFPR documents that only 59.3% of individuals aged 18 years or older underwent DXA during 2015 to 2019.[79] Ongoing studies aim to improve both patient and CF Center compliance with the guidelines.

Research into Mechanisms of Cystic Fibrosis-Related Bone Disease

Briefly stated, CFBD is an example of a multifactorial disorder, with contributions from vitamin D deficiency, malnutrition, hypogonadism, increased inflammatory cytokines, and glucocorticoid therapies.[80–91] Additionally, male gender, advanced lung disease, malnutrition, and low fat-free body mass are established additional risk factors for CFBD.[80,92–94] Furthermore, emerging data suggest a direct genetic component to the development of low bone density. The F508del-*CFTR* mutation is the most common mutation resulting in CF in the United States, with almost 85.3% of CF individuals having at least 1 copy and 44.4% homozygous for this genotype.[95] More severe mutations, and especially the F508del-*CFTR* genotype, are more commonly associated with reduced bone density.[96]

Although many factors associated with CFBD are established, other disease states provide insights into additional contributors. Bone health is maintained through a dynamic bone turnover process. In CF, uncoupled bone turnover (a state of decreased bone formation in the presence of increased osteoclast bone resorption) is present.

A well-described contributor to CFBD in the literature, vitamin D deficiency with resultant reduced calcium gut absorption, continues to be confounding bone health today. Guidelines can assist with vitamin D absorption difficulties in CF patients, proposing target concentrations of 25-hydroxy vitamin D and approaches to meet these. Reduced 25-hydroxy vitamin D and calcium concentrations induce release of parathyroid hormone (PTH) and consequently osteoclastic bone turnover to restore circulating calcium and the body's immediate needs.

Corticosteroid therapy has long been appreciated as a contributor to CFBD, especially in the posttransplant population. Corticosteroids impact bone health through multiple mechanisms: (1) reduced gastrointestinal calcium absorption, (2) increased urinary calcium excretion, and (3) increased osteoclast-driven bone resorption (via production of receptor activator of nuclear factor-kappa B ligand or RANKL).[84] Through similar mechanisms, increased and chronic inflammation (IL-8 and others) upregulates the same pathway, and correlates with BMC.[85–87,96,97]

The chronic insulin deficient state found in CF and CFRD is a less-recognized contribution to CFBD. Insulin (an anabolic hormone) is a potent stimulator of osteoblast proliferation and function. Rana and colleagues compared DXA outcomes by CFRD status in 81 youth aged 18 years or younger, demonstrating an association with reduced bone density.[92] Other proanabolic hormones, such as insulin-like growth factor 1 (IGF-1) and sex hormones (testosterone and estrogen) directly affect bone health. Although reduced IGF-1 concentrations are repeatedly documented in CF individuals and animal models of CF, serum IGF-1 correlates with bone density in CF. The contributions of testosterone and estrogen are more theoretic in CF, based on their contributions in healthy individuals. One retrospective study by Wu and colleagues demonstrated higher BMD in women who had been treated with supplemental estrogen before age 21.[98] Ongoing studies are examining the influence of estrogen supplementation upon CF bone health.

Studies also identify a direct contribution of CFTR to CFBD. Multiple animal studies in CF deficient mice (CFTR knockout and the F508del-CFTR models) demonstrate reduced bone density, and a study of CF rats found reduced bone content. Notably, the rodent model does not develop overt lung manifestations (prior to these findings in the CF rat).[99–102] Reduced bone mineral content was found in the newborn CF piglets compared with wild-type littermates (and simultaneously lower IGF-1 concentrations).[103] At the cellular level, *Cftr* mRNA expression and immunohistochemistry staining of CFTR have been documented in murine osteoblasts, but not murine osteoclasts. Reduced bone formation and fewer osteoblasts but increased osteoclasts were also found in CFTR-deficient murine cell cultures. Osteoblast–osteoclast cell signaling in dynamic cell cultures revealed reduced expression of the RANKL competitive inhibitor, osteoprotegerin (OPG) and an increased *Rankl* to *OPG* ratio that drives osteoclastogenesis.

The use of novel CFTR modulators has added to the evidence of a direct CFTR contribution (or at least a systemic one). Recently, improvements in cortical microarchitecture, as measured by high-resolution peripheral quantitative computed tomography, were found in adults with the G551D-CFTR genotype and treated with ivacaftor, but no differences in children were found.[104]

Research Studies of Cystic Fibrosis-Related Bone Disease Treatment

The CFRD treatment paradigm for CFBD has largely focused on disease prevention or interrupting disease progression. The prevention arm focuses on vitamin D, calcium, and vitamin K supplementation although newer studies focus on factors like insulin (in CFRD) and sex hormone replacement. The CFF guidelines suggest the following for vitamin D supplementation: 400 to 500 IU/day for children 12 months and younger, 800 to 1000 IU/day for 1 to 10 years of age, and 800 to 2000 IU/day for 11 years and older. Additionally, a serum 25-hydroxyvitamin D concentration at least 30 ng/mL is recommended.[105] CFBD treatment is limited to bisphosphonate medications in adults with DXA BMD Z-scores less than 2. These medications increase BMD in CFBD but the impact upon fracture risk is not known.[106] Newer therapies, such as teriparatide (which stimulates osteoblast activity) could address the uncoupled nature of bone disease. Growth hormone may also improve bone content in CF,[107] but studies have focused more on the linear growth potential. IGF-1 therapy and oxandrolone, which also stimulate osteoblast activity, have yet to be studied in CFBD. Finally, other antiresorptive agents such as denosumab (monoclonal antibody against RANKL) are attractive for targeting the increased inflammatory contribution to CFBD.[108]

GROWTH RESTRICTION IN CYSTIC FIBROSIS
Introduction

Linear bone growth and bone health are intimately related. Growth, as a function of weight and BMI, has long been associated with improved health and lung function in CF. Issues of weight gain and the direct contribution of nutrition are beyond the scope of this review; therefore we focus here on the issue of linear growth itself. However, it is notable that a limited focus on height, and more focus on weight and BMI, may have led to an underrecognized linear growth problem in CF. Recently, investigators have discovered that despite improvements in weight and BMI to that of the 50th% or better, 20% of individuals had a height less than the 10th%.[109] More alarming, impaired linear growth can be an early indicator of pulmonary disease, even before spirometry can be reliably obtained.[110] In a study by Sanders and colleagues, maintaining a height for age above the 50th percentile was a predictor for pulmonary function despite BMI.[111] The more dramatic depiction of stunting, defined as height below the 5th percentile, is a predictor of mortality in CF.[112] In our brief discussion, we will review the potential role of CFTR itself in linear growth, and the expected benefits of a new era of therapies.

Mechanisms of Linear Growth Impairment

Much like bone health, linear growth is multifactorial with many positive and negative contributors. In CF, the weight of these confounders is unbalanced to a less productive endpoint. Unfortunately some clinical treatments that are used in CF may impair growth further (such as corticosteroids).[113] The GH hormone and IGF-1 axis contributing to linear growth has been studied clinically and in animal models.[103,114,115] Controversies over GH secretion exist, but consistently IGF-1 concentrations are low, believed to reflect the impact of chronic inflammation on this axis.[116,117] This factor lowers the anabolic drive of the growing child. Other nonhormonal factors that negatively impact growth such as chronic inflammation, inflammatory cytokines, and corticosteroid usage can directly interfere with the growth plate itself.[113]

However, poor growth in CF begins very early in life and may be linked to the degree of CFTR deficiency (or severity of the genotype). In the BONUS study, an MCT of infants with CF diagnosed by newborn screen, weight for age and length for age had already declined by 1 to 3 months of age (**Fig. 4**).[118] While weight for age recovers by 8 to 10 months of age with the general population, length for age does not by 1 year in CF. In that particular study, the investigators discovered that the presence of pancreatic insufficiency was a predictor of whether infants would meet their expected length for age by 1 year.

Additionally, the animal models discussed above in bone health and CFBD demonstrate growth restriction despite a lack of pulmonary manifestations and/or pancreatic disease. In an early paper by Rosenberg and colleagues, the authors studied growth in the CFTR-deficient mouse.

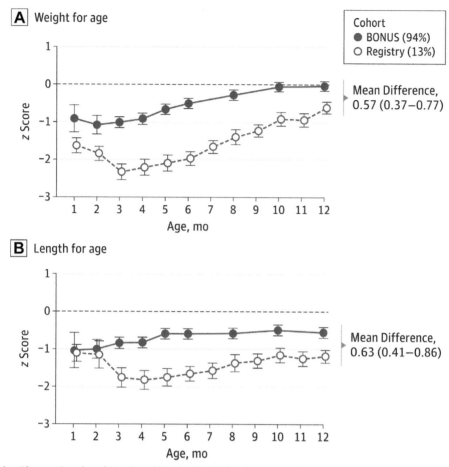

Fig. 4. Baby Observational and Nutrional Study (BONUS) Cohort and Historic Infant Cohort z Scores for Growth During the First Year of Life. (A) Weight for age, (B) Length for age. (*From* Leung DH, Heltshe SL, Borowitz D, Gelfond D, Kloster M, Heubi JE, Stalvey M, Ramsey BW; Baby Observational and Nutrition Study (BONUS) Investigators of the Cystic Fibrosis Foundation Therapeutics Development Network. Effects of Diagnosis by Newborn Screening for Cystic Fibrosis on Weight and Length in the First Year of Life. JAMA Pediatr. 2017 Jun 1;171(6):546-554.)

CFTR-deficient mice had reduced weight and length compared with their wild-type counterparts. Additionally, the CF mice had reduced IGF-1 concentrations.[114] A similar finding was detected by Rogan and colleagues in the CF newborn piglets, in which even at birth they had shorter humeral lengths and IGF-1 levels than non-CF pigs.[103] Lastly, the CF rat model was found to have analogous findings of reduced femoral length, weight, and IGF-1.[115] These discoveries led to some of the early evidence that CFTR may directly contribute to linear growth. However, a better understanding of the contribution to growth by CFTR is needed, and whether it occurs as a systemic or direct effect.

Clinical evidence that linear growth is potentially impacted directly by CFTR dysfunction in childhood was first demonstrated by improvements in growth following ivacaftor treatment in pre-pubertal CF children with at least one copy of the G551D-CFTR genotype.[119] In that report, children (ages 6–11 years) in the multi-center observational study GOAL and the placebo-controlled study ENVISION, demonstrated an improvement in height Z-scores as well as annualized growth velocities following treatment with ivacaftor. Ongoing and future studies are attempting to evaluate the changes in growth following the initiation of newer HEMT in both infants and toddlers, as well as prepubertal and pubertal children with CF. These newer modulators under investigation target the F508del genotype which will encompass a much broader clinical base and may have a larger effect on the CF population.

Treatment Approaches to Linear Growth Impairment

Unfortunately, despite the advances to date, interventions to optimize growth have been limited, that is outside of the nutritional recommendations. Multiple studies through the past couple of decades have examined the use of human growth hormone (hGH) as a supplemental therapy. In a randomized MCT, treatment with hGH in prepubertal CF children demonstrated a 0.5 SDS improvement in height over 1 year, and mean height velocity of 8.2 cm/y compared to 5.3 cm/y in the observation group.[120] However, growth hormone treatment-related improvements in linear growth, bone mineral density, weight, and lean body mass did not translate into dramatic improvements in pulmonary function. Additionally, growth hormone carries the theoretic risk of worsening or precipitating CFRD, however data from the above MC trial did not support that concern.

Research Efforts to Treat Linear Growth Impairment

A study by Zhang in 2013 reviewed peak height velocity and adult height in CF,[121] the authors found about a 6-month delay and 15% reduction in peak height velocity. This delay in peak height velocity may represent a second-hit following the early restriction seen in infants. As pubertal delays in CF improve in the HEMT era, these delay may be further attenuated in the future. In a more recent paper by Zysman-Colman, peak height velocity already shows a more consistent timing with the general pediatric population, although remaining still shorter than their peers.[122]

Current data from the CFF Patient Registry Annual Report documents the average length of individuals under the age of 24 months to be 30th percentile, and those between the ages of 2 and 19 years to be 38.4th percentile.[79] Regardless, we have seen improvements over the past 15 years, with height less than 5th percentile decreasing from 15% of individuals to 10%. As growth restriction affects individuals with severe genotypes and those who are pancreatic insufficient to a greater extent,[118] we could predict that if HEMT does improve growth, we would see much improvement in the years to come.

SUMMARY

As we celebrate highly effective modulator therapy and longevity, endocrine comorbidities are becoming increasingly important considerations in the care of people with CF. Insights into the pathophysiology of CF-related endocrinopathies from the *PROMISE* study and improvements in the overall health among people using highly effective modulator therapy may lead to radical changes in the prevalence of and management options for CFRD, CFBD, and linear growth.

CLINICS CARE POINTS

- Progressive insulin secretion defects underlie abnormal glucose tolerance in cystic fibrosis (CF).
- Leveraging diabetes technologies and type 2 diabetes therapeutics may advance care in youth and adults with CF-related abnormal glucose tolerance.
- Advances in care and the introduction of highly effective modulator therapies may challenge traditional paradigms that focus on the nutritional compromise that accompanies insulin secretion defects in CF.
- The complexity of clinical care in CF confounds and may worsen bone health, thus close supervision is warranted to exacerbate an existing problem.
- When possible, prevention of bone disease is the best course.
- Growth restriction in CF can be a prognostic indicator and should not be overlooked for the sake of focusing weight and BMI.

DISCLOSURE

A. Kelly has nothing to disclose. B. Marks has received investigator initiated research support from Tandem Diabetes Care and Dexcom. M. Stalvey has nothing to disclose.

REFERENCES

1. Kwong E, Desai S, Chong L, et al. The impact of cystic fibrosis-related diabetes on health-related quality of life. J Cystic Fibrosis 2019;7–9.
2. Moran A, Brunzell C, Cohen RC, et al. Clinical care guidelines for cystic fibrosis-related diabetes: a position statement of the American Diabetes Association and a clinical practice guideline of the Cystic Fibrosis Foundation, endorsed by the Pediatric Endocrine Society. Diabetes Care 2010;33(12): 2697–708.
3. Chan CL. Cystic fibrosis related diabetes: Revisiting the OGTT and alternate screening tests. J Cyst Fibros 2020;19(5):671–2.

4. Burgess JC, Bridges N, Banya W, et al. HbA1c as a screening tool for cystic fibrosis related diabetes. J Cyst Fibros 2016;15(2):251–7.

5. Boudreau V, Coriati A, Desjardins K, et al. Glycated hemoglobin cannot yet be proposed as a screening tool for cystic fibrosis related diabetes. J Cyst Fibros 2016;15(2):258–60.

6. Gilmour JA, Sykes J, Etchells E, et al. Cystic fibrosis-related diabetes screening in adults: a Gap analysis and evaluation of accuracy of Glycated hemoglobin levels. Can J Diabetes 2019;43(1):13–8.

7. Sheikh S, Localio AR, Kelly A, et al. Abnormal glucose tolerance and the 50-gram glucose challenge test in Cystic fibrosis. J Cyst Fibros 2020;19(5):696–9.

8. Taylor-Cousar JL, Janssen JS, Wilson A, et al. Glucose >200 mg/dL during continuous glucose monitoring identifies adult patients at risk for development of cystic fibrosis related diabetes. J Diabetes Res 2016;2016:1527932.

9. Chan CL, Pyle L, Vigers T, Zeitler PS, Nadeau KJ.J Clin Endocrinol Metab. The Relationship Between Continuous Glucose Monitoring and OGTT in Youth and Young Adults With Cystic Fibrosis. 2022 Jan 18;107(2):e548-e560. doi: 10.1210/clinem/dgab692.PMID: 34537845.

10. Clemente Leon M, Bilbao Gasso L, Moreno-Galdo A, et al. Oral glucose tolerance test and continuous glucose monitoring to assess diabetes development in cystic fibrosis patients. Endocrinol Diabetes Nutr (Engl Ed 2018;65(1):45–51.

11. Elidottir H, Diemer S, Eklund E, et al. Abnormal glucose tolerance and lung function in children with cystic fibrosis. Comparing oral glucose tolerance test and continuous glucose monitoring. J Cyst Fibros 2021;20(5):779–84.

12. Gojsina B, Minic P, Todorovic S, et al. Continuous glucose monitoring as a valuable tool in the early detection of diabetes related to cystic fibrosis. Front Pediatr 2021;9:659728.

13. Chan CL, Vigers T, Pyle L, et al. Continuous glucose monitoring abnormalities in cystic fibrosis youth correlate with pulmonary function decline. J Cyst Fibros 2018;17(6):783–90.

14. Inman TB, Proudfoot JA, Lim M, et al. Continuous glucose monitoring in a cystic fibrosis patient to predict pulmonary exacerbation? J Cyst Fibros 2017;16(5):628–30.

15. Leclercq A, Gauthier B, Rosner V, et al. Early assessment of glucose abnormalities during continuous glucose monitoring associated with lung function impairment in cystic fibrosis patients. J Cyst Fibros 2014;13(4):478–84.

16. Colomba J, Boudreau V, Lehoux-Dubois C, et al. The main mechanism associated with progression of glucose intolerance in older patients with cystic fibrosis is insulin resistance and not reduced insulin secretion capacity. J Cyst Fibros 2019;18(4):551–6.

17. Hart NJ, Aramandla R, Poffenberger G, et al. Cystic fibrosis-related diabetes is caused by islet loss and inflammation. JCI Insight 2018;3(8).

18. Bogdani M, Blackman SM, Ridaura C, et al. Structural abnormalities in islets from very young children with cystic fibrosis may contribute to cystic fibrosis-related diabetes. Sci Rep 2017;7(1):17231.

19. Sun X, Yi Y, Xie W, et al. CFTR influences beta cell function and insulin secretion through non-cell Autonomous exocrine-derived factors. Endocrinology 2017;158(10):3325–38.

20. Uc A, Olivier AK, Griffin MA, et al. Glycaemic regulation and insulin secretion are abnormal in cystic fibrosis pigs despite sparing of islet cell mass. Clin Sci (Lond) 2015;128(2):131–42.

21. Hull RL, Gibson RL, McNamara S, et al. Islet interleukin-1beta Immunoreactivity is an early feature of cystic fibrosis that may contribute to beta-cell Failure. Diabetes Care 2018;41(4):823–30.

22. Lam AN, Aksit MA, Vecchio-Pagan B, et al. Increased expression of anion transporter SLC26A9 delays diabetes onset in cystic fibrosis. J Clin Invest 2020;130(1):272–86.

23. Segerstolpe A, Palasantza A, Eliasson P, et al. Single-cell Transcriptome Profiling of human pancreatic islets in health and type 2 diabetes. Cell Metab 2016;24(4):593–607.

24. Baron M, Veres A, Wolock SL, et al. A single-cell Transcriptomic Map of the human and mouse pancreas Reveals inter- and Intra-cell population Structure. Cell Syst 2016;3(4):346–360 e4.

25. Edlund A, Esguerra JL, Wendt A, et al. CFTR and Anoctamin 1 (ANO1) contribute to cAMP amplified exocytosis and insulin secretion in human and murine pancreatic beta-cells. BMC Med 2014;12:87.

26. Bellin MD, Laguna T, Leschyshyn J, et al. Insulin secretion improves in cystic fibrosis following ivacaftor correction of CFTR: a small pilot study. Pediatr Diabetes 2013;14(6):417–21.

27. Kelly A, De Leon DD, Sheikh S, et al. Islet hormone and incretin secretion in cystic fibrosis after Four Months of ivacaftor therapy. Am J Respir Crit Care Med 2019;199(3):342–51.

28. Volkova N, Moy K, Evans J, et al. Disease progression in patients with cystic fibrosis treated with ivacaftor: data from national US and UK registries. J Cyst Fibros 2020;19(1):68–79.

29. Misgault B, Chatron E, Reynaud Q, et al. Effect of one-year lumacaftor-ivacaftor treatment on glucose tolerance abnormalities in cystic fibrosis patients. J Cyst Fibros 2020;19(5):712–6.

30. Ballmann M, Prinz N, Glass A, et al. Comment on "Effect of one-year lumacaftor-ivacaftor treatment

on glucose tolerance abnormalities in cystic fibrosis patients. J Cyst Fibros 2020;19(5):839.

31. Moheet A, Beisang D, Zhang L, et al. Lumacaftor/ivacaftor therapy fails to increase insulin secretion in F508del/F508del CF patients. J Cyst Fibros 2021;20(2):333–8.

32. Scully KJ, Marchetti P, Sawicki GS, Uluer A, Cernadas M, Cagnina RE, Kennedy JC, The effect of elexacaftor/tezacaftor/ivacaftor (ETI) on glycemia in adults with cystic fibrosis. Putman MS.J Cyst Fibros. 2022 Mar;21(2):258-263. doi: 10.1016/j.jcf.2021.09.001. Epub 2021 Sep 14.PMID: 34531155.

33. Nichols DP, Donaldson SH, Frederick CA, et al. PROMISE: Working with the CF community to understand emerging clinical and research needs for those treated with highly effective CFTR modulator therapy. J Cyst Fibros 2021;20(2):205–12.

34. Aksit MA, Pace RG, Vecchio-Pagan B, et al. Genetic modifiers of cystic fibrosis-related diabetes have extensive Overlap with type 2 diabetes and related Traits. J Clin Endocrinol Metab 2020;105(5).

35. Blackman SM, Commander CW, Watson C, et al. Genetic modifiers of cystic fibrosis-related diabetes. Diabetes 2013;62(10):3627–35.

36. Sun L, Rommens JM, Corvol H, et al. Multiple apical plasma membrane constituents are associated with susceptibility to meconium ileus in individuals with cystic fibrosis. Nat Genet 2012;44(5):562–9.

37. Lin YC, Keenan K, Gong J, et al. Cystic fibrosis-related diabetes onset can be predicted using biomarkers measured at birth. Genet Med 2021;23(5):927–33.

38. Nyirjesy SC, Sheikh S, Hadjiliadis D, et al. beta-Cell secretory defects are present in pancreatic insufficient cystic fibrosis with 1-hour oral glucose tolerance test glucose >/=155 mg/dL. Pediatr Diabetes 2018;19(7):1173–82.

39. Tommerdahl KL, Brinton JT, Vigers T, et al. Delayed glucose peak and elevated 1-hour glucose on the oral glucose tolerance test identify youth with cystic fibrosis with lower oral disposition index. J Cyst Fibros 2021;20(2):339–45.

40. Tschritter O, Fritsche A, Shirkavand F, et al. Assessing the shape of the glucose curve during an oral glucose tolerance test. Diabetes Care 2003;26(4):1026–33.

41. Abdul-Ghani MA, Abdul-Ghani T, Ali N, et al. One-hour plasma glucose concentration and the metabolic syndrome identify subjects at high risk for future type 2 diabetes. Diabetes Care 2008;31(8):1650–5.

42. Boudreau V, Coriati A, Hammana I, et al. Variation of glucose tolerance in adult patients with cystic fibrosis: what is the potential contribution of insulin sensitivity? J Cyst Fibros 2016;15(6):839–45.

43. Harindhanavudhi T, Wang Q, Dunitz J, et al. Prevalence and factors associated with overweight and obesity in adults with cystic fibrosis: a single-center analysis. J Cyst Fibros 2020;19(1):139–45.

44. Hanna RM, Weiner DJ. Overweight and obesity in patients with cystic fibrosis: a center-based analysis. Pediatr Pulmonol 2015;50(1):35–41.

45. Middleton PG, Mall MA, Drevinek P, et al. Elexacaftor-Tezacaftor-Ivacaftor for Cystic Fibrosis with a Single Phe508del Allele. N Engl J Med 2019;381(19):1809–19.

46. Moran A, Pillay K, Becker D, et al. ISPAD Clinical Practice Consensus Guidelines 2018: management of cystic fibrosis-related diabetes in children and adolescents. Pediatr Diabetes 2018;19(Suppl 27):64–74.

47. Milla CE, Warwick WJ, Moran A. Trends in pulmonary function in patients with cystic fibrosis correlate with the degree of glucose intolerance at baseline. Am J Respir Crit Care Med 2000;162(3 Pt 1):891–5.

48. Lanng S, Thorsteinsson B, Nerup J, et al. Influence of the development of diabetes mellitus on clinical status in patients with cystic fibrosis. Eur J Pediatr 1992;151(9):684–7.

49. Peraldo M, Fasulo A, Chiappini E, et al. Evaluation of glucose tolerance and insulin secretion in cystic fibrosis patients. Horm Res 1998;49(2):65–71.

50. Kilberg MJ, Harris C, Sheikh S, Stefanovski D, Cuchel M, Kubrak C, Hadjiliadis D, Rubenstein RC, Rickels MR, Kelly A. Hypoglycemia and Islet Dysfunction Following Oral Glucose Tolerance Testing in Pancreatic-Insufficient Cystic Fibrosis. J Clin Endocrinol Metab. 2020 Oct 1;105(10):3179-89. doi: 10.1210/clinem/dgaa448. PMID: 32668452; PMCID: PMC7755140.

51. Kilberg MJ, Sheikh S, Stefanovski D, et al. Dysregulated insulin in pancreatic insufficient cystic fibrosis with post-prandial hypoglycemia. J Cyst Fibros 2020;19(2):310–5.

52. Marks BE, Wolfsdorf JI. Monitoring of pediatric type 1 diabetes. Front Endocrinol (Lausanne) 2020;11:128.

53. O'Riordan SM, Hindmarsh P, Hill NR, et al. Validation of continuous glucose monitoring in children and adolescents with cystic fibrosis: a prospective cohort study. Diabetes Care 2009;32(6):1020–2.

54. Battelino T, Danne T, Bergenstal RM, et al. Clinical targets for continuous glucose monitoring data Interpretation: recommendations from the International Consensus on time in range. Diabetes Care 2019;42(8):1593–603.

55. Beck RW, Bergenstal RM, Cheng P, et al. The relationships between time in range, hyperglycemia Metrics, and HbA1c. J Diabetes Sci Technol 2019;13(4):614–26.

56. Marks BE, Kilberg MJ, Aliaj E, et al. Perceptions of diabetes technology Use in cystic fibrosis-related diabetes management. Diabetes Technol Ther 2021;23(11):753–9.

57. Hardin DS, Rice J, Rice M, et al. Use of the insulin pump in treat cystic fibrosis related diabetes. J Cyst Fibros 2009;8(3):174–8.
58. Pinsker JE, Deshpande S, McCrady-Spitzer S, et al. Use of the Interoperable Artificial pancreas system for type 1 diabetes management during Psychological stress. J Diabetes Sci Technol 2021;15(1):184–5.
59. Brown SA, Kovatchev BP, Raghinaru D, et al. Six-month randomized, Multicenter trial of Closed-Loop control in type 1 diabetes. N Engl J Med 2019;381(18):1707–17.
60. Sherwood JS, Jafri RZ, Balliro CA, et al. Automated glycemic control with the bionic pancreas in cystic fibrosis-related diabetes: a pilot study. J Cyst Fibros 2020;19(1):159–61.
61. Dobson L, Hattersley AT, Tiley S, et al. Clinical improvement in cystic fibrosis with early insulin treatment. Arch Dis Child 2002;87(5):430–1.
62. Bizzarri C, Lucidi V, Ciampalini P, et al. Clinical effects of early treatment with insulin glargine in patients with cystic fibrosis and impaired glucose tolerance. J Endocrinol Invest 2006;29(3):RC1–4.
63. Mozzillo E, Franzese A, Valerio G, et al. One-year glargine treatment can improve the course of lung disease in children and adolescents with cystic fibrosis and early glucose derangements. Pediatr Diabetes 2009;10(3):162–7.
64. Moran A, Pekow P, Grover P, et al. Insulin therapy to improve BMI in cystic fibrosis-related diabetes without fasting hyperglycemia: results of the cystic fibrosis related diabetes therapy trial. Diabetes Care 2009;32(10):1783–8.
65. Minicucci L, Haupt M, Casciaro R, et al. Slow-release insulin in cystic fibrosis patients with glucose intolerance: a randomized clinical trial. Pediatr Diabetes 2012;13(2):197–202.
66. Ballmann M, Hubert D, Assael BM, et al. Repaglinide versus insulin for newly diagnosed diabetes in patients with cystic fibrosis: a multicentre, open-label, randomised trial. Lancet Diabetes Endocrinol 2018;6(2):114–21.
67. Kelly A, Sheikh S, Stefanovski D, Peleckis AJ, Nyirjesy SC, Eiel JN, Sidhaye A, Localio R, Gallop R, De Leon DD, Hadjiliadis D, Rubenstein RC, Effect of Sitagliptin on Islet Function in Pancreatic Insufficient Cystic Fibrosis With Abnormal Glucose Tolerance. Rickels MR.J Clin Endocrinol Metab. 2021 Aug 18;106(9):2617-2634. doi: 10.1210/clinem/dgab365. Epub 2021 May 22.PMID: 34406395.
68. Beaudoin N, Bouvet GF, Coriati A, et al. Combined exercise training improves glycemic control in adult with cystic fibrosis. Med Sci Sports Exerc 2017;49(2):231–7.
69. Monteiro KS, Azevedo MP, Jales LM, et al. Effects of aerobic interval training on glucose tolerance in children and adolescents with cystic fibrosis: a randomized trial protocol. Trials 2019;20(1):768.
70. Kuo P, Stevens JE, Russo A, et al. Gastric emptying, incretin hormone secretion, and postprandial glycemia in cystic fibrosis–effects of pancreatic enzyme supplementation. J Clin Endocrinol Metab 2011;96(5):E851–5.
71. Perano SJ, Couper JJ, Horowitz M, et al. Pancreatic enzyme supplementation improves the incretin hormone response and attenuates postprandial glycemia in adolescents with cystic fibrosis: a randomized crossover trial. J Clin Endocrinol Metab 2014;99(7):2486–93.
72. Sun X, Yi Y, Liang B, et al. Incretin dysfunction and hyperglycemia in cystic fibrosis: role of acyl-ghrelin. J Cyst Fibros 2019;18(4):557–65.
73. Geyer MC, Sullivan T, Tai A, et al. Exenatide corrects postprandial hyperglycaemia in young people with cystic fibrosis and impaired glucose tolerance: a randomized crossover trial. Diabetes Obes Metab 2019;21(3):700–4.
74. Olatunbosun ST. Chronic incretin-based therapy in cystic fibrosis-related diabetes: A tale of 3 patients treated with sitagliptin for over 5 years. J Cyst Fibros. 2021 Nov;20(6):e124-e128. doi: 10.1016/j.jcf.2021.02.005. Epub 2021 Mar 2. PMID: 33674210.
75. Mischler EH, Chesney PJ, Chesney RW, et al. Demineralization in cystic fibrosis detected by direct photon absorptiometry. Am J Dis Child 1979;133(6):632–5.
76. Aris RM, Renner JB, Winders AD, et al. Increased rate of fractures and severe kyphosis: sequelae of living into adulthood with cystic fibrosis. Ann Intern Med 1998;128(3):186–93.
77. Rovner AJ, Zemel BS, Leonard MB, et al. Mild to moderate cystic fibrosis is not associated with increased fracture risk in children and adolescents. J Pediatr 2005;147(3):327–31.
78. Latzin P, Griese M, Hermanns V, et al. Sternal fracture with fatal outcome in cystic fibrosis. Thorax 2005;60(7):616.
79. Foundation CF. Cystic Fibrosis Foundation Patient Registry 2019 Annual Data Report. Bethesda (MD): 2020.
80. Aris RM, Merkel PA, Bachrach LK, et al. Guide to bone health and disease in cystic fibrosis. J Clin Endocrinol Metab 2005;90(3):1888–96.
81. Aris RM, Ontjes DA, Buell HE, et al. Abnormal bone turnover in cystic fibrosis adults. Osteoporos Int 2002;13(2):151–7.
82. Aris RM, Lester GE, Dingman S, et al. Altered calcium homeostasis in adults with cystic fibrosis. Osteoporos Int 1999;10(2):102–8.
83. Hall WB, Sparks AA, Aris RM. Vitamin d deficiency in cystic fibrosis. Int J Endocrinol 2010;2010:218691.
84. Hofbauer LC, Gori F, Riggs BL, et al. Stimulation of osteoprotegerin ligand and inhibition of

osteoprotegerin production by glucocorticoids in human osteoblastic lineage cells: potential paracrine mechanisms of glucocorticoid-induced osteoporosis. Endocrinology 1999;140(10):4382–9.

85. DiMango E, Ratner AJ, Bryan R, et al. Activation of NF-kappaB by adherent Pseudomonas aeruginosa in normal and cystic fibrosis respiratory epithelial cells. J Clin Invest 1998;101(11):2598–605.

86. Ionescu AA, Nixon LS, Evans WD, et al. Bone density, body composition, and inflammatory status in cystic fibrosis. Am J Respir Crit Care Med 2000; 162(3 Pt 1):789–94.

87. Haworth CS, Selby PL, Webb AK, et al. Inflammatory related changes in bone mineral content in adults with cystic fibrosis. Thorax 2004;59(7):613–7.

88. Shead EF, Haworth CS, Barker H, et al. Osteoclast function, bone turnover and inflammatory cytokines during infective exacerbations of cystic fibrosis. J Cyst Fibros 2010;9(2):93–8.

89. Shead EF, Haworth CS, Gunn E, et al. Osteoclastogenesis during infective exacerbations in patients with cystic fibrosis. Am J Respir Crit Care Med 2006;174(3):306–11.

90. Stead RJ, Hodson ME, Batten JC, et al. Amenorrhoea in cystic fibrosis. Clin Endocrinol (Oxf) 1987;26(2):187–95.

91. Leifke E, Friemert M, Heilmann M, et al. Sex steroids and body composition in men with cystic fibrosis. Eur J Endocrinol 2003;148(5):551–7.

92. Rana M, Munns CF, Selvadurai H, et al. The impact of dysglycaemia on bone mineral accrual in young people with cystic fibrosis. Clin Endocrinol (Oxf) 2013;78(1):36–42.

93. Gordon CM, Binello E, LeBoff MS, et al. Relationship between insulin-like growth factor I, dehydroepiandrosterone sulfate and proresorptive cytokines and bone density in cystic fibrosis. Osteoporos Int 2006;17(5):783–90.

94. Rossini M, Del Marco A, Dal Santo F, et al. Prevalence and correlates of vertebral fractures in adults with cystic fibrosis. Bone 2004;35(3):771–6.

95. Foundation CF. Cystic fibrosis Foundation patient Registry, 2019. Bethesda, MD: Annual Data Report; 2020.

96. King SJ, Topliss DJ, Kotsimbos T, et al. Reduced bone density in cystic fibrosis: DeltaF508 mutation is an independent risk factor. Eur Respir J 2005; 25(1):54–61.

97. Lam GY, Desai S, Fu J, et al. IL-8 correlates with reduced baseline femoral neck bone mineral density in adults with cystic fibrosis: a single center retrospective study. Sci Rep 2021;11(1):15405.

98. Wu M, Bettermann EL, Arora N, et al. Relationship between estrogen treatment and Skeletal health in women with cystic fibrosis. Am J Med Sci 2020;360(5):581–90.

99. Dif F, Marty C, Baudoin C, et al. Severe osteopenia in CFTR-null mice. Bone 2004;35(3):595–603.

100. Haston CK, Li W, Li A, et al. Persistent osteopenia in adult cystic fibrosis transmembrane conductance regulator-deficient mice. Am J Respir Crit Care Med 2008;177(3):309–15.

101. Pashuck TD, Franz SE, Altman MK, et al. Murine model for cystic fibrosis bone disease demonstrates osteopenia and sex-related differences in bone formation. Pediatr Res 2009;65(3): 311–6.

102. Le Henaff C, Gimenez A, Haÿ E, et al. The F508del mutation in cystic fibrosis transmembrane conductance regulator gene impacts bone formation. Am J Pathol 2012;180(5):2068–75.

103. Rogan MP, Reznikov LR, Pezzulo AA, et al. Pigs and humans with cystic fibrosis have reduced insulin-like growth factor 1 (IGF1) levels at birth. Proc Natl Acad Sci U S A 2010;107(47):20571–5.

104. Putman MS, Greenblatt LB, Bruce M, et al. The effects of ivacaftor on bone density and microarchitecture in children and adults with cystic fibrosis. J Clin Endocrinol Metab 2021;106(3): e1248–61.

105. Tangpricha V, Kelly A, Stephenson A, et al. An update on the screening, diagnosis, management, and treatment of vitamin D deficiency in individuals with cystic fibrosis: evidence-based recommendations from the Cystic Fibrosis Foundation. J Clin Endocrinol Metab 2012;97(4):1082–93.

106. Conwell LS, Chang AB. Bisphosphonates for osteoporosis in people with cystic fibrosis. Cochrane Database Syst Rev 2012;4:CD002010.

107. Hardin DS, Ahn C, Prestidge C, et al. Growth hormone improves bone mineral content in children with cystic fibrosis. J Pediatr Endocrinol Metab 2005;18(6):589–95.

108. Putman MS, Anabtawi A, Le T, et al. Cystic fibrosis bone disease treatment: Current knowledge and future directions. J Cyst Fibros 2019;18(Suppl 2): S56–65.

109. Konstan MW, Pasta DJ, Wagener JS, et al. BMI fails to identify poor nutritional status in stunted children with CF. J Cyst Fibros 2017;16(1):158–60.

110. Assael BM, Casazza G, Iansa P, et al. Growth and long-term lung function in cystic fibrosis: a longitudinal study of patients diagnosed by neonatal screening. Pediatr Pulmonol 2009; 44(3):209–15.

111. Sanders DB, Slaven JE, Maguiness K, et al. Early-life height Attainment in cystic fibrosis is associated with pulmonary function at age 6 Years. Ann Am Thorac Soc 2021;18(8):1335–42.

112. Vieni G, Faraci S, Collura M, et al. Stunting is an independent predictor of mortality in patients with cystic fibrosis. Clin Nutr 2013;32(3):382–5.

113. Wong SC, Dobie R, Altowati MA, et al. Growth and the growth hormone-insulin like growth factor 1 Axis in children with chronic inflammation: Current evidence, Gaps in knowledge, and future directions. Endocr Rev 2016;37(1):62–110.

114. Rosenberg LA, Schluchter MD, Parlow AF, et al. Mouse as a model of growth retardation in cystic fibrosis. Pediatr Res 2006;59(2):191–5.

115. Stalvey MS, Havasi V, Tuggle KL, et al. Reduced bone length, growth plate thickness, bone content, and IGF-I as a model for poor growth in the CFTR-deficient rat. PLoS One 2017;12(11): e0188497.

116. Pascucci C, De Biase RV, Savi D, et al. Deregulation of the growth hormone/insulin-like growth factor-1 axis in adults with cystic fibrosis. J Endocrinol Invest 2018;41(5):591–6.

117. Gifford AH, Nymon AB, Ashare A. Serum insulin-like growth factor-1 (IGF-1) during CF pulmonary exacerbation: trends and biomarker correlations. Pediatr Pulmonol 2014;49(4):335–41.

118. Leung DH, Heltshe SL, Borowitz D, et al. Effects of diagnosis by newborn screening for cystic fibrosis on weight and length in the first Year of life. JAMA Pediatr 2017;171(6):546–54.

119. Stalvey MS, Pace J, Niknian M, et al. Growth in prepubertal children with cystic fibrosis treated with ivacaftor. Pediatrics 2017;139(2).

120. Stalvey MS, Anbar RD, Konstan MW, et al. A multicenter controlled trial of growth hormone treatment in children with cystic fibrosis. Pediatr Pulmonol 2012;47(3):252–63.

121. Zhang Z, Lindstrom MJ, Lai HJ. Pubertal height velocity and associations with prepubertal and adult heights in cystic fibrosis. J Pediatr 2013;163(2): 376–82.

122. Zysman-Colman ZN, Kilberg MJ, Harrison VS, et al. Genetic potential and height velocity during childhood and adolescence do not fully account for shorter stature in cystic fibrosis. Pediatr Res 2021;89(3):653–9.

Management of Mental Health in Cystic Fibrosis

Christina Jayne Bathgate, PhD[a],*, Michelle Hjelm, MD[b], Stephanie S. Filigno, PhD[c], Beth A. Smith, MD[d], Anna M. Georgiopoulos, MD[e]

KEYWORDS

- Cystic fibrosis • Mental health • Psychological treatment • Medication
- Psychopharmacological treatment • Depression • Anxiety • ADHD

KEY POINTS

- Mental health concerns are common among persons with cystic fibrosis (pwCF).
- Recognizing mental health symptoms can prepare providers across disciplines to identify and address concerns within their role.
- Empirically supported psychological and pharmacologic treatments can effectively treat mental health concerns; more research on the impact of such treatments among pwCF is warranted.
- Psychological interventions reduce mental health symptoms by addressing underlying and perpetuating causes of such symptoms while promoting positive coping strategies.
- Psychopharmacologic treatments on their own or in conjunction with psychological interventions can also reduce mental health symptoms.

BACKGROUND

Mental health concerns are common among persons with cystic fibrosis (pwCF). If left untreated, unfavorable physical and emotional outcomes may ensue, such as decreased lung function, increased pulmonary exacerbations, lower body mass index, poorer health-related quality of life, higher health care utilization, and earlier mortality.[1–3] The current median predicted life expectancy is 46 years for those born between 2015 and 2019.[4] As the lifespan of pwCF continues to improve in the era of highly effective modulator therapy (HEMT), the psychosocial stressors and challenges pwCF encounter have become more complex and chronic. These challenges can include promoting normal childhood development alongside chronic disease management, evolving nutritional needs and feeding challenges, changes in family dynamics, adherence to complex and potentially burdensome treatment regimens, disclosure of disease to peers, schools, and/or employers, disruptions in education and work due to health challenges, shifts in roles and expectations based on health status, sexual and reproductive health concerns, and lung transplant considerations.[5] In addition, HEMT has been shown to affect mental health in pwCF. Adverse mental health and neurocognitive events were seen among all 4 HEMT in postclinical trial studies.[6] After initiating lumacaftor/ivacaftor, researchers observed worsening symptoms of depression and anxiety,[7,8] suicidal ideation,[7] and suicide attempts requiring psychiatric hospitalization.[7] After initiating elexacaftor/texacaftor/ivacaftor (ETI), researchers observed worsening symptoms of depression and anxiety,[9,10] "mental

[a] Department of Medicine, National Jewish Health, 1400 Jackson Street, Denver, CO 80206, USA; [b] University of Cincinnati College of Medicine; Division of Pulmonary Medicine, Cincinnati Children's Hospital Medical Center, 3333 Burnet Avenue, Cincinnati, OH 45229, USA; [c] University of Cincinnati College of Medicine; Division of Behavioral Medicine and Clinical Psychology, Cincinnati Children's Hospital Medical Center, 3333 Burnet Avenue, Cincinnati, OH 45229, USA; [d] Jacobs School of Medicine and Biomedical Sciences, Children's Psychiatry Clinic, 1028 Main Street, Buffalo, NY 14202, USA; [e] Part-Time, Harvard Medical School; Department of Psychiatry, Massachusetts General Hospital, Yawkey 6900, 55 Fruit Street, Boston, MA 02114, USA
* Corresponding author.
E-mail address: bathgatec@njhealth.org

Clin Chest Med 43 (2022) 791–810
https://doi.org/10.1016/j.ccm.2022.06.014
0272-5231/22/© 2022 Elsevier Inc. All rights reserved.

fogginess,"[10,11] and discontinuation of ETI due to mental health side effects.[10] On the other hand, there have also been reports of positive psychological and social effects after initiating ETI.[12]

The aim of this article is to introduce CF team members to mental health concerns they may encounter; how they might uniquely present in pwCF; and ways to manage such symptoms with risk assessment, psychological interventions, and/or psychotropic medications. Although our focus is on pwCF, providers working with caregivers of pwCF should be mindful that untreated mental health symptoms in caregivers may negatively affect the care they are able to provide.[1,3,13]

CLINICAL RELEVANCE
Cystic Fibrosis Mental Health Guidelines Focus on Depression and Generalized Anxiety

Depression is a common and serious medical illness that negatively affects thoughts, feelings, and behaviors. Depression is caused by a combination of genetic, biological, environmental (eg, exposure to violence, poverty), and psychological factors (eg, low self-esteem). Central to the diagnosis is depressed mood and/or loss of interest or pleasure in activities.[14] Some of the physical symptoms pwCF may experience, such as loss of appetite, fatigue, and insomnia, can overlap or even mimic symptoms of depression, which is why it can be important to place emphasis on identifying other psychological symptoms of depression, such as an inability to derive joy from previously enjoyed activities, guilt, and impairments in self-esteem. CF symptoms and treatments should be routinely considered in the assessment and differential diagnosis of pwCF with neuropsychiatric symptoms of any type.[3] In particular, close monitoring is recommended when pwCF initiate use of an HEMT,[8] given reports of temporally associated changes in mood, anxiety, sleep, and neurocognition.[6,11]

Anxiety is characterized by feelings of tension, worried thoughts, and physical changes such as increased heart rate. Individuals with anxiety disorders usually experience intense, excessive, and persistent worry, which may lead to avoidance.[14] Generalized anxiety disorder (GAD) is excessive anxiety and worry about a range of concerns accompanied by restlessness, fatigue, impaired concentration, muscle tension, and sleep disruptions.[14] Individuals with anxiety disorders often have unrealistic anxiety, such as fear of a situation that will likely never happen. However, pwCF often have rational anxiety and fear related to their health (eg, worries about disease progression, disability, or death) that can affect daily CF care.

The International Depression/Anxiety Epidemiologic Study (TIDES) found rates of depression and anxiety 2 to 3 times higher in pwCF and caregivers than those reported in community samples.[1] Furthermore, 5-year survival data were evaluated in 1005 adults with CF from TIDES, and a positive depression screen was associated with increased mortality.[2] The negative consequences of depression and anxiety on CF management and outcomes led to the development of International Mental Health Guidelines. These guidelines recommend annual depression and anxiety screenings for pwCF aged 12 years or older and caregivers of children with CF, using the Patient Health Questionnaire-9[15] and Generalized Anxiety Disorder 7-Item Scale,[16] with stepped care models for the treatment of depression and anxiety that can be incorporated into routine CF care.[3,17] Collaborative care models integrating mental health screening and treatment have now been widely implemented into CF Centers internationally.[18–20] Some CF Centers may have the capacity to expand screening to younger age groups or other mental health conditions.[21] For example, the Preschool Pediatric Symptom Checklist (ages 18 months–5 years) and the Pediatric Symptom Checklist-17 (ages 4–17 years) can be used to detect a broad range of symptoms, prompting further assessment and treatment as needed.[22–24]

Some forms of depression and anxiety develop under circumstances requiring special management, such as peripartum or in association with psychotic symptoms. People with bipolar disorder may report depressive episodes or anxiety but also experience extreme highs with euphoric or irritable moods.[14] Individuals with borderline personality disorder may have co-occurring major depression or GAD; however, mood instability presents prominently with an unstable sense of self, difficulties in interpersonal relationships, and often suicidal and self-harming behaviors.[14] Because these conditions typically require expertise beyond that of the CF team, their management was considered outside the scope of the CF mental health guidelines, but they should be considered in the differential diagnosis of depression and anxiety symptoms.

Other Anxiety-Related Conditions Affecting People with Cystic Fibrosis

Social anxiety involves intense anxiety or fear of being negatively evaluated or rejected in social and/or performance situations, leading to avoidance of these experiences.[14] Intense physical symptoms, such as rapid heart rate, nausea, sweating, and difficulty breathing, may occur during a panic attack. Social anxiety can lead to difficulties in communication and relationship building with CF medical teams, seeking out appropriate social support, and can affect the school and workplace when pwCF believe other people have negative evaluations of their CF.

Obsessive-compulsive disorder (OCD) causes distress and anxiety through persistent obsessions (intrusive and unwanted thoughts, images, or urges) and compulsions (behaviors that are difficult to control and often result in a consequent reduction in anxiety and temporary elimination of the obsession).[14] Germ contamination is a common obsession and may be protective when managing CF; however, if the washing/cleaning compulsion causes disruption in functioning, treatment of OCD is warranted. OCD is more prevalent in adults than children, given the cognitive nature of the condition.[14] If distress related to OCD symptoms is reported, assessment of functional impairment might include time spent occupied by obsessive thoughts and/or compulsive behaviors, how much effort they spend trying to resist such thoughts and behaviors, and how successful they are at reducing the impact of thoughts and behaviors.

Procedural anxiety (PAnx) is experienced by individuals when there is worry related to negative anticipation of a future medical procedure and acute distress leading up to and/or during the procedure. PwCF undergo numerous routine and unplanned medical procedures across the lifespan when managing their disease. The experience of PAnx is common for children and adults, particularly for procedures that are associated with anticipation of pain. PAnx presents differently based on age, coping style, and severity of the anxiety. Young children may demonstrate more externalizing behavior (ie, crying, screaming, resistance), whereas teens and adults may internalize anxiety and avoid recommended medical care. Limited research exists for procedural distress and screening tools specifically in CF.[25]

Medical traumatic stress (MTS) can develop when an individual directly experiences medical trauma and/or when they observe the trauma of someone else in a medical setting. MTS contributes to the development of heightened stress responses to environmental cues including fear, worry, and body symptoms, which consequently lead to impaired functioning in environments that may be safe, yet be perceived as unsafe.[21] Because CF care requires frequent medical environment interactions, the likelihood of having a negative experience in the medical environment is increased.

Nonmedical trauma occurs when an individual experiences a potentially life-threatening event including, but not limited to, serious injury, violence, and/or death of a loved one. Within the first 4 weeks of exposure to such trauma, an acute stress disorder may emerge with features of anxiety, intense fear or helplessness, reexperiencing the event, avoidance behaviors, and dissociative symptoms.[14] When these trauma reactions are prolonged and impairing (ie, >4 weeks), providers might consider a diagnosis of posttraumatic stress disorder. The experience of MTS can put individuals with CF at risk for increased trauma reactions to subsequent negative nonmedical experiences if the MTS is not adequately addressed.[21] If distress associated with medical or nonmedical trauma is observed or reported, referral to a licensed mental health provider with trauma expertise can provide more thorough assessment and assistance to the care team.

Other Behavioral Disorders that can Emerge in Childhood Among People with Cystic Fibrosis

Attention-deficit hyperactivity disorder (ADHD) is a neurobiological, familial disorder with childhood onset featuring pervasive symptoms of inattention, hyperactivity, and/or impulsivity.[14] In prospective, controlled studies, children with ADHD demonstrate impairment in educational, occupational, legal, and interpersonal functioning into adulthood.[26] ADHD is associated with comorbid learning disabilities; the onset of mental health conditions including depression, anxiety, personality disorder, suicidality, and substance misuse; and adverse physical health outcomes; one study found childhood ADHD diagnosis conferred a 9- to 10-year decrease in adult life expectancy.[26] ADHD is 2 to 4 times more common in pwCF than in the general population, and attentional difficulties are also reported in CF parents and siblings.[21] When pwCF or their caregivers have ADHD, difficulty registering and retaining information, disorganization, and task avoidance may complicate navigating the health care system and disease self-management.[21]

Autism spectrum disorder (ASD) is an early onset, neurodevelopmental disorder with varied phenotypes reflecting impaired social interactions (reciprocity, nonverbal communication, relationship building) and behavior patterns.[14] The repetitive/restricted behaviors, inflexibility, and sensory dysregulation associated with ASD can interfere with CF care and nutrition.[21]

Children with oppositional defiant disorder (ODD) display persistent anger and defiance, attributable to both temperament and environment.[14] ODD often co-occurs with ADHD and confers risk for conduct disorder, substance misuse, depression, and anxiety.[14] Argumentativeness may undermine caregiver relationships and lead to CF treatment refusal.[21]

If a clinician suspects ADHD, ASD, or ODD is present and affecting daily functioning, referral to a licensed mental health provider with expertise in the assessment of ADHD, ASD, or ODD is recommended.

Sleep Disturbances May Manifest in People with Cystic Fibrosis as a Part of or Separate from Mental Health Concerns

Sleep disturbances are a frequent comorbidity of mental health and behavioral disorders.[27] Symptoms can include daytime somnolence, frequent nocturnal awakenings, excessive sleep times, and insomnia. Although these symptoms may be secondary to inadequate sleep time or quality, they may also be associated with medical sleep disorders such as hypoxemia, sleep apnea, restless leg syndrome, circadian rhythm disorder, narcolepsy, and hypoventilation.[28]

Sleep disruption and impaired sleep quality have been reported as high as 50% in pwCF.[29,30] Medical conditions associated with sleep disturbances in pwCF include mental health disorders, behavioral disorders, CF-related diabetes, overnight tube feeds, asthma, and severe obstructive lung disease.[29] In addition, changes in sleep have been reported with CFTR modulator use.[6,11]

It is important to consider screening pwCF for medical sleep disorders when there are persistent mental health concerns, behavioral health concerns, or new sleep disturbances. Sleep screening should begin by asking pwCF and/or their caregivers if they have a "concern or problem with sleep," and for an explanation of the symptoms if a concern is identified. Additional questions to help guide screening may include asking about total sleep time, ease of falling asleep, nighttime awakenings, daytime sleepiness, and snoring. If significant concerns are identified, a referral to a sleep medicine specialist should be considered.

Problematic Eating Patterns in People with Cystic Fibrosis

PwCF are at increased risk for several types of disordered eating patterns. This increased risk for disordered eating is often attributed to the inherent risk factors for weight and growth disturbances and the persistent focus placed on nutrition due to its impact on overall health and lung function. In addition, mental health conditions, such as anxiety and depression, are common comorbid conditions in people with eating disturbances.[31]

In early childhood, there can be increased prevalence of avoidant or symptomatic behaviors (gagging/retching) around meals as well as overt food refusal. In later childhood, adolescence, and adulthood, pwCF may have restrictive eating behaviors, body image disorders, or preoccupation with meals. In addition, pwCF are more likely to use excessive exercise or misuse medications, such as pancreatic enzymes, as part of weight control when compared with other chronic disease populations.[32] Insulin restriction is common and associated with medical complications in people with type 1 diabetes, but it has not been well studied in people with CF-related diabetes.[33]

Although no screening tools exist for disordered eating in pwCF, if clinical concerns exist it is important to consider asking questions about food avoidance, food scarcity, preoccupation with food or meals, and medication use to help guide the need for further evaluation. These questions may be of additional benefit in patients with significant changes in weight with initiation or ongoing CFTR modulator therapy. Partnering with a CF dietician can be incredibly useful for addressing such concerns.

Impact of Substance Misuse in People with Cystic Fibrosis

Substance misuse is defined as cognitive, behavioral, and physiologic symptoms resulting from continued use of a substance despite significant substance-related problems.[14] Commonly misused substances include alcohol, tobacco, marijuana, benzodiazepines, and opioids. Key clinical symptoms and useful questions for screening problematic use include longer use or larger amounts of use than expected, unsuccessful efforts to cut back, excessive time spent obtaining the substance, craving, tolerance, and/or withdrawal symptoms.[14]

Substance misuse is of particular concern in pwCF because of the significant impacts it can have on financial well-being, physical health, and emotional health. Commonly misused substances have associations with increased pulmonary symptoms, lung injury, and respiratory failure.[34] In addition, they can have negative impacts on common medical comorbidities in pwCF including CF-related liver disease, CF-related diabetes, and lung transplantation. Studies in the general population have noted the association of mental health disorders with substance misuse,[35] which supports concerns for substance misuse in pwCF, given higher rates of symptoms of anxiety and depression.[1]

Recent literature investigating substance misuse in pwCF suggests that rates are similar to or higher than the general population. Self-reported data in pwCF demonstrate increased excessive alcohol use on average, as well as an increased risk of hospitalization with excessive alcohol use.[36] Another study looking at self-reported marijuana use revealed that 15% of respondents used marijuana in the past 12 months, with use ranging from edible products to vaping or smoking.[37] Similarly, general lung transplant data not limited to pwCF suggest chronic opioid use, defined as 3 consecutive months of use more than 1 year posttransplant, may be associated with reduced lung function and survival posttransplant.[38]

As the percentage of adults with CF (awCF) continues to expand, so should the consideration of substance misuse. Recent data demonstrate that the average age of pwCF being hospitalized is increasing, with more than 65% of hospitalizations occurring among awCF. When comparing hospitalization data from pwCF younger than 18 years to hospitalization data from awCF, the prevalence of substance misuse was 10 times higher in awCF,[39] which suggests there may be an increasing need for screening and treatment strategies for substance misuse in pwCF.

THERAPEUTIC OPTIONS
Risk Assessment

Assessing risk includes a pwCF's narrative about their own risk, a careful history and mental status examination, and information from other sources (eg, family, other providers working with the patient). Factors to consider include previous self-harm, whether such harm was attributed to suicidal or nonsuicidal motivations, suicide attempts, violence, alcohol or substance use, and/or recent stressors, and protective factors (eg, coping skills, connections to others, supports). Psychiatric consultation is recommended when there is a risk for self-harm or violence. If risk is imminent, crisis mental health services should be accessed (eg, psychiatric urgent care/emergency room, mobile crisis team, or a general emergency room when a community lacks crisis mental health services).

Referral is recommended for pwCF with complex presentations, such as bipolar disorder, psychosis, or mental health conditions refractory to first-line interventions. Decisions about the level of care and referral sources can be made with a mental health provider. Levels of psychiatric and substance use disorder treatment include the following:

- *Self-help*, such as the National Alliance on Mental Illness (NAMI) support groups, Alcoholics Anonymous (AA), or Narcotics Anonymous (NA);
- *Outpatient services*, such as individual/group/family psychotherapy or pharmacologic treatment;
- *Intensive outpatient care*, such as a day program or partial hospitalization;
- *Inpatient care*, such as acute psychiatric care, medically managed intensive inpatient or detoxification, or residential treatment facility; or
- *Crisis intervention*, such as safety assessment/planning or need for a psychiatric hold.

Psychological and Pharmacological Treatments

Brief supportive therapies and targeted evidence-based psychological therapies are first-line treatments recommended for pwCF experiencing mental health symptoms.[3,17,40,41] **Table 1** provides a summary of common psychological treatments and uses. Psychotropic medications are also appropriate for some mental health concerns. Summary tables for psychotropic medications are provided for guidance in using selective serotonin reuptake inhibitors (SSRIs) for depression and anxiety in pwCF (**Table 2**), selected SSRI alternatives for depression and anxiety in pwCF (**Table 3**), potential dose adjustments when using selected SSRIs and CF medications (**Table 4**), and medications for ADHD in pwCF (**Table 5**).

Commonly used treatments for depression and generalized anxiety disorder in people with cystic fibrosis

The International Mental Health Guidelines for CF recommend supportive interventions and psychoeducation for pwCF reporting mild symptoms of depression and/or generalized anxiety and a more thorough clinical assessment to determine what evidence-based psychological and/or pharmacologic interventions would be best suited for someone reporting moderate to severe symptoms.[17] Pilot studies among awCF have found promising results suggesting that cognitive behavioral therapy (CBT),[42,43] stress management,[44] and acceptance and commitment therapy[45] may be effective at reducing symptoms of depression and anxiety. Larger randomized controlled trials examining the effectiveness of these CF-specific therapies with adolescents and adults are currently underway.

Table 1
Common psychological treatments and uses

Type of Psychological Treatment	What is It?	Commonly Recommended for:
Acceptance and Commitment Therapy (ACT)	Mindfulness-based skills aimed at encouraging committed actions consistent with personal values, developing psychological flexibility, and learning to accept and experience the range of human emotions with a kind and open perspective.	Depression, anxiety, eating disorders, substance use, chronic pain, psychosis
Applied behavior analysis (ABA)	Teaches family, care providers, and educators how to use principles of reinforcement and managing antecedents and consequences to structure environments to promote learning and behavior change (increasing/decreasing frequency of behavior). ABA therapy is intensive and uses repetition and practice of skills to reach behavioral goals.	Language and communication, behavioral challenges, learning self-care skills, social skills, academics
Cognitive behavioral therapy (CBT)	Structured treatment aimed at helping identify and challenge unhelpful ways of thinking that may lead to problematic emotional responses and behavioral patterns. Techniques involve cognitive restructuring, role play, and relaxation strategies.	Depression, anxiety disorders, substance misuse, eating disorders, chronic pain, posttraumatic stress disorder (PTSD), adherence
Cognitive behavioral therapy for insomnia (CBTi)	Short-term multicomponent therapy aimed at improving sleep through (1) psychoeducation focused on homeostatic sleep drive, circadian rhythms, and sleep-interfering arousal patterns; (2) behavioral interventions, such as stimulus control, sleep restriction, and relaxation; and (3) cognitive interventions aimed at changing inaccurate or unhelpful thoughts about sleep.	Poor sleep, insomnia, depression

(continued on next page)

Table 1
(continued)

Type of Psychological Treatment	What is It?	Commonly Recommended for:
Dialectical behavioral therapy (DBT)	Skills-based training aimed at creating a life worth living by improving coping skills in the areas of emotion regulation, mindfulness, distress tolerance, and interpersonal effectiveness.	Borderline personality disorder, suicidality or nonsuicidal self-injury, nonsuicidal risk behaviors, eating disorders, chronic pain, substance use
Existential therapy	Evidence-based approaches aimed at reducing suffering and restoring hope, resilience, sense of purpose, and social engagement by addressing key existential conflicts—death, choice, isolation, and meaning—that disrupt identity formation and consolidation, including • Dignity therapy • Logotherapy • Meaning-centered psycho-therapy (MCP)	Depression, anxiety, trauma/PTSD, adjustment disorders, especially coping with changes in health and end-of-life
Exposure therapies	Systematic desensitization pairs progressively anxiety-inducing situations (imagined or in-vivo) with relaxation techniques. Exposure and response prevention (ERP) uses controlled exposure to feared a stimulus, experiencing the body's natural physiological response, and staying with that discomfort until it naturally subsides via parasympathetic nervous system activation. Achieving homeostasis in the face of a feared stimulus allows incorporation of corrective information into one's cognitive schema.	Procedural anxiety, phobias, OCD, social anxiety
Family systems therapy (FT)	Addresses psychological concerns resulting from problematic, collective interactions among individuals in a family system. Skills include improving emotion expression, validation, active listening, perspective-taking, assertiveness, and collaborative problem solving. Practice of skills in the home environment is encouraged.	Family functioning problems (communication, partnership), anxiety, mood, adjustment disorders, ADHD, behavioral concerns, trauma, chronic pain, disordered eating

(continued on next page)

Table 1
(continued)

Type of Psychological Treatment	What is It?	Commonly Recommended for:
Group therapy	Involves one or more therapists who typically meet with 5–15 individuals who are addressing a common struggle and likely have a shared experience. The group promotes a supportive social setting where skills can be practiced with others while receiving coaching and guidance from therapists. Given infection control considerations, there should not be more than one person with CF in a group unless the group is being delivered through telemedicine.	Social skills, anxiety, mood, trauma, substance misuse, interpersonal functioning, grief, adjustment disorders, parenting, coping with chronic illness or pain, healthy habits (nutrition, physical activity)
Interpersonal therapy (IPT)	Time-limited therapy informed by attachment and communication theory addressing psychological distress by targeting grief, loss, interpersonal disputes, and role transitions.	Depression (including perinatal), eating disorders
Motivational interviewing (MI)	Directive approach aimed at addressing ambivalence and resistance to change by enhancing motivation. Techniques include developing discrepancies between goals, values, and current behaviors, rolling with resistance, increasing confidence, supporting self-efficacy, and expressing empathy through reflective listening.	Substance use, risky behaviors, improving adherence, encouraging healthy behaviors
Parent management training (PMT)	Teaching caregivers to acquire and use skills to help a child engage in more positive prosocial behaviors and less oppositional, dysregulated, dangerous, and/or defiant behaviors. Skills include identifying "the ABCs" (antecedents, behaviors, and consequences) in the home environment to more effectively prompt response to behaviors through positive attending, removing attention for problem behaviors, and using safe and effective discipline.	Behavioral concerns associated with ADHD, ODD, and adjustment disorders

(continued on next page)

Table 1
(continued)

Type of Psychological Treatment	What is It?	Commonly Recommended for:
Psychodynamic therapy (PDT)	Addressing distress and persistent, maladaptive patterns of behavior, especially in the face of developmental adversity and attachment trauma, by changing understanding and experiences of self and others via accessing emotions, exploring meanings, and attending to in-session process. There are many evidence-based, manualized forms of PDT, which vary in structure and duration, including • Internet-based psychodynamic therapy (IPDT) • Mentalization-based treatment (MBT) • Time-limited dynamic therapy (TLDT) • Short-term psychoanalytic psychotherapy (STPP)	Personality disorders, depression, anxiety, trauma, eating disorders
Stress management and self-help	Focus on the mind-body connection, increasing relaxation, reworking unhelpful thoughts, expanding social support and communication, prioritizing self-care, adopting healthy nutrition and movement habits, improving coping and problem solving, and setting effective goals.	Stress, subclinical psychological symptoms, adjustment disorders, role/life changes, depression, anxiety disorders, adherence
Supportive therapy	Prevention and early treatment of mood-related symptoms by increasing resiliency through active coping strategies such as problem solving, seeking and accepting social support, realistic goal setting, outlook modification, and self-care.	Stress, subclinical psychological symptoms, adjustment disorders, role/life changes

(continued on next page)

Table 1 (continued)		
Type of Psychological Treatment	**What is It?**	**Commonly Recommended for:**
Trauma therapies	Common therapies include cognitive processing therapy (CPT), which focuses on challenging and modifying beliefs related to the trauma to reduce its negative effects on one's present experience, and eye movement desensitization and reprocessing (EMDR), which uses bilateral eye movements alongside reviewing thoughts, emotions, and bodily sensations associated with the trauma in a controlled environment to encourage adaptive resolution.	PTSD, anxiety, medical- and nonmedical-related trauma

Table 2
Selective serotonin reuptake inhibitors for depression and anxiety in children, adolescents, and adults with cystic fibrosis

Medication	Starting Dose	Titration	Target Dose	General Comments	CYP Metabolism of SSRI and Interactions
General guidance	Start low Low starting dose suggested for PwCF Hepatic impairment? Keep dose lower	Go slow Titrate up every 1–4 wk if partial or no response Side effects? Maintain dose longer or reduce dose	Treat-to-target dose When PHQ-9, GAD-7, and functioning return to normal, continue target dose for 1 y, then consider taper off SSRI	For recurrent symptoms off an SSRI: consider longer term treatment	Examples in CF: Risk of serotonin syndrome with linezolid and SSRIs; use with clinical monitoring only if no safer alternatives
Citalopram (Celexa)	5–10 mg/d	By 5–10 mg	< 12 y: 10–40 mg/d ≥ 12 y: 20–40 mg/d	QTc prolongation	CYP450 Major substrates: 2C19 and 3A4
Escitalopram (Lexapro)	2.5–5 mg/d	By 2.5–5 mg	< 12 y: 5–20 mg/d ≥ 12 y: 10–20 mg/d	S-isomer of citalopram	CYP450 Major substrates: 2C19 and 3A4
Fluoxetine (Prozac)	5–10 mg/d	By 5–10 mg	< 12 y: 10–60 mg/d ≥ 12 y: 20–80 mg/d	Long half-life prevents withdrawal symptoms if a dose is missed	CYP450 minor substrates: 3A4, 2C9, 2C19, 2D6
Sertraline (Zoloft)	12.5–25 mg/d	By 12.5–25 mg	< 12 y: 25–200 mg/d ≥ 12 y: 50–200 mg/d	Sedating	CYP450 minor substrates: 3A4, 2C9, 2C19, 2D6

Abbreviation: CYP450, cytochrome P-450 enzyme.

Table 3
Selected selective serotonin reuptake inhibitor alternatives for depression and anxiety in children, adolescents, and adults with cystic fibrosis[a]

Category/Generic Name	Typically Used for:	When to Consider	Comments
Serotonin- Norepinephrine Reuptake Inhibitors (SNRIs)			
Duloxetine Milnacipran Venlafaxine ER	Anxiety, depression	Ongoing use: • Comorbid pain (especially duloxetine) • Switch for inadequate response to SSRI • Duloxetine is approved in children	Start low and titrate slowly (with particular caution in children) to minimize initiation and discontinuation syndromes—headache, dizziness, GI distress, jitteriness, or fatigue Side effects similar to SSRIs: monitor for sexual side effects, serotonin toxicity, mania, and suicidality Venlafaxine may elevate blood pressure
Noradrenergic and Specific Serotonergic Antidepressant (NaSSA)			
Mirtazapine	Anxiety (off-label), depression	Intermittent/short-term or ongoing use: • Insomnia • Low appetite Ongoing use: • Switch or augmentation for inadequate response or intolerability of SSRI/SNRI/NDRI	Take at night Monitor for daytime sedation, unwelcome weight gain, mania, and suicidality Few drug-drug interactions No monoamine reuptake inhibition Fewer GI side effects than SSRIs/SNRIs; may improve nausea/vomiting by blocking 5HT3 receptors Sexual side effects less common
Norepinephrine and Dopamine Reuptake Inhibitors (NDRI)			
Bupropion SR or XL	Depression	Ongoing use: • Fatigue • Poor concentration • Switch or augmentation for inadequate response to or intolerability of SSRI/SNRI/NaSSA	Monitor for low appetite, constipation, insomnia, vivid dreams, hypertension, mania, suicidality Sexual side effects uncommon
Methylphenidate	Depression (off-label)	Intermittent/short-term or ongoing use: • Fatigue • Poor concentration • Need for rapid response Ongoing use: • Comorbid ADHD	Controlled substance, caution with history of substance misuse Monitor for low appetite, insomnia, irritability, anxiety, psychosis

(continued on next page)

Table 3
(continued)

Category/Generic Name	Typically Used for:	When to Consider	Comments
		• Augmentation for partial response to SSRI/SNRI/NaSSA	
Serotonin Antagonist and Reuptake Inhibitor (SARI)			
Trazodone	Anxiety (off-label), depression	Intermittent/short-term use (low dose/off-label): • Insomnia • Agitation	Rarely used at full dose for depression due to sedation Monitor for priapism, orthostasis
Serotonin Receptor Partial Agonist			
Buspirone	Anxiety, depression (off-label)	Ongoing use: • Switch or augmentation for anxiety or depression refractory to SSRI/SNRI/NaSSA	Side effects similar to SSRIs: monitor for serotonin toxicity, mania, and suicidality Sexual side effects less common
Tricyclic Antidepressants			
Amitriptyline Nortriptyline	Depression, anxiety	Intermittent/short-term use (low dose, off-label): • Insomnia Ongoing use: • Comorbid pain Switch for inadequate response to SSRI/SNRI/NDRI	Use limited by cardiac toxicity in overdose (QRS widening, ventricular tachycardia) Monitor for anticholinergic side effects, sedation, weight gain, serotonin toxicity, mania, suicidality Monitor blood levels and EKG
Benzodiazepines			
Lorazepam Clonazepam	Anxiety	Intermittent/shortterm use: • Procedural anxiety • Panic attack • Insomnia • To augment SSRI/SNRI/NDRI during early titration phase Ongoing use: • Contraindication or intolerance of SSRI/SNRI (eg, history of serotonin syndrome or mania) • Switch or augmentation for anxiety refractory to SSRI/SNRI/NaSSA	Controlled substance; caution with history of substance misuse Physical dependence; requires down titration to safely discontinue with chronic use due to seizure risk Use with alcohol, opiates, or other CNS depressants may increase risk of respiratory depression Monitor for sedation, cognitive side effects, tachyphylaxis, delirium Caution with peri-transplant use

(continued on next page)

Table 3
(continued)

Category/Generic Name	Typically Used for:	When to Consider	Comments
Gabapentinoids			
Gabapentin Pregabalin	Anxiety (off-label)	Intermittent/short-term use (gabapentin): • Panic attack • Insomnia Ongoing use: • Comorbid pain, especially neuropathic • Contraindication or intolerance of SSRI/SNRI (eg, history of serotonin syndrome or mania) • Augmentation for partial response to SSRI/SNRI	Not controlled substances, but monitor for misuse Use with alcohol, opiates, or other CNS depressants may increase risk of respiratory depression Monitor for sedation

Abbreviations: CNS, central nervous sytem; EKG, electrocardiogram; GI, gastrointestinal.

[a] Duloxetine is approved in children ≥7 years with generalized anxiety disorder; lorazepam is approved in children ≥12 years for anxiety; other medications listed are off-label to treat pediatric depression/anxiety.

Table 4
Potential dose adjustments when using selected selective serotonin reuptake inhibitors and cystic fibrosis medications

	Inhibitors	Inducers	Substrates
	Decreases CYP450 enzyme activity; may need to reduce SSRI dose	Increases CYP450 enzyme activity; may need to increase SSRI dose	Metabolized by the CYP450 enzyme
CYP3A4	Clarithromycin, erythromycin, fluconazole, itraconazole, ivacaftor (weak), ketoconazole, posaconazole, tezacaftor (weak), voriconazole	Lumacaftor, rifabutin, rifampin	*Citalopram* (major), *escitalopram* (major), *fluoxetine* (minor), *sertraline* (minor), elexacaftor, ivacaftor, lumacaftor, tezacaftor
CYP2C9	*Fluoxetine* (weak to moderate), *sertraline* (weak to moderate), fluconazole, miconazole, tezacaftor (weak), voriconazole	Lumacaftor, rifabutin, rifampin	*Fluoxetine* (minor), *sertraline* (minor), ibuprofen (minor)
CYP2C19	*Fluoxetine* (moderate), *sertraline* (weak to moderate), cimetidine, fluconazole, proton pump inhibitors (eg, esomeprazole, omeprazole), tezacaftor (weak), voriconazole	Lumacaftor, rifampin	*Citalopram* (major), *escitalopram* (major), *fluoxetine* (minor), ibuprofen (minor), *sertraline* (minor)
CYP2D6	*Fluoxetine* (strong), *escitalopram* (weak), *citalopram* (weak), *sertraline* (weak), cimetidine, methadone, metoclopramide, tezacaftor (weak)	—	*fluoxetine* (minor), *sertraline* (minor)

Note: SSRI medications are given in italics.

Table 5
Medications for attention-deficit hyperactivity disorder in children, adolescents, and adults with cystic fibrosis

Category/Generic Name	US Trade Names	Typical Dose	Comments
Stimulants			
Methylphenidate derivatives	Adhansia XR, Aptensio XR, Concerta, Cotempla XR-ODT, Daytrana, Focalin, Focalin XR, Jornay PM, Metadate CD/ER, Methylin, QuilliChew ER, Quillivant XR, Ritalin, Ritalin LA	*Methylphenidate:* 0.3–2 mg/kg/d *Dexmethylphenidate:* 0.15–1 mg/kg/d	Avoid OROS-methylphenidate (Concerta) capsules in pancreatic insufficiency due to risk of bowel obstruction Appetite suppression; monitor growth Insomnia Monitor pulse and blood pressure
Amphetamine derivatives	Adderall, Adderall XR, Adzenys XR-ODT, Dexedrine, Dexedrine Spansules XR, Dyanavel XR, Evekeo, Mydayis, ProCentra, Vyvanse, Zenzedi	*Mixed amphetamine salts or dextroamphetamine:* 0.15–1 mg/kg/d *Other:* See product labeling	Antacids/proton pump inhibitors can increase levels Appetite suppression; monitor growth Insomnia Monitor pulse and blood pressure
Nonstimulants: Alpha-2 Agonists			
Guanfacine ER	Intuniv	Start: 1 mg qam or qpm (0.05 mg qd or bid for immediate release) Target: 1–4 mg/d (0.05–0.12 mg/kg/d)	Do not administer with high-fat meals due to increased exposure Major CYP3A4 substrate; administration with strong inhibitors or inducers requires dose adjustment Significant renal or hepatic impairment may require dose reduction Less likely to cause appetite suppression Initial trial of immediate release (off-label) required by some insurance formularies; more likely to cause sedation, dizziness, and hypotension Monitor pulse and blood pressure

Clonidine ER	Kapvay	Start: 0.1 mg qhs Target: 0.1–0.4 mg/d (divided bid)	Renal impairment may require dose reduction Less likely to cause appetite suppression Initial trial of immediate release (off-label) required by some insurance formularies; more likely to cause sedation, dizziness, and hypotension Transdermal clonidine also available Monitor pulse and blood pressure

Nonstimulants: Selective Norepinephrine Reuptake Inhibitors (SNRIs)

Atomoxetine	Strattera	Start: • Up to 70 kg: ≤0.5 mg/kg once daily • ≥70 kg or adult: 40 mg/d Target: • Up to 70 kg: 1.2–1.4 mg/kg/d • ≥70 kg or adult: 80–100 mg/d	Use with CYP2D6 inhibitors (eg, fluoxetine) or by those with 2D6 slow metabolism requires dose reduction Hepatic impairment requires dose reduction Less likely to cause appetite suppression Titrate gradually to minimize GI distress and sedation Monitor pulse, blood pressure, and mood Discontinue if liver function tests increase
Viloxazine	Qelbree	Start: • 6–11 y: 100 mg/d • 12–17 y: 200 mg/d Target: may titrate to maximum of 400 mg/d	Strong CYP1A2 inhibitor (eg, avoid with tizanidine, duloxetine) Weak CYP2D6 and CYP3A4 inhibitor Severe renal impairment requires dose reduction Less likely to cause appetite suppression Titrate gradually to minimize GI distress and sedation Monitor pulse, blood pressure, and mood Can sprinkle on applesauce

Note: Selection may be based on factors including personal and family history of response, drug-drug interactions, and side-effect profile.
Data from Georgiopoulos AM, Christon LM, Filigno SS, et al. Promoting emotional wellness in children with CF, part II: Mental health assessment and intervention. Pediatric pulmonology. 2021;56 Suppl 1:S107-s122.

Although there has been less research on treating symptoms of depression and anxiety in younger children with CF, evidence more broadly focused on children with long-term physical conditions suggests that children may benefit from adaptations of these interventions.[21,46]

Antidepressants are not typically prescribed to pwCF reporting mild depression or anxiety unless they are experiencing significant functional impairment or distress. For those reporting moderate to severe depression or anxiety, antidepressants should typically be prescribed in combination with evidence-based psychological interventions but may be considered on their own when therapy is not feasible or fully effective.[17] The CF Mental Health Guidelines recommend the SSRIs citalopram, escitalopram, sertraline, and fluoxetine as appropriate first-line antidepressants for most pwCF aged 12 years or older reporting anxiety and depression that require pharmacotherapy.[17] However, SSRIs may also be appropriate for pre-adolescents when psychological approaches are not feasible or fully effective.[21,47] **Table 2** provides guidance on CF-specific SSRI management strategies,[17] and **Table 3** provides a summary of SSRI alternatives commonly used to treat depression and anxiety.[48] The potential for drug-drug interactions should also be assessed when prescribing other SSRIs (fluvoxamine, paroxetine) or newer medications with SSRI plus additional serotonin modulating activity (vilazodone, vortioxetine); **Table 4** presents potential dose adjustments when using selected SSRIs and CF medications.[49] Of note, the dose of citalopram, escitalopram, and sertraline may require an increase when used with a CFTR modulator containing lumacaftor.[8] In addition, the strong CYP3A4 inducers, such as St. John's Wort, a supplement commonly used to treat depression, and carbamazepine, an anticonvulsant also used for mood stabilization, are expected to substantially reduce exposure to ETI and should not be used with this CFTR modulator.[50]

For complex conditions, such as treatment-resistant depression, bipolar disorder, or schizophrenia, mood stabilizers or antipsychotics are often required and should be prescribed in collaboration with a psychiatric provider.

Commonly used treatments for other anxiety-related conditions that affect people with cystic fibrosis

Social anxiety, OCD, procedural anxiety, and trauma all tend to elicit significant distress and commonly emerge in childhood. Adverse childhood experiences are likely to contribute to worse outcomes in pwCF,[51] with a dose-dependent relationship seen between the number of maltreatments in childhood and poorer social and health outcomes as an adult.[52] The aforementioned concerns are typically addressed using prevention and preparedness techniques or more structured interventions, such as trauma-focused CBT, eye movement desensitization and reprocessing, and play-based interventions for younger children.[21]

For those fearing specific situations or procedures, having a detailed conversation using age-appropriate, supportive language about what to expect before, during, and after can go a long way. Graded exposure, systematic desensitization, and exposure and response prevention are techniques used to help promote relaxation responses through parasympathetic nervous system activation, building habituation to anxiety-provoking stimuli, and increasing self-efficacy. Other useful techniques include anesthetizing a procedure site, comfort positioning by a caregiver,[53] active distraction (eg, favorite toy, watching videos, vibrational tool such as the "Buzzy Bee"), referencing and reinforcing positive coping and cooperation, considering postprocedure incentives, and creating a procedural care plan outlining the pwCF's preferences of what they need from medical staff to maximize cooperation and their ability to cope.[21] The CF Mental Health Guidelines recommend short-term use of lorazepam for distressing procedural anxiety that has not adequately responded to behavioral interventions.[17]

Commonly used treatments for other behavioral disorders that may emerge in childhood among people with cystic fibrosis

Behavioral disorders that present in childhood among youth with CF, including ADHD, ASD, and ODD, warrant proactive assessment and intervention.[14] The behavioral aspects of these disorders can contribute to difficulty in daily functioning (mood, anxiety, and behavior) and nighttime sleep. They might also interfere specifically in parent-child interactions around CF daily care.

The first-line treatment of ADHD is often psychopharmacology based on presenting concerns in conjunction with behaviorally based parent management training (PMT) techniques. PMT helps parents increase their use of effective parenting skills to encourage more prosocial behaviors in their children.[54] PwCF with ADHD may be treated with stimulant or nonstimulant monotherapy or combination strategies (see **Table 5**). For those taking stimulant medications such as methylphenidate or amphetamine derivatives, it remains to be determined how HEMT may affect the salience of appetite suppression and weight loss, particularly for children with CF. The side effect of low appetite can be managed with a variety of strategies including increasing calorie density, medication "holidays" to allow for compensatory intake (eg, use only on school or work days), dose reduction, or alternative ADHD medication trials. When feasible, these methods should be considered before the addition of appetite stimulants (eg, cyproheptadine).[21]

Applied behavior analysis[55] services are recommended for children with ASD to help home and school environments support learning adaptive behavior, including activities of daily living, following instructions, social skills, and self-regulation. Establishing compliance and instructional control early can be especially important, given the importance of the parent-child relationship in effectively managing CF, as well as the child compliance needed during the multiple additional health care tasks required each day. Finally, PMT is considered a first-line treatment of ODD to help a child engage in more positive prosocial behaviors and less oppositional, dysregulated, dangerous, and/or defiant behaviors through the improvement of effective parenting skills.[54] PMT can be delivered through family therapy and/or group therapy formats.[54]

Commonly used treatments for insomnia in people with cystic fibrosis

The recommended first-line intervention for insomnia is cognitive behavioral therapy for insomnia (CBT-I). CBT-I has similar outcomes compared with pharmacotherapy and is effective via telehealth, which may help alleviate patient and care center burden related to travel, clinic space, and infection control considerations.[56,57] In the general population, CBT-I has been shown to improve anxiety and depression symptoms that exist with comorbid insomnia and could be an additional consideration for pwCF who have increased mental health symptoms.[58]

Little data exist for pharmacologic management of insomnia in pwCF. Some medications used to treat insomnia such as benzodiazepines and non-benzodiazepine hypnotics have been associated with respiratory side effects and should be used with caution.[59] When insomnia presents as a manifestation of a mental health condition such as depression or anxiety, pharmacotherapy should generally be directed at treating the underlying disorder.

Commonly used treatments to address problematic eating patterns in people with cystic fibrosis

Early detection and intervention of problematic eating behaviors have been shown to reduce the frequency of disordered eating and delay artificial supplementation needs in pwCF.[32] Disordered eating can be compounded by mental health disorders, lung disease, parent or caregiver mental health disorders, food security, and degree of nutrition burden. Young children may benefit from nutritional planning and education, and behavioral therapy to target disordered eating. Adolescents and adults who struggle with eating disorders may benefit from nutritional interventions with family-based treatment or CBT.[60] Psychological treatments for pwCF with pancreatic enzyme or insulin misuse have not been studied. Adjunctive pharmacotherapy for people with eating disorders most often targets comorbid conditions (eg, depression, GAD, OCD, ADHD). Evidence supports using SSRIs, stimulants, or topiramate to reduce episodes of binge eating,[60] but the possibility of weight loss related to stimulants and topiramate must be considered in the risk-benefit analysis for pwCF. Conversely, medications with appetite-stimulating properties are sometimes used to help restore weight.

Commonly used treatments to address substance misuse in people with cystic fibrosis

Treatments for substance misuse in pwCF are not well studied. Psychological therapies helpful for treatment and relapse prevention include CBT, contingency management, motivational interviewing/enhancement, 12-step groups, family therapy, and combinations of these interventions.[61] Substance withdrawal syndromes are uncomfortable and, especially in the case of alcohol, benzodiazepine, and opiate dependence, place individuals at medical risk, requiring timely identification and medical treatment. Medication-assisted treatments (MAT) are often underutilized and are substance specific. For example, nicotine misuse can be treated with bupropion, varenicline, and nicotine replacement and alcohol misuse with disulfiram, acamprosate, or naltrexone. MAT for opiate misuse (buprenorphine/naloxone, methadone, naltrexone) decreases mortality, and naloxone should be kept on hand to reverse overdose.[62]

DISCUSSION

Mental health concerns among pwCF are common. These concerns may emerge in childhood or adolescence and can persist into adulthood. Untreated and inadequately treated mental health symptoms may result in negative health outcomes[1,2]; therefore, it is crucial to engage pwCF proactively and responsively when it comes to emotional wellness. Therapeutic advances, such as HEMT, antibiotics, and mucolytics, have increased lifespan expectancy among pwCF,[4] which may also result in both positive and negative psychosocial stressors. Although most CF centers are following the international consensus guidelines to screen pwCF annually for symptoms of depression and GAD, there are other mental health concerns that are not captured by these measures. It is important to consider other conditions such as procedural anxiety, personality disorders, trauma, ADHD, sleep disorders, neurodevelopmental disorders, and substance misuse when evaluating patients. Collaborating with a psychosocial provider (eg, social worker, psychologist, psychiatrist, psychiatric nurse practitioner, palliative and holistic health care workers, child life specialists) can provide more in-depth evaluation of these concerns, as well as determine what type of therapeutic intervention might work best.

When discussing potential options, it is important to consider a pwCF's preferences and ability to engage in treatment. Psychological interventions might be preferred over medication by some pwCF to minimize the risk of side effects and drug-drug interactions, but barriers including time, expenses, and availability of psychotherapists trained in evidence-based interventions must also be considered. Because therapy tends to focus on underlying causes and perpetuating factors associated with mental health concerns, learning new ways to cope and building up self-efficacy with such coping strategies can make the effects of therapy persist long after therapy has ended. On the other hand, medications tend only to work as long as they are being taken. In some cases, such as severe depression, bipolar disorder, psychosis, or ADHD, medications are often the first line of treatment, ideally in conjunction with psychological intervention. In addition, pharmacotherapy is often added to augment treatment when psychological interventions are not fully effective. Setting appropriate expectations for desired results is recommended, such as reminding individuals that it may take time to start seeing changes in their mood on initiating treatment and that consistent engagement/use is critical for success. Our goal as providers is to improve and prolong the health of pwCF. Physical and mental health are inextricably linked, and when we become more comfortable discussing and normalizing mental health concerns, it opens the door for more candid conversations about treatment planning and finding the best strategy to improve the health and quality of life of pwCF.

CLINICS CARE POINTS

- Mental health concerns are common among pwCF and should be addressed during routine CF clinic visits to support the promotion of improved overall health and wellness.
- Psychotherapeutic interventions are first-line treatments for many mental health conditions because they address underlying causes and perpetuating factors, learning new ways to cope, and building self-efficacy, all of which can persist after therapy has ended.
- CF Mental Health Guidelines recommend the SSRIs citalopram, escitalopram, sertraline, and fluoxetine as appropriate first-line antidepressants for most pwCF aged 12 years or older who require pharmacotherapy.
- SSRIs may also be appropriate for preadolescents when psychological approaches are not feasible or fully effective.
- Certain mental health conditions, as well as mental health concerns refractory to first-line treatment, should be treated in conjunction with a psychiatric provider.

DISCLOSURE

C.J. Bathgate, S.S. Filigno, M. Hjelm, and B.A. Smith receive funding from the Cystic Fibrosis Foundation. A.M. Georgiopoulos reports grant funding and personal fees from Vertex Pharmaceuticals, United States and the Cystic Fibrosis Foundation; grant funding from the Dutch Cystic Fibrosis Foundation, the Netherlands; and personal fees from Cystic Fibrosis Australia, Johns Hopkins University/DKBmed, and Saudi Pediatric Pulmonology Association.

REFERENCES

1. Quittner AL, Goldbeck L, Abbott J, et al. Prevalence of depression and anxiety in patients with cystic fibrosis and parent caregivers: results of the International Depression Epidemiological Study across nine countries. Thorax 2014;69(12):1090–7.

2. Schechter MS, Ostrenga JS, Fink AK, et al. Decreased survival in cystic fibrosis patients with a positive screen for depression. J Cyst Fibros 2021; 20(1):120–6.

3. Smith BA, Georgiopoulos AM, Quittner AL. Maintaining mental health and function for the long run in cystic fibrosis. Pediatr Pulmonol 2016;51(S44): S71–8.

4. Cystic Fibrosis Foundation Patient Registry 2020 Annual Data Report Bethesda, Maryland ©2021, Cystic Fibrosis Foundation.

5. Muther EF, Polineni D, Sawicki GS. Overcoming psychosocial challenges in cystic fibrosis: promoting resilience. Pediatr Pulmonol 2018;53(S3):S86–92.

6. Dagenais RVE, Su VCH, Quon BS. Real-world safety of CFTR modulators in the treatment of cystic fibrosis: a systematic review. J Clin Med 2021;10(1):23.

7. McKinzie CJ, Goralski JL, Noah TL, et al. Worsening anxiety and depression after initiation of lumacaftor/ivacaftor combination therapy in adolescent females with cystic fibrosis. J Cyst Fibros 2017;16(4):525–7.

8. Talwalkar JS, Koff JL, Lee HB, et al. Cystic fibrosis transmembrane regulator modulators: implications for the management of depression and anxiety in cystic fibrosis. Psychosomatics 2017;58(4):343–54.

9. Tindell W, Su A, Oros SM, et al. Trikafta and psychopathology in cystic fibrosis: a case report. Psychosomatics 2020;61(6):735–8.

10. Bathgate CJ, Barboa C. Mental health and neurocognitive side effects after initiating elexacaftor/tezacaftor/ivacaftor. J Cyst Fibros 2021;20S2:S130.

11. Heo S, Young DC, Safirstein J, et al. Mental status changes during elexacaftor/tezacaftor/ivacaftor therapy. J Cyst Fibros 2021;21(2):339–43.

12. Martin C, Burnet E, Ronayette-Preira A, et al. Patient perspectives following initiation of elexacaftor-tezacaftor-ivacaftor in people with cystic fibrosis and advanced lung disease. Respir Med Res 2021;80:100829.

13. Prieur MG, Christon LM, Mueller A, et al. Promoting emotional wellness in children with cystic fibrosis, Part I: child and family resilience. Pediatr Pulmonol 2021;56(Suppl 1):S97–106.

14. American Psychiatric Association. Diagnostic and statistical manual of mental disorders. 5th edition. Washington, DC: Author; 2013.

15. Kroenke K, Spitzer RL, Williams JB. The PHQ-9: validity of a brief depression severity measure. J Gen Intern Med 2001;16(9):606–13.

16. Spitzer RL, Kroenke K, Williams JB, et al. A brief measure for assessing generalized anxiety disorder: the GAD-7. Arch Intern Med 2006;166(10):1092–7.

17. Quittner AL, Abbott J, Georgiopoulos AM, et al. International Committee on mental health in cystic fibrosis: cystic fibrosis Foundation and European cystic fibrosis Society consensus statements for screening and treating depression and anxiety. Thorax 2015;71(1):26–34.

18. Quittner AL, Abbott J, Hussain S, et al. Integration of mental health screening and treatment into cystic fibrosis clinics: evaluation of initial implementation in 84 programs across the United States. Pediatr Pulmonol 2020;55(11):2995–3004.

19. Abbott J, Havermans T, Jarvholm S, et al. Mental Health screening in cystic fibrosis centres across Europe. J Cyst Fibros 2019;18(2):299–303.

20. Smith BA, Georgiopoulos AM, Mueller A, et al. Impact of COVID-19 on mental health: effects on screening, care delivery, and people with cystic fibrosis. J Cyst Fibros 2021;20(Suppl 3):31–8.

21. Georgiopoulos AM, Christon LM, Filigno SS, et al. Promoting emotional wellness in children with CF, part II: mental health assessment and intervention. Pediatr Pulmonol 2021;56(Suppl 1):S107–22.

22. Sheldrick RC, Henson BS, Merchant S, et al. The Preschool Pediatric Symptom Checklist (PPSC): development and initial validation of a new social/emotional screening instrument. Acad Pediatr 2012;12(5):456–67.

23. Jellinek MS, Murphy JM, Robinson J, et al. Pediatric Symptom Checklist: screening school-age children for psychosocial dysfunction. J Pediatr 1988;112(2):201–9.

24. Murphy JM, Bergmann P, Chiang C, et al. The PSC-17: Subscale Scores, reliability, and factor structure in a new national sample. Pediatrics 2016;138(3):e20160038.

25. Ayers S, Muller I, Mahoney L, et al. Understanding needle-related distress in children with cystic fibrosis. Br J Health Psychol 2011;16(Pt 2):329–43.

26. Cherkasova MV, Roy A, Molina BSG, et al. Review: adult outcome as seen through controlled prospective Follow-up studies of children with attention-deficit/hyperactivity disorder followed into adulthood. J Am Acad Child Adolesc Psychiatry 2021;61(3):378–91.

27. Freeman D, Sheaves B, Waite F, et al. Sleep disturbance and psychiatric disorders. Lancet Psychiatry 2020;7(7):628–37.

28. American Academy of Sleep Medicine. International classification of sleep disorders. 3rd edition. Darien, IL: Author; 2014.

29. Shakkottai A, O'Brien LM, Nasr SZ, et al. Sleep disturbances and their impact in pediatric cystic fibrosis. Sleep Med Rev 2018;42:100–10.

30. Perin C, Fagondes SC, Casarotto FC, et al. Sleep findings and predictors of sleep desaturation in adult cystic fibrosis patients. Sleep Breath 2012;16(4):1041–8.

31. Godart NT, Perdereau F, Rein Z, et al. Comorbidity studies of eating disorders and mood disorders. Critical review of the literature. J affective Disord 2007;97(1–3):37–49.

32. Quick V, Byrd-Bredbenner C. Disordered eating and body image in cystic fibrosis. Diet and exercise in cystic fibrosis. San Diego (CA): Academic Press; 2015. p. 11–8.

33. Winston AP. Eating disorders and diabetes. Curr Diabetes Rep 2020;20(8):32.

34. Mégarbane B, Chevillard L. The large spectrum of pulmonary complications following illicit drug use: features and mechanisms. Chem Biol Interact 2013;206(3):444–51.

35. Grant BF, Stinson FS, Dawson DA, et al. Prevalence and co-occurrence of substance use disorders and

independent mood and anxiety disorders: results from the National Epidemiologic Survey on Alcohol and Related Conditions. Arch Gen Psychiatry 2004;61(8):807–16.

36. Lowery EM, Afshar M, West N, et al. Self-reported alcohol use in the cystic fibrosis community. J Cyst Fibros 2020;19(1):84–90.

37. Stephen MJ, Chowdhury J, Tejada LA, et al. Use of medical marijuana in cystic fibrosis patients. BMC Complement Med therapies 2020;20(1):323.

38. Drees D, Tumin D, Miller R, et al. Chronic opioid use and clinical outcomes in lung transplant recipients: a single-center cohort study. Clin Respir J 2018;12(9).2446–53.

39. Ramsey ML, Lara LF, Gariepy CE, et al. National trends of hospitalizations in cystic fibrosis highlight a need for pediatric to adult transition clinics. Pancreas 2021;50(5):704–9.

40. Castellani C, Duff AJA, Bell SC, et al. ECFS best practice guidelines: the 2018 revision. J Cyst Fibros 2018;17(2):153–78.

41. Bell SC, Robinson PJ. Cystic fibrosis standards of care, Australia. Sydney, NSW: North Ryde; 2008.

42. Friedman D, Quittner AL, Smith B, et al. Preventing depression and anxiety: results of a pilot study of a CF-specific CBT intervention for adults with CF. Pediatr Pulmonol 2019;54(S2):397.

43. Graziano S, Boldrini F, Righelli D, et al. Psychological interventions during COVID pandemic: telehealth for individuals with cystic fibrosis and caregivers. Pediatr Pulmonol 2021;56(7):1976–84.

44. Bathgate CJ, Kilbourn KM, Murphy NH, et al. Pilot RCT of a telehealth intervention to reduce symptoms of depression and anxiety in adults with cystic fibrosis. J Cyst Fibros 2022;21(2):332–8.

45. O'Hayer CV, O'Loughlin CM, Nurse CN, et al. ACT with CF: a telehealth and in-person feasibility study to address anxiety and depressive symptoms among people with cystic fibrosis. J Cyst Fibros 2021;20(1):133–9.

46. Thabrew H, Stasiak K, Hetrick SE, et al. Psychological therapies for anxiety and depression in children and adolescents with long-term physical conditions. Cochrane Database Syst Rev 2018;12(12):Cd012488.

47. Jane Garland E, Kutcher S, Virani A, et al. Update on the use of SSRIs and SNRIs with children and adolescents in clinical practice. J Can Acad Child Adolesc Psychiatry 2016;25(1):4–10.

48. Georgiopoulos A, Friedman D, Sher Y. Best practice guide: Management of depression and anxiety Improving Life with CF: A Primary Palliative Care Partnership 2021. Available at: improvinglifewithCF.org. Accessed October 28, 2021.

49. Jordan CL, Noah TL, Henry MM. Therapeutic challenges posed by critical drug-drug interactions in cystic fibrosis. Pediatr Pulmonol 2016;51(S44):S61–70.

50. Vertex Pharmaceuticals. Trikafta prescribing information. 2019. https://pi.vrtx.com/files/uspi_elexacaftor_tezacaftor_ivacaftor.pdf. Accessed February 6, 2022.

51. McGarry ME, Williams WA 2nd, McColley SA. The demographics of adverse outcomes in cystic fibrosis. Pediatr Pulmonol 2019;54 Suppl 3(Suppl 3):S74–83.

52. Felitti VJ, Anda RF, Nordenberg D, et al. Relationship of childhood abuse and household dysfunction to many of the leading causes of death in adults. The Adverse Childhood Experiences (ACE) Study. Am J Prev Med 1998;14(4):245–58.

53. Eull D, Postier A, Hermes D, et al. Children's Comfort Promise; successfully implementing an evidence based pain protocol for needle procedures throughout a large children's hospital and clinic system. J Pain 2016;17(4):S43.

54. Kazdin AE. Parent management training and problem-solving skills training for child and adolescent conduct problems. In: Weisz JR, Kazdin AE, editors. Evidence-based psychotherapies for children and adolescents. 3rd edition. New York: Guilford Press; 2017. p. 142–58.

55. National Center on Birth Defects and Developmental Disabilities. Treatment and intervention services for autism Spectrum disorder 2019. Available at: https://www.cdc.gov/ncbddd/autism/treatment.html. Accessed October 28, 2021.

56. Okajima I, Komada Y, Inoue Y. A meta-analysis on the treatment effectiveness of cognitive behavioral therapy for primary insomnia. Sleep Biol Rhythms 2011;9:24–34.

57. Gehrman P, Gunter P, Findley J, et al. Randomized noninferiority trial of telehealth delivery of cognitive behavioral treatment of insomnia compared to in-person care. J Clin Psychiatry 2021;82(5):20m13723.

58. Taylor DJ, Pruiksma KE. Cognitive and behavioural therapy for insomnia (CBT-I) in psychiatric populations: a systematic review. Int Rev Psychiatry (Abingdon, England) 2014;26(2):205–13.

59. Chung WS, Lai CY, Lin CL, et al. Adverse respiratory events associated with hypnotics use in patients of chronic obstructive pulmonary disease: a population-based case-control study. Medicine 2015;94(27):e1110.

60. Klein DA, Sylvester JE, Schvey NA. Eating disorders in primary care: diagnosis and management. Am Fam Physician 2021;103(1):22–32.

61. Drake RE, O'Neal EL, Wallach MA. A systematic review of psychosocial research on psychosocial interventions for people with co-occurring severe mental and substance use disorders. J Subst Abuse Treat 2008;34(1):123–38.

62. National Institute on Drug Abuse. Effective treatments for opioid addiction. 2016. Available at: https://www.drugabuse.gov/publications/effective-treatments-opioid-addiction. Accessed October 28, 2021.

Family Planning and Reproductive Health in Cystic Fibrosis

Lauren N. Meiss, MD, MS[a], Raksha Jain, MD, MSCI[b],
Traci M. Kazmerski, MD, MS[c,d],*

KEYWORDS

- Cystic fibrosis • Family planning • Contraception • Fertility • Pregnancy

KEY POINTS

- Cystic fibrosis (CF) care teams should routinely partner with people with CF in reproductive goals conversations.
- It is imperative to assess for sexual functioning concerns in all people with CF.
- Pregnancy planning in CF is recommended as health status at the time of conception can serve as an important prognostic indicator of obstetric and neonatal outcomes.
- Most of the men and some women with CF will need to consider assisted reproductive technology (ART) as an option due to fertility concerns.
- With advances in care, rates of pregnancy and parenthood among people with CF are increasing.

INTRODUCTION

Family planning is defined broadly by the World Health Organization (WHO) as the process that "allows people to attain their desired number of children, if any, and to determine the spacing of their pregnancies…[as] achieved through use of contraceptive methods and the treatment of infertility."[1] It is an increasingly important consideration for people with cystic fibrosis (CF) as they live longer and healthier lives.[2] Notably, family planning is often viewed narrowly in health care circles as access to and use of contraceptive and abortion services. However, a recent qualitative study uncovered that people with CF define family planning as inclusive of all options for family-building along with pregnancy prevention.[3] This review will thus address contraceptive use, pregnancy, fertility, disease-specific sexual functioning concerns, use of assisted reproductive technologies (ART),

parenthood, and the importance of patient-centered reproductive goals counseling and care for people with CF.

SEXUAL ACTIVITY AND FUNCTION

Compared with the general population, people with CF have a similar age of onset of sexual activity, sexual activity rate, and number of partners[4] and are equally likely to engage in risky sexual behaviors.[5,6]

Consequences of CF transmembrane conductance regulator (CFTR) dysfunction may impair sexual function. Common CF symptoms include frequent cough and constipation, increase pressure on the pelvic floor, and are potentially detrimental to proper muscle tone.[7] This leads to pelvic floor dysfunction and may result in bladder/bowel dysfunction, sexual dysfunction, and prolapse of pelvic organs.[8–11]

[a] Department of Obstetrics, Gynecology, and Reproductive Sciences, Yale School of Medicine, 20 York Street, New Haven, CT 06510, USA; [b] Department of Medicine, University of Texas Southwestern Medical Center, 5323 Harry Hines Blvd., Dallas, TX 75390-8558, USA; [c] Department of Pediatrics, University of Pittsburgh School of Medicine, Pittsburgh, PA, USA; [d] Center for Innovative Research on Gender Health Equity (CONVERGE), University of Pittsburgh, Pittsburgh, PA, USA
* Corresponding author. University Center, 120 Lytton Avenue Suite M060, Pittsburgh, PA 15213.
E-mail address: traci.kazmerski@chp.edu

Clin Chest Med 43 (2022) 811–820
https://doi.org/10.1016/j.ccm.2022.06.015

In women with CF, dyspareunia and coital incontinence rates are higher than a non-CF sample of nulliparous women of similar age.[8] Among sexually active 15 to 24-year-old women with CF, 16% reported sexual dysfunction.[5] In one survey, 65% of men with CF reported sexual dysfunction, and the most prevalent reported symptom was reduced ejaculation.[8] This is likely caused by decreased ejaculate due to congenital bilateral absence of the vas deferens (CBAVD), present in greater than 98% of men with CF.[12]

Embarrassment and lack of awareness of treatment options may cause hesitancy in seeking care for sexual concerns.[13–15] Thus, it is imperative to assess for sexual functioning concerns in all people with CF. Although they may be reluctant to initiate such conversations, most people with CF are comfortable discussing these concerns with their CF team when asked.[8]

SEXUALLY TRANSMITTED INFECTIONS AND CONTRACEPTION

People with CF have the same risks of sexually transmitted infections (STIs) and unplanned pregnancies as individuals without CF.

Men with CF report suboptimal condom use, caused in part by knowledge of male infertility leading to the assumed lack of need for barrier protection,[16] thus increasing STI risk. Prevalence of STIs in women with CF is reported to be similar to the general population and guidance for screening follows recommendations for non-CF peers, yet they report lower rates of STI screening.[5,17]

Organ transplantation and immunosuppression are associated with increased risk of cervical dysplasia,[18] but data suggest that both transplanted and nontransplanted women with CF had a high proportion of abnormal cervical screening tests.[19] Despite this, women with CF have lower lifetime rates of ever obtaining a Pap smear compared with the general population.[5,20] High-grade cervical dysplasia can be efficiently prevented through HPV vaccination.[21] While women with CF in the United States (US) report similar rates of HPV vaccination compared with the general population, these numbers are still suboptimal (43% vs 44%).[5] Current guidelines recommend that women with CF follow guidelines for the general population and those with solid organ transplant follow the current CDC guidelines for HIV-infected women.[22]

Women with CF in the US report lower rates of lifetime contraception use than the general population.[5] Several reports indicate that women with CF have a lack of knowledge regarding their fertility,[4,23–25] which may lead to the underutilization of contraception.

Limited data exist exploring the use and efficacy of various types of contraception in CF[26–28]; however, current literature suggests that there is no method of contraception either contraindicated or recommended. Disease-specific risk factors must be considered, including, but not limited to, active liver disease, severe pulmonary hypertension, osteoporosis/osteopenia, and cholelithiasis. For example, caution is advised for the use of depot medroxyprogesterone acetate, a hormonal injection associated with accelerated, but potentially reversible, loss of bone mineral density[29] due to concern for premature osteopenia in people with CF.[30] Additionally, some preparations of combined oral contraception are associated with an increased risk of venous thromboembolism, which should be considered for those with implantable vascular access devices or other increased risks for thromboembolism.[29,31] Any potential risk associated with a method of contraception must be compared with the risks of pregnancy.

Hormonal contraceptives may be affected by medications commonly used in CF. Of the CFTR modulator drugs, ivacaftor/lumacaftor has unclear interactions with hormonal contraceptive methods,[32] and, therefore, current product information states that the hormonal contraceptives should not be relied on as effective contraception when coadministered.[33] In contrast, ivacaftor, tezacaftor/ivacaftor and elexacaftor/tezacaftor/ivacaftor (ETI) are not expected to have an impact on the efficacy of hormonal contraceptives.[34–36]

PREGNANCY PLANNING

Pregnancy planning in CF is recommended as health status at the time of conception can serve as an important prognostic indicator of obstetric and neonatal outcomes.[37–40] Collaboration between the CF care team and high-risk obstetrics specialists is ideal. In CF, aspects of maternal health that contribute to pregnancy outcomes include preconception nutrition, pulmonary function, CF-related diabetes control, and bacterial colonization.[38,39,41]

While data are limited and largely relies on retrospective and often single-center observational studies, there are a few clinical features that pose higher risk for adverse pregnancy outcomes in CF. Malnutrition is a known risk for poor fetal outcomes, including premature and low birth weight babies.[42,43] Importantly, a more optimal prepregnancy body mass index (BMI) correlates with better maternal health outcomes and a BMI of at least 22 kg/m^2 is recommended before pregnancy.[44] Additionally, fat-soluble vitamin levels should be monitored and adjusted based on serum and plasma micronutrient levels.[45] Vitamin A levels, in particular, should be monitored closely in the pre-conception period if giving doses higher than 10,000 IU per day as high doses can be associated with increased risk of miscarriage and congenital malformations.[46] Iron and folate supplementation is similar to that of people without CF.

An additional key indicator of maternal health in CF is lung function. Low percent predicted forced expiratory volume in 1 second (ppFEV$_1$) carries a higher risk of both maternal and neonatal adverse outcomes, including the destabilization of maternal health and premature delivery, delivery by cesarean section, and low birthweight. Several studies demonstrate that a ppFEV1 less than 50% is associated with poorer outcomes.[37,39,47] In the era of highly effective CFTR modulator therapy, lung health is stabilizing and preliminary data are showing that women with lower lung function are having successful pregnancies,[48] but this has not yet been evaluated longitudinally. Pulmonary hypertension is a rare CF complication and, while it has not been uniquely studied in pregnancy in CF, data show that pregnant people with pulmonary hypertension have an increased risk for maternal mortality, eclampsia, preterm delivery, and intrauterine fetal demise.[49]

Approximately 30% of people with CF have CF-related diabetes (CFRD).[2] Hyperglycemia related to inadequate diabetic control can cause major fetal anomalies.[50,51] An oral glucose tolerance test is recommended to screen for diabetes before pregnancy in people with CF.

Finally, an additionally important aspect of pre-pregnancy planning for people with CF includes genetic testing. As CF is an autosomal recessive disorder, an infant born to a mother with CF will be an obligate carrier of one CFTR mutation. Preconception carrier screening for reproductive partners should be offered to discuss the risk of having a child with CF.[52] As there are more than 3000 disease-causing CFTR mutations, next-generation sequencing is recommended for partners regardless of race or ethnicity.[53,54] If the reproductive partner is identified as a CF carrier, additional genetic counseling should include discussion of reproductive options, including sperm or ovum donation, preimplantation genetic testing, and prenatal diagnostic testing.

If feasible, preconception health assessment allows for attempts at the optimization of nutritional status, vitamin levels, lung function, and glycemic control to prevent maternal and fetal morbidity and mortality.

FERTILITY

Infertility is nearly universal in men with CF, with approximately 98% affected by CBAVD and subsequent obstructive azoospermia.[55,56] Despite this anatomic obstruction, men with CF have the option to have biological children through ART as outlined later in discussion.

Most women with CF are fertile and able to conceive naturally.[43] However, subfertility in women with CF is likely multifactorial.[55,57] The reproductive female anatomy in CF is structurally normal, but mutations in the CFTR gene can affect the function of reproductive epithelial cells.[58,59] CFTR channels are present in the endometrial epithelium after puberty,[60] and the cervix.[61,62] Abnormal function of CFTR can result in viscous, dehydrated cervical mucus, which may impair the infiltration of sperm and result in a pH-imbalanced intrauterine setting limiting sperm capacitation, effectively preventing fertilization.[59,63–65]

CFTR modulator therapy does not reverse CBAVD, and therefore will not impact male infertility,[66] but the effect on female fertility remains unknown. In animal models, CFTR modulators show no adverse impact on fertility.[33–36] They may favorably change cervical mucus viscosity and pH[32,67] and there have been reports of both improved fertility and unplanned pregnancies in women using CFTR modulators.[32,68] Care teams should routinely advise women who are starting CFTR modulators about the potential for increased fecundity to prevent unplanned pregnancies.

ASSISTED REPRODUCTIVE TECHNOLOGY

Most of the men and some women with CF will need to consider ART as an option to become pregnant for reasons outlined in the section above. These techniques largely include IVF and intrauterine insemination (IUI) (**Fig. 1**), but other options are available.

For men with CF, the first step involves surgical sperm retrieval or testicular sperm aspiration (also known as percutaneous epididymal sperm extraction [PESA], testicular sperm extraction [TESA], microsurgical epididymal sperm aspiration [MESA], or testicular sperm extraction [TESE]). These procedures are office-based and performed using local anesthesia and a needle attached to a syringe to extract sperm from the testicle or epididymis. The same procedure is used for partners of women with CF to harvest sperm for IUI or IVF. For obstructive azoospermia, sperm retrieval rates are typically as high as 100%.[69,70]

In IUI, sperm is inserted directly into the uterus.[71] IVF, on the other hand, uses the process of combining an egg and sperm in a laboratory dish and transferring the formed embryo into the uterus. Both are reasonable options for women

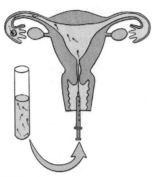
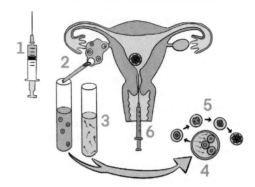

Fig. 1. Intrauterine insemination (IUI) involves direct insertion of sperm into the uterus. In vitro fertilization (IVF) is a multistep procedure, involving (1) ovarian stimulation, (2) oocyte aspiration, (3) sperm preparation, (4) egg fertilization, (5) embryonic development, and (6) embryo transfer to intrauterine environment.

with CF. In IUI, the sperm is implanted in the uterus past the thickened cervical mucus using a catheter. No adjuvant hormonal supplementation is required. Rarely, the procedure can be associated with infection. For IVF, the sperm fertilizes the egg outside of the body and is implanted into the uterus. Hormone stimulation is required for IVF, but this allows for embryos to be stored for later use and for preimplantation genetic testing. Success rates for pregnancies using IUI are estimated to be 5% to 25%, whereas IVF success rates are typically 20% to 40%.[59,72] Meta-analysis has also shown that IVF is associated with a significantly higher live birth rate than IUI with no significant difference in multiple pregnancy rate.[73]

PREGNANCY

Over the past several years, there has been a notable rise in the number of pregnancies in people with CF (**Fig. 2**). The US CFF Patient Registry reported more than 600 pregnancies in 2020, nearly doubling the incidence reported in the prior year.[74]

Several recent review articles have been published related to pregnancy in CF.[75–77] Here we detail the impact and use of CFTR modulators in pregnancy. Further details about the importance of coordinated care during pregnancy between obstetric and CF teams, pregnancy and lung transplant in CF, management of routine CF medications during pregnancy, and other considerations are summarized separately.

In the US, highly effective CFTR modulator therapy is available for approximately 90% of people with CF and, thus, a major consideration for people with CF is the use and safety of CFTR modulators during pregnancy. While known to be associated with improved lung function and weight and decreased pulmonary exacerbations,[33–36,78–82] there are case series reporting health decline and even death in both nonpregnant and pregnant people who discontinued CFTR modulators.[33–36] There is currently little long-term data available, so the decision to continue or stop modulators is complicated.

Data currently available regarding the use of CFTR modulators in pregnancy come from animal models and case series. Animal models have not demonstrated fetal harm at typical human doses of CFTR modulators.[33–36] CFTR modulators are described to cross the placenta and into breast

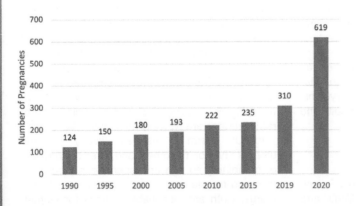

Fig. 2. Annual number of pregnancies in people with CF.

milk.[83] In 2 multi-center surveys, data in pregnant people using CFTR modulators did not show a pattern to suggest harm to the fetus/infant.[84,85] Nash and colleagues reported maternal and infant outcome data from 44 pregnancies associated with modulator exposure to ivacaftor, lumacaftor/ivacaftor, and tezacaftor/ivacaftor.[84] There were 2 maternal complications considered related to CFTR modulator therapy. The miscarriage rate for those on modulator therapy was 4.7% (lower than that reported in the general population). Nine cases had a decline in health with the cessation of modulator therapy. No infant complications were thought to be associated with modulator use. In a study of 45 mothers exposed to ETI, Taylor-Cousar and colleagues reported one maternal complication deemed related to ETI; 2 complications deemed unknown in relatedness to ETI.[85] Three infant complications were deemed unknown in relatedness to ETI and 2 complications were deemed unrelated to ETI use. Two of the infants had severe congenital malformations; however, based on maternal history, providers reported both instances of congenital malformations as unrelated to ETI.[85] The use of CFTR modulator therapy by men with CF during conception and during their partner's pregnancy has yet to be studied. In combination, the limited available clinical data are reassuring for the overall safety of the use of CFTR modulators during pregnancy. Larger and ideally prospective studies are needed to further understand the safety of CFTR modulator use in pregnancy. A prospective observational clinical trial in the US supported by the CF Foundation and Therapeutics Development Network studying pregnancies with and without CFTR modulator exposure has begun and intends to enroll more than 250 pregnant people with CF (Maternal and Fetal Outcomes in the Era of Modulators – MAYFLOWERS; NCT04828382).

PARENTHOOD

There remains limited CF-specific data on the experience and impact of parenting for people with CF. Prior qualitative evidence suggests that the decision of whether to become a parent is complex, and CF is a major factor in reproductive decision making.[86] People with CF express concerns around the balance of caring for themselves and their children and reflect on parenting with both a limited life expectancy and complex daily treatments, and the necessity to prioritize these often-conflicting needs.[87,88] They also worry about communication with children about CF care and prognosis and the potential impacts of health decline, recurrent illness, or parental death on their children.[87]

People with CF can pursue many paths to parenthood, including pregnancy (potentially via ART), adoption, foster parenting, and step-parenthood.[76] The ART options discussed above are also viable if considering surrogacy or a gestational carrier.

The impact of parenthood on the physical health of people with CF remains largely unknown. A 2003 retrospective study found that women with CF who became pregnant had better survival at 10 years compared with women with CF who did not.[89] Subsequently, it was shown that pregnant women with CF did not experience worse disease progression at 1.5 years after pregnancy, but were treated for more pulmonary exacerbations and had more illness-related outpatient visits compared with women who did not become pregnant.[90] A study of French fathers with CF in the first 3 years of parenthood had a trend toward increased outpatient visits, but did not experience clinical deterioration in lung function or BMI.[91] Recently, fathers with CF in the United Kingdom (UK) demonstrated a significant decline in weight and a trend toward declining lung function in the first year of fatherhood.[92]

Large, multicenter studies describing the impact of parenthood on health outcomes are lacking. Furthermore, investigations of the impacts of CFTR modulators on the effects of parenthood are needed.

CONCLUSIONS AND CARE RECOMMENDATIONS

People with CF often experience fragmented and limited family planning and reproductive health care.[93] Research has identified critical gaps in current CF reproductive health care delivery models, which include a failure to proactively identify reproductive health needs and, thus, address preventable adverse outcomes.

Historically, people with CF were discouraged from becoming pregnant due to fears of the potential impact on respiratory health and survival. While this has not been the case for many decades, people with CF continue to express reticence to disclose their reproductive plans to their CF team for fear of judgment or lack of support.[23]

For most of the men with CF, planning is a necessity given the need for ART or the pursuit of other options for family-building. Among women, reproductive planning in CF is important to optimize prepregnancy health, undergo genetic counseling and testing, avoid potential teratogenic exposures, and develop support systems and strategies for times of illness while pregnant or during parenthood.

However, a reproductive planning framework is limited and may ignore those who do not hold clear intentions regarding pregnancy timing or have complex feelings about achieving or avoiding pregnancy.[94,95] When counseling people with CF related to their reproductive goals, providers should recognize that pregnancy and parenthood intentions are not strictly binary and many either cannot or do not want to plan such decisions.[96] Indeed, counseling focused on planning may create harm from equity and reproductive justice perspectives, as structural factors may make such planning unattainable or irrelevant. As such, not all unplanned pregnancies are unwelcome and not all ambivalence related to reproductive plans can and should be resolved. Importantly for those with CF, CF teams should avoid personally judging people's reproductive choices or desires and allowing those biases to impact their care. Finally, it should not be assumed that everyone wants preconception counseling and care.[97]

CF teams should partner with people with CF in routine reproductive goals conversations guided by relationship-centered language to elicit emotional thoughts and preferences (rather than planning-based questions and intentions).[98] Use of derivatives of questions or scales to assess such thoughts may be helpful to guide open reproductive health conversations.[99] Given the important health considerations for people with CF related to pregnancy, contraception, and parenthood, continued discussion of the reasons for encouraged reproductive planning and preconception counseling is reasonable, but such conversations should be infused with respect for the range of realities and desires of the person with CF. Reproductive health and family planning services should be universally offered in comprehensive CF care and referrals to reproductive health providers familiar with modern CF care is crucial. Firm situation of such counseling and care using a reproductive justice lens assures that all people with CF are met whereby they are in relation to their reproductive goals.[100]

CLINICS CARE POINTS

- CF teams should partner with people with CF in routine reproductive goals conversations guided by relationship-centered language to elicit emotional thoughts and preferences (rather than planning-based questions and intentions).
- Reproductive planning should be encouraged among people with CF to optimize prepregnancy health and support. Reproductive health and family planning services should be universally offered in comprehensive CF care.
- CF teams should build partnerships with reproductive health providers familiar with modern CF care.

DISCLOSURE

T.M. Kazmerski and R. Jain receive grant support from the Cystic Fibrosis Foundation (KAZM-ER21Y3, JAIN21Y3) to support the CF Foundation TDN Sexual Health, Reproduction, and Gender Research Working Group (SHARING), which directly supports this work. No conflicts of interest are applicable to this work.

REFERENCES

1. World Health Organization (WHO). Contraception. Available at: https://www.who.int/health-topics/contraception#tab=tab_1. Accessed October 5, 2021.
2. Cystic Fibrosis Foundation patient Registry report 2019. 2019. Available at: https://www.cff.org/Research/Researcher-Resources/Patient-Registry/2019-Patient-Registry-Annual-Data-Report.pdf. Accessed October 5, 2021.
3. Leech MM, Stransky OM, Talabi MB, et al. Exploring the reproductive decision support needs and preferences of women with cystic fibrosis. Contraception 2021;103(1):32–7.
4. Sawyer SM, Phelan PD, Bowes G. Reproductive health in young women with cystic fibrosis: knowledge, behavior and attitudes. J Adolesc Health 1995;17(1):46–50.
5. Kazmerski TM, Sawicki GS, Miller E, et al. Sexual and reproductive health behaviors and experiences reported by young women with cystic fibrosis. J Cyst Fibros 2018;17(1):57–63.
6. Britto MT, Garrett JM, Dugliss MAJ, et al. Risky behavior in teens with cystic fibrosis or sickle cell disease: a multicenter study. Pediatrics 1998;101(2):250–6.
7. Dodd ME, Langman H. Urinary incontinence in cystic fibrosis. J R Soc Med 2005;98(Suppl 45):28–36.
8. Chambers R, Lucht A, Reihill A, et al. Prevalence and impact of pelvic floor dysfunction in an adult cystic fibrosis population: a questionnaire survey. Int Urogynecol J 2017;28(4):591–604.
9. Mariani A, Gambazza S, Carta F, et al. Prevalence and factors associated with urinary incontinence in females with cystic fibrosis: an Italian single-centre

cross-sectional analysis. Pediatr Pulmonol 2021. https://doi.org/10.1002/ppul.25723.

10. Kazmerski TM, Nelson E, Newman LR, et al. Talking about sex: the training wants and needs of the CF interprofessional team. Conference Abstract. Pediatr Pulmonol 2018;53(Supplement 2):444–5.

11. Neemuchwala F, Ahmed F, Nasr SZ. Prevalence of pelvic incontinence in patients with cystic fibrosis. Glob Pediatr Health 2017;4. 2333794x17743424.

12. Wilschanski M, Corey M, Durie P, et al. Diversity of reproductive tract abnormalities in men with cystic fibrosis. JAMA 1996;276(8):607–8.

13. Orr A, McVean RJ, Webb AK, et al. Questionnaire survey of urinary incontinence in women with cystic fibrosis. BMJ 2001;322(7301):1521.

14. Moran F, Bradley JM, Boyle L, et al. Incontinence in adult females with cystic fibrosis: a Northern Ireland survey. Int J Clin Pract 2003; 57(3):182–3.

15. Gumery L, Lee J, Whitehouse J, et al. The prevalence of urinary incontinence in adult cystic fibrosis males. J Cyst Fibros 2005;4(suppl 1):S97.

16. Sawyer SM, Farrant B, Cerritelli B, et al. A survey of sexual and reproductive health in men with cystic fibrosis: new challenges for adolescent and adult services. Thorax 2005;60(4):326–30.

17. Kazmerski TM, Prushinskaya OV, Hill K, et al. Sexual and reproductive health of young women with cystic fibrosis: a concept mapping study. Acad Pediatr 2019;19(3):307–14.

18. Malouf MA, Hopkins PM, Singleton L, et al. Sexual health issues after lung transplantation: importance of cervical screening. J Heart Lung Transplant 2004;23(7):894–7.

19. Rousset-Jablonski C, Reynaud Q, Nove-Josserand R, et al. High proportion of abnormal pap smear tests and cervical dysplasia in women with cystic fibrosis. Eur J Obstet Gynecol Reprod Biol 2018;221:40–5.

20. Rousset Jablonski C, Reynaud Q, Perceval M, et al. Contraceptive practices and cervical screening in women with cystic fibrosis. Hum Reprod 2015; 30(11):2547–51.

21. Arbyn M, Xu L, Simoens C, et al. Prophylactic vaccination against human papillomaviruses to prevent cervical cancer and its precursors. Cochrane Database Syst Rev 2018;5:CD009069.

22. Moscicki AB, Flowers L, Huchko MJ, et al. Guidelines for cervical cancer screening in immunosuppressed women without HIV infection. J Low Genit Tract Dis 2019;23(2):87–101.

23. Kazmerski TM, Gmelin T, Slocum B, et al. Attitudes and decision making related to pregnancy among young women with cystic fibrosis. Matern child Health J 2017;21(4):818–24.

24. Korzeniewska A, Grzelewski T, Jerzynska J, et al. Sexual and reproductive health knowledge in cystic fibrosis female patients and their parents. J Sex Med 2009;6(3):770–6.

25. Ashley Gage L. What deficits in sexual and reproductive health knowledge exist among women with cystic fibrosis? a systematic review. Health Social Work 2012;37(1):29–36.

26. Jain R, Kazmerski TM, Aitken ML, et al. Challenges faced by women with cystic fibrosis. Clin Chest Med 2021;42(3):517–30.

27. Roe AH, Traxler S, Schreiber CA. Contraception in women with cystic fibrosis: a systematic review of the literature. Review. Contraception. 2016;93(1): 3–10.

28. Whiteman MK, Oduyebo T, Zapata LB, et al. Contraceptive safety among women with cystic fibrosis: a systematic review. Review. Contraception. 2016;94(6):621–9.

29. Curtis KM, Tepper NK, Jatlaoui TC, et al. U.S. Medical eligibility criteria for contraceptive use, 2016. Mmwr Recommendations Rep 2016;65(3):1–103.

30. Conway SP. Impact of lung inflammation on bone metabolism in adolescents with cystic fibrosis. Paediatr Respir Rev 2001;2(4):324–31.

31. Deerojanawong J, Sawyer SM, Fink AM, et al. Totally implantable venous access devices in children with cystic fibrosis: incidence and type of complications. Thorax 1998;53(4):285–9.

32. Jones GH, Walshaw MJ. Potential impact on fertility of new systemic therapies for cystic fibrosis. Paediatr Respir Rev 2015;16(Suppl 1):25–7.

33. Incorporated VP. Lumacaftor/ivacaftor (Orkambi) United States prescribing information 2018. Available at: https://pi.vrtx.com/files/uspi_lumacaftor_ivacaftor.pdf. Accessed October 5, 2021.

34. Incorporated VP. Elexacaftor/tezacaftor/ivacaftor (Trikafta) United States prescribing information. Updated October 2021. Available at: https://pi.vrtx.com/files/uspi_elexacaftor_tezacaftor_ivacaftor.pdf. Accessed October 5, 2021.

35. Incorporated VP. Tezacaftor/ivacaftor (Symdeko) United States prescribing information. Available at: https://pi.vrtx.com/files/uspi_tezacaftor_ivacaftor.pdf. Accessed October 5, 2021.

36. Incorporated VP. Ivacaftor (Kalydeco) United States prescribing information updated 9/2020. Available at: https://pi.vrtx.com/files/uspi_ivacaftor.pdf. Accessed October 5, 2021.

37. Thorpe-Beeston JG, Madge S, Gyi K, et al. The outcome of pregnancies in women with cystic fibrosis-single centre experience 1998-2011. BJOG 2013;120(3):354–61.

38. Edenborough FP, Borgo G, Knoop C, et al. Guidelines for the management of pregnancy in women with cystic fibrosis. J Cyst Fibros 2008;7(SUPPL. 1):S2–32.

39. Cohen-Cymberknoh M, Gindi Reiss B, Reiter J, et al. Baseline Cystic fibrosis disease severity has

an adverse impact on pregnancy and infant outcomes, but does not impact disease progression. J Cyst Fibros 2021;20(3):388–94.

40. Reynaud Q, Rousset Jablonski C, Poupon-Bourdy S, et al. Pregnancy outcome in women with cystic fibrosis and poor pulmonary function. J Cyst Fibros 2020;19(1):80–3.

41. Canny GJ, Corey M, Livingstone RA, et al. Pregnancy and cystic fibrosis. Obstet Gynecol 1991; 77(6):850–3.

42. Kotloff RM, FitzSimmons SC, Fiel SB. Fertility and pregnancy in patients with cystic fibrosis. Review. Clin Chest Med 1992;13(4):623–35.

43. McArdle JR. Pregnancy in cystic fibrosis. Review. Clin Chest Med 2011;32(1):111–20.

44. McDonald CM, Alvarez JA, Bailey J, et al. Academy of nutrition and Dietetics: 2020 cystic fibrosis evidence analysis center evidence-based nutrition practice guideline. J Acad Nutr Diet 2021;121(8): 1591–636.e3.

45. Cheng EY, Goss CH, McKone EF, et al. Aggressive prenatal care results in successful fetal outcomes in CF women. J Cyst Fibros 2006;5(2):85–91.

46. Rothman KJ, Moore LL, Singer MR, et al. Teratogenicity of high vitamin A intake. N Engl J Med 1995; 333(21):1369–73.

47. Ashcroft A, Chapman SJ, Mackillop L. The outcome of pregnancy in women with cystic fibrosis: a UK population-based descriptive study. BJOG 2020;127(13):1696–703.

48. Raksha Jain AK, MinJae Lee, Natalie West, Traci M. Kazmersk, Moira Aitke, Andrea H. Roe, Denis Hadjiliadis, Ahmet Uluer, Sheila Mody, Patrick Flume, Leigh Ann Bray, Jennifer Taylor-Cousar. Effect of pregnancy on lung function: impact of CFTR modulators. presented at: NACFC; 2021; North American CF Conference, held virtually, October 2021.

49. Thomas E, Yang J, Xu J, et al. Pulmonary hypertension and pregnancy outcomes: Insights from the National Inpatient sample. J Am Heart Assoc 2017; 6(10). https://doi.org/10.1161/JAHA.117.006144.

50. Ludvigsson JF, Neovius M, Soderling J, et al. Periconception glycaemic control in women with type 1 diabetes and risk of major birth defects: population based cohort study in Sweden. BMJ 2018;362: k2638.

51. Guerin A, Nisenbaum R, Ray JG. Use of maternal GHb concentration to estimate the risk of congenital anomalies in the offspring of women with pre-pregnancy diabetes. Diabetes Care 2007;30(7): 1920–5.

52. Committee Opinion No. 691: carrier screening for genetic conditions. Obstet Gynecol 2017;129(3): e41–55.

53. Beauchamp KA, Johansen Taber KA, Grauman PV, et al. Sequencing as a first-line methodology for

cystic fibrosis carrier screening. Genet Med 2019; 21(11):2569–76.

54. Deignan JL, Astbury C, Cutting GR, et al. CFTR variant testing: a technical standard of the American College of Medical Genetics and Genomics (ACMG). Genet Med 2020;22(8):1288–95.

55. Boyd JB, Mehta A, Murphy DJ. Fertility and pregnancy outcomes in men and women with cystic fibrosis in the United Kingdom. Hum Reprod 2004;19(10):2238–43.

56. Gazvani R, Lewis-Jones DI. Cystic fibrosis mutation screening before assisted reproduction. Review. Int J Androl 2004;27(1):1–4.

57. Sueblinvong V, Whittaker LA. Fertility and pregnancy: common concerns of the aging cystic fibrosis population. Review. Clin Chest Med 2007; 28(2):433–43.

58. Edenborough FP. Women with cystic fibrosis and their potential for reproduction. Thorax 2001; 56(8):649–55.

59. Ahmad A, Ahmed A, Patrizio P. Cystic fibrosis and fertility. Review. Curr Opin Obstet Gynecol 2013; 25(3):167–72.

60. Tizzano EF, Silver MM, Chitayat D, et al. Differential cellular expression of cystic fibrosis transmembrane regulator in human reproductive tissues. Clues for the infertility in patients with cystic fibrosis. Am J Pathol 1994;144(5):906–14.

61. Hayslip CC, Hao E, Usala SJ. The cystic fibrosis transmembrane regulator gene is expressed in the human endocervix throughout the menstrual cycle. Fertil Steril 1997;67(4):636–40.

62. Ismail N, Giribabu N, Muniandy S, et al. Estrogen and progesterone differentially regulate the levels of cystic fibrosis transmembrane regulator (CFTR), adenylate cyclase (AC), and cyclic adenosine mono-phosphate (cAMP) in the rat cervix. Mol Reprod Dev 2015;82(6):463–74.

63. Kopito LE, Kosasky HJ, Shwachman H. Water and electrolytes in cervical mucus from patients with cystic fibrosis. Fertil Steril 1973;24(7):512–6.

64. Lyon A, Bilton D. Fertility issues in cystic fibrosis. Review. Paediatr Respir Rev 2002;3(3):236–40.

65. Chan HC, Shi QX, Zhou CX, et al. Critical role of CFTR in uterine bicarbonate secretion and the fertilizing capacity of sperm. Mol Cell Endocrinol 2006;250(1–2):106–13.

66. Khan FN, Tangpricha V, Hughan KS, et al. Men's health in the modern era of cystic fibrosis. J Cyst Fibros 2020. https://doi.org/10.1016/j.jcf.2020.12. 013.

67. Heltshe SL, Godfrey EM, Josephy T, et al. Pregnancy among cystic fibrosis women in the era of CFTR modulators. J Cyst Fibros 2017;16(6): 687–94.

68. Ladores S, Kazmerski TM, Rowe SM. A case report of pregnancy during use of Targeted Therapeutics

for cystic fibrosis. J Obstet Gynecol neonatal Nurs 2017;46(1):72–7.

69. Coward RM, Mills JN. A step-by-step guide to office-based sperm retrieval for obstructive azoospermia. Transl Androl Urol 2017;6(4):730–44.

70. Esteves SC, Miyaoka R, Agarwal A. Sperm retrieval techniques for assisted reproduction. Int Braz J Urol 2011;37(5):570–83.

71. Kredentser JV, Pokrant C, McCoshen JA. Intrauterine insemination for infertility due to cystic fibrosis. Fertil Sterility 1986;45(3):425–6.

72. Medical Advisory S. In vitro fertilization and multiple pregnancies: an evidence-based analysis. Ont Health Technol Assess Ser 2006;6(18):1–63.

73. Nandi A, Raja G, White D, et al. Intrauterine insemination + controlled ovarian hyperstimulation versus in vitro fertilisation in unexplained infertility: a systematic review and meta-analysis. Arch Gynecol Obstet 2021. https://doi.org/10.1007/s00404-021-06277-3.

74. Cystic fibrosis Foundation patient Registry report 2020. 2020. Available at: https://www.cff.org/sites/default/files/2021-11/Patient-Registry-Annual-Data-Report.pdf. Accessed October 5, 2021.

75. Middleton PG, Gade EJ, Aguilera C, et al. ERS/TSANZ Task Force Statement on the management of reproduction and pregnancy in women with airways diseases. Eur Respir J 2020;55(2) (no pagination)1901208.

76. Kazmerski TM, West NE, Jain R, et al. Family-building and parenting considerations for people with cystic fibrosis. Review. Pediatr Pulmonol 2021. https://doi.org/10.1002/ppul.25620.

77. Jain R, Kazmerski TM, Zuckerwise LC, et al. Pregnancy in cystic fibrosis: review of the literature and expert recommendations. Review. J Cyst Fibros 2021. https://doi.org/10.1016/j.jcf.2021.07.019.

78. Ramsey BW, Davies J, McElvaney NG, et al. A CFTR potentiator in patients with cystic fibrosis and the G551D mutation. N Engl J Med 2011; 365(18):1663–72.

79. Middleton PG, Mall MA, Drevinek P, et al. Elexacaftor-Tezacaftor-Ivacaftor for Cystic Fibrosis with a Single Phe508del Allele. N Engl J Med 2019; 381(19):1809–19.

80. Heijerman HGM, McKone EF, Downey DG, et al. Efficacy and safety of the elexacaftor plus tezacaftor plus ivacaftor combination regimen in people with cystic fibrosis homozygous for the F508del mutation: a double-blind, randomised, phase 3 trial. Lancet 2019;394(10212):1940–8.

81. Accurso FJ, Rowe SM, Clancy JP, et al. Effect of VX-770 in persons with cystic fibrosis and the G551D-CFTR mutation. N Engl J Med 2010; 363(21):1991–2003.

82. Rowe SM, Daines C, Ringshausen FC, et al. Tezacaftor-ivacaftor in residual-function heterozygotes with cystic fibrosis. N Engl J Med 2017;377(21):2024–35.

83. Trimble A, McKinzie C, Terrell M, et al. Measured fetal and neonatal exposure to Lumacaftor and Ivacaftor during pregnancy and while breastfeeding. J Cyst Fibros 2018;17(6):779–82.

84. Nash EF, Middleton PG, Taylor-Cousar JL. Outcomes of pregnancy in women with cystic fibrosis (CF) taking CFTR modulators - an international survey. J Cyst Fibros 2020;19(4):521–6.

85. Taylor-Cousar JL, Jain R. Maternal and fetal outcomes following elexacaftor-tezacaftor-ivacaftor use during pregnancy and lactation. J Cyst Fibros 2021;20(3):402–6.

86. Jacob A, Journiac J, Fischer L, et al. How do cystic fibrosis patients experience parenthood? A systematic review. J Health Psychol 2021;26(1):60–81.

87. Hailey CE, Tan JW, Dellon EP, et al. Pursuing parenthood with cystic fibrosis: reproductive health and parenting concerns in individuals with cystic fibrosis. Pediatr Pulmonol 2019;54(8):1225–33.

88. Barker H, Moses J, O'Leary C. 'I've got to prioritise': being a parent with cystic fibrosis. Psychol Health Med 2017;22(6):744–52.

89. Goss CH, Rubenfeld GD, Otto K, et al. The effect of pregnancy on survival in women with cystic fibrosis. Chest 2003;124(4):1460–8.

90. Schechter MS, Quittner AL, Konstan MW, et al. Long-term effects of pregnancy and motherhood on disease outcomes of women with cystic fibrosis. Ann Am Thorac Soc 2013;10(3):213–9.

91. Dugueperoux I, Hubert D, Dominique S, et al. Paternity in men with cystic fibrosis: a retrospective survey in France. J Cyst Fibros 2006;5(4):215–21.

92. Bianco B, Horsley A, Brennan A. Implications of fatherhood in cystic fibrosis. Review. Paediatr Respir Rev 2019;31:18–20.

93. West NE, Kazmerski TM, Taylor-Cousar JL, et al. Optimizing sexual and reproductive health across the lifespan in people with cystic fibrosis. Pediatr Pulmonol 2021. https://doi.org/10.1002/ppul.25703.

94. Callegari LS, Aiken AR, Dehlendorf C, et al. Addressing potential pitfalls of reproductive life planning with patient-centered counseling. Am J Obstet Gynecol 2017;216(2):129–34.

95. Borrero S, Nikolajski C, Steinberg JR, et al. It just happens": a qualitative study exploring low-income women's perspectives on pregnancy intention and planning. Contraception 2015;91(2):150–6.

96. Callegari LS, Aiken ARA, Dehlendorf C, et al. Reproductive life planning and patient-centered

care: can the Inconsistencies be reconciled? Matern Child Health J 2019;23(7):869–70.

97. Aiken AR, Borrero S, Callegari LS, et al. Rethinking the pregnancy planning paradigm: unintended conceptions or unrepresentative concepts? Perspect Sex Reprod Health 2016;48(3):147–51.

98. Family Planning: Cystic Fibrosis and Reproductive Goals, Cystic Fibrosis Foundation; Bethesda, MD.

99. Stulberg DB, Datta A, White VanGompel E, et al. One key Question(R) and the desire to avoid pregnancy scale: a comparison of two approaches to asking about pregnancy preferences. Contraception 2020;101(4):231–6.

100. Ross LJ. Reproductive justice as Intersectional Feminist activism. Souls 2017;19(3):286–314.

Update on Lung Transplantation for Cystic Fibrosis

Joseph M. Pilewski, MD

KEYWORDS

- Lung transplant • Advanced CF lung disease • CFTR modulators

KEY POINTS

- Lung Transplant is an important treatment option for Advanced Cystic Fibrosis lung disease, as survival is improving over time and criteria for transplant have evolved.
- Early discussion regarding lung transplant and timely referral for transplant evaluation are critical to maximizing opportunities and optimizing outcomes.
- CF providers should not unilaterally deem that an individual is not a viable transplant candidate, rather discuss with one or more transplant programs.
- Shared care between CF and lung transplant providers improves the transplant journey from referral to evaluation to listing to after transplant care.

INTRODUCTION

Lung transplantation is an attractive treatment option for many patients with end-stage lung disease, particularly individuals with cystic fibrosis (CF). Since inception in the 1980s, increasing numbers of adult lung transplantations have been performed worldwide, and more than 4,000 are performed annually, according to the most recent International Society of Heart and Lung Transplantation registry report.[1] Despite the development of newer CF therapies and improved median survival for patients with CF,[2] most individuals with CF succumb to respiratory failure. For those who progress to advanced lung disease, lung transplantation provides an opportunity for a better quality of life and prolonged survival. Despite the changes in lung allocation policies, 10% to 20% of individuals with CF die while waiting for lung transplantation.[3]

Among the challenges for transplant as a treatment option, inability to predict survival has made it difficult to identify the optimal time for individuals to pursue transplant. Historically, the fraction of expiratory volume in 1 second (FEV_1) has been the most often used functional variable to predict prognosis, with early reports of FEV_1 30% predicted being associated with a 2-year mortality of 50%.[4] A more recent analysis of the Cystic Fibrosis Foundation Patient Registry determined that the median survival of individuals with CF and FEV_1 less than 30% predicted has improved in recent decades, to 6.6 years,[5] and the development of highly effective CFTR modulators is likely to extend survival further.[6,7] In addition to FEV_1, other variables associated with a high risk of death from CF are hypoxia, hypercapnia, pulmonary hypertension, reduced 6-min walk distance and female sex.[4] From these variables, a few predictive models of survival in patients with CF have been developed; however, predicting survival for patients with CF is imprecise at best.[5,8,9] The goal of lung transplantation in patients with CF is to not only extend survival, but also to improve quality of life. In comparison to other patients with end-stage lung disease, individuals with CF face unique challenges when considering lung transplantation, yet the median survival of

Lung Transplant Program, Pulmonary, Allergy and Critical Care Medicine Division, University of Pittsburgh Medical Center (UPMC); Cystic Fibrosis Program, UPMC Presbyterian and UPMC Children's Hospital, NW 628 MUH, 3459 Fifth Avenue, Pittsburgh, PA 15213, USA
E-mail address: pilewskijm@upmc.edu

Clin Chest Med 43 (2022) 821–840
https://doi.org/10.1016/j.ccm.2022.07.002
0272-5231/22/© 2022 Published by Elsevier Inc.

Table 1
Controversial comorbidities in CF and their Impact on Transplant Outcomes

Comorbidity	Impact on Outcomes
• Multiple-drug resistant *Pseudomonas aeruginosa*	• None
• Gram-negative CF pathogens other than *Burkholderia gladioli* and *Burkholderia cenocepacia*	• None
• *Burkholderia cenocepacia*	• Approximately 40% decrease in 1-year survival; minimal effect on 5-year survival
• *Mycobacterium abscessus*	• Increase in perioperative morbidity; no appreciable effect on mortality
• *Aspergillus fumigatus*	• None
• Cirrhosis	• None with Child-Pugh A and perhaps B
• Malnutrition	• Debated but worst case estimate 10% lower survival at 3 and 5 y with BMI < 18
• Mechanical support with invasive ventilation or ECMO • HIV and Hepatitis C	• Increase morbidity; no appreciable decrease in short-term survival and unknown impact on long-term survival • Unknown but likely none if viral infection cleared before transplant

10 years for individuals with CF after transplant exceeds those of individuals transplanted for other end-stage lung diseases.[1]

Highly effective CF transmembrane conductance regulator (CFTR) modulators have significantly impacted the number of individuals with CF who are referred, listed, and undergo lung transplant. In the US in 2020, more than 80% of individuals 12 or older were prescribed a modulator (2020 Cystic Fibrosis Foundation Patient Registry), most frequently elexacaftor/tezacaftor/ivacaftor (ETI). Based on the demonstrated pulmonary and nutritional benefits, and the potential for preventing infections, diabetes, and other CF complications, the collective transformative experience in children and adults with CF suggests that long-term survival will improve significantly for those on effective modulators. However, adverse events may limit use for some individuals, and some do not respond. While the number of individuals with CF needing transplant will decline for the foreseeable future, numbers will increase as individuals survive longer and eventually develop advanced lung disease. This demographic change will create new challenges for CF and transplant providers as the population requiring transplant will be older with more comorbidities. Despite these challenges, modulators will offer the population of individuals with CF an opportunity for improved quality and quantity of life before the need for transplant, and potentially better posttransplant survival.

Overview of the Journey to Lung Transplant

Due to complexities in patient selection, comorbidities, and availability of suitable organ donors, the journey to lung transplant typically requires significant time—rarely weeks, and more typically months to years. The journey can be broken into phases and transitions to highlight the processes and requirements (**Fig. 1**). The initial phase is a discussion with the individual with CF and her or his psychosocial support system regarding the risk of death from lung disease, trajectory of disease, and difficulties predicting survival with CF. Ideally, lung transplant is presented in the context of other CF treatment options, from routine airway clearance and exercise to inhaled mucolytics, inhaled and systemic antibiotics, CFTR modulators, and respiratory support with oxygen and noninvasive ventilation. Because transplant is a complex intervention, the introduction of transplant as a treatment is best conducted well before the onset of respiratory failure to allow for education and timely referral to a transplant program. Initial discussions are often most effective over the course of several clinic visits and incorporate discussions of survival and quality of life with and without a lung transplant, as well as educational materials from sources such as the United Network for Organ Sharing (https://transplantliving.org/organ-facts/lung/) and the Cystic Fibrosis Foundation in the US (https://www.cff.org/Life-With-CF/Treatments-and-Therapies/Lung-Transplantation/) or the country of residence

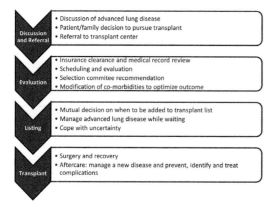

Fig. 1. Phases of the lung transplant journey.

(https://www.cysticfibrosis.ca/; https://www.ecfs. eu/). The goal of these discussions is to assess the individual with CF or their parents' interest in the second phase of the journey – referral for the consideration of lung transplant as a future treatment option. Referral to a transplant center involves the identification of a specific lung transplant program and sending pertinent demographic and medical records to the transplant center. Referral is the beginning of a transition of care, as the CF team engages with the transplant team to share information and allow the transplant team to make an educated decision of when a transplant evaluation should be scheduled.

Guidelines for Referral and Evaluation

To date, there are no prospective, randomized, well-powered studies that define the optimal timing of transplant referral and listing, particularly for CF. Contributing to the challenge of when to refer is that the data regarding survival with advanced CF lung disease are limited. For many years, CF clinicians relied on data published in the early 1990s that reported median survival for individuals with CF and FEV_1 less than 30% predicted while clinically stable was 2 years.[4] A subsequent attempt to develop a multi-variable model identified variables associated with 2-year mortality but had no better positive or negative predictive value for survival than FEV_1 alone.[8] Analysis of a more contemporary data set provides important insight to survival with advanced CF lung disease. Ramos and colleagues, using the US CF Foundation Patient Registry, reported that for individuals with CF and FEV_1 less than 30% predicted during periods of clinical stability, median survival is 6.6 years, markedly improved compared with the earlier study. However, 10% of those with FEV_1 less than 30% predicted died each year.[5] In the US, a significant percentage —

approximately one-third of individuals with CF and FEV_1 less than 30% predicted between 2003 and 2013 died without a lung transplant,[3] due to patient preference, failure of the CF provider to refer before the development of respiratory failure, and/or misperceptions regarding transplant criteria, particularly with respect to resistant pathogens.[10] Due to significant variability in criteria among transplant centers, CF providers are encouraged to defer decisions on transplant candidacy to transplant programs. Early referral to a lung transplant center, before the anticipated need for listing, is highly encouraged to optimize patient and family education, and to identify and correct potential barriers to lung transplantation (eg, malnutrition, substance abuse, poor psychosocial support).

Expert consensus recommendations for CF lung transplant referral were published in 2019,[11] and highlight several key areas: (1) the need to discuss lung transplant as a treatment option early in the course of CF lung disease; (2) approaches to identify modifiable risk factors that can be addressed before transplant to maximize transplant benefit and reduce morbidity; (3) the variability in criteria among transplant programs and need to consult multiple programs if an initial center declines the individual as a transplant candidate; and (4) the benefit of frequent communication between CF and transplant centers from time of initial referral through listing, transplant, and postoperative care.

Discussing Lung Transplant as a Treatment Option for Cystic Fibrosis

The consensus guidelines recommended the introduction of lung transplant as a routine part of CF care, and formal referral for transplant based on variables that predict shortened survival. As death without lung transplant occurs for significant numbers of individuals with CF, and as lung transplant has become more available with improved posttransplant survival, the guidelines recommend general discussion of lung transplant as a treatment option as part of an annual assessment of disease trajectory, and no later than when the FEV_1 falls below 50% predicted; formal transplant referral should occur no later than when the FEV_1 is less than 30% predicted. For individuals with FEV_1 30% to 40% predicted, and for selected individuals with $FEV_1 > 40\%$ predicted, a referral is encouraged for individuals with risk factors that have been shown to increase mortality, including hypoxemia, hypercapnia, life-threatening hemoptysis, frequent infectious exacerbations, and pulmonary hypertension.[10] Discussion of transplant should focus on general principles and not include preconceived ideas based on CF clinician experiences because lung transplant outcomes are improving and determination of which patients are suitable lung transplant candidates should be deferred to the transplant program. Facts that are helpful for discussion regarding lung transplant are summarized in **Box 1**.

Impact of Cystic Fibrosis Transmembrane Conductance Regulator Modulators on Lung Transplant Referral

The development of CFTR modulators has been a remarkable story in respiratory medicine. Defining the genetic, molecular, and cellular biology of CF mutations enabled high throughput screening to identify compounds that partially restore CFTR function. The first highly effective CFTR modulator became available in 2012 when the FDA approved ivacaftor (Kalydeco, IVA) for individuals with the G551D CFTR mutation. IVA substantially decreased sweat chloride, increased respiratory function, promoted weight gain, reduced exacerbation frequency, and improved the quality of life for patients with an FEV_1 of 40% to 90% predicted.[105,106] Since that time, IVA was approved for several other gating mutations, providing opportunity by early 2020 for ~20% of individuals with CF to be treated with a disease-modifying oral medication. Several studies have examined the effect of IVA on patients with advanced lung disease and demonstrated similar improvements to that which was observed in patients with modest lung disease.[13–16]

In late 2019, the second highly effective CFTR modulator therapy, elexacaftor/tezacaftor/ivacaftor (Trikafta, ETI) was approved for individuals with the F508del CFTR mutation. ETI also dramatically improves sweat chloride, FEV_1 (by ~14% absolute predicted), nutritional status, exacerbation frequency, and quality of life for individuals with an FEV_1 of 40% to 90% predicted.[110–112] Because F508del is the most common CFTR mutation, now ~90% of individuals with CF have access to an efficacious disease-modifying therapy.

In early 2021, the effect of ETI for individuals with CF and advanced lung disease who received ETI through an early access program in France was reported.[113] Consistent with prior studies,

ETI was well tolerated in individuals with an $FEV_1 <$ 40% predicted, and there were dramatic improvements in lung function and weight. The 15% mean increases in absolute %predicted FEV_1 was consistent with the subset of patients in the Phase 3 studies whose FEV_1 was just below 40% predicted.[111] This study provided additional evidence for a transformative effect of ETI for individuals with severe lung disease, as ETI use reduced the need for supplemental O_2 by 50%, noninvasive ventilation (NIV) by 30%, and enteral tube feeding by 50%. Perhaps more important for lung transplant programs, before the initiation of ETI in this population, 16 patients were on the lung transplant waiting list and 37 were undergoing transplant evaluation. Although somewhat confounded by the COVID-19 pandemic, 2 patients underwent lung transplantation, 1 died, and only 5 remained on the path to transplant. Given the duration of the study, these results are extraordinary and sustained[118], and have contributed to a marked reduction in the number of individuals with CF referred for lung transplant, and in the number of lung transplants for CF in countries whereby ETI is available.

Long-term studies recently demonstrated that IVA significantly reduced the progression of CF lung disease over 5 years.[114] This decrease in progression, coupled with the short-term effects of both IVA,[106-109,115] and ETI[113,118] for individuals with CF and advanced disease, suggests that survival with advanced CF lung disease will increase significantly. Although additional studies are needed, experience thus far suggests that those on ETI are less likely to suffer rapid progression to respiratory failure and death. ETI may slow the progression of lung disease such that individuals with CF on ETI will progress more like individuals with bronchiectasis due to diseases other than CF, such as PCD or immune deficiency. Progression with advanced CF lung disease is likely to occur slowly, suggesting that for this population, decisions on listing for transplant should be made carefully to avoid early transplants that may decrease life span. In contrast, for the ~10% of individuals with CF who are not on IVA or ETI, disease progression is likely to approximate the 6.6-year median survival when FEV_1 is < 30% predicted, with up to 10% of individuals dying or undergoing transplant each year after going below that threshold during periods of clinical stability.[5] For this subgroup of individuals with CF, decisions on transplant listing do not require practice change.

CFTR modulators have improved the nutritional status of many with CF, and fewer individuals with CF will approach transplant malnourished. In fact, obesity is an emerging challenge in CF. Moreover, with slowing of the decline in lung function, individuals with CF will come to transplant older, perhaps with additional comorbidities like a coronary disease that historically have rarely been an issue in CF.

Selection of Candidates for Lung Transplantation

Lung transplantation should be considered for patients who have advanced lung disease despite maximal medical therapy. Candidates should have a high risk of death from lung disease (>50%) within 2 years without lung transplantation and a high likelihood of 5-year posttransplant survival in the setting of acceptable graft function.[23-30] To determine the severity of disease and appropriateness for lung transplantation, several studies are performed during the evaluation process (**Box 2**). The ideal candidate is free of significant extra-pulmonary comorbidities; however, the other systemic manifestations of CF rarely preclude lung transplantation. The absolute and relative contraindications for lung transplantation have changed as surgical techniques and management of complications have improved over the past decade. In general, patients with CF should be free from malignancy within the past 2 years; however, decisions regarding cancer-free interval before transplant are increasingly based on tumor biology and prognosis rather than absolute timelines. Ideally, lung transplant candidates do not have significant heart, renal or hepatic dysfunction, but coronary interventions, a viable plan for renal replacement, liver disease with preserved synthetic function, or combined heart-lung or liver–lung transplant may overcome seemingly unsurmountable extrapulmonary disease in younger individuals. Other challenges may also be acceptable in some transplant programs, such as significant chest wall deformity or bleeding disorders. In contrast, uncontrolled psychiatric, psychosocial or financial issues may not be remedied and preclude adherence to a complex post-transplant medical regimen and compliance with follow-up care. Candidates should demonstrate an ability to partner with health care providers and be adherent to medical therapies, have good insight and a reliable social support system, have the potential for physical rehabilitation and be free of any recent substance abuse or dependence.[23] Practices on use of cannabinoids and chronic opioids, in the absence of abuse, vary among transplant programs so should be addressed proactively. As some barriers to transplant are modifiable before the development of respiratory failure, early referral is important to

Box 2
Studies performed during lung transplant evaluation for CF

- Chest X-ray
- Computed Tomography of the Chest
- Complete Pulmonary Function Tests
- 6-min Walk
- Quantitative Ventilation/Perfusion scan
- Barium Swallow
- Electrocardiogram
- Transthoracic Echocardiogram
- Right ± left Heart Catheterization
- Bone Densitometry
- Age-appropriate Health Maintenance Exams
- Complete Blood Count
- Renal Function Panel
- Hepatic Function Panel
- Arterial Blood gas
- Sputum Culture
- 24-h Urine for Creatinine Clearance
- Thrombosis Risk Panel
- HLA Molecular typing
- HLA antibody Screen
- Blood Group type
- Hemoglobin A1C
- Urinalysis
- PPD/Quantiferon Gold TB Test
- Serologies o HIV
  - o Hepatitis B
  - o Hepatitis C
  - o Syphilis
  - o Herpes Simplex Virus
  - o Varicella Zoster Virus
  - o Cytomegalovirus
  - o Epstein Barr Virus
  - o Toxoplasmosis

allow sufficient time to address barriers and optimize the opportunity for a successful transplant.

Comorbidities in Cystic Fibrosis and Impact on Transplant Candidacy and Outcomes

An important consideration for lung transplantation is the impact of comorbidities on outcomes. Several reports of single-center outcomes for patients with CF have been published and identify risk factors for worse transplant outcomes;

however, to date, there are no predictive models that allow the estimation of risk associated with multiple comorbidities. CF-specific comorbidities and their individual impact on survival are listed in Table 1, **Box 3** Candidacy for lung transplant is based largely on center experience and level of risk aversion, which varies widely among transplant programs. Higher volume transplant centers will often offer transplant to patients previously declined at less experienced centers. For this reason, it is imperative that CF clinicians be familiar with the criteria at their regional transplant centers to maximize the opportunity for motivated individuals with CF, and to explore referral to multiple transplant centers when necessary to overcome barriers to transplant.

Prior Thoracic Procedures

Historically, prior thoracic procedures were a major contraindication to lung transplantation. Pneumothoraces are a risk factor for mortality in patients with CF,[31] and for the transplant surgeon, less aggressive measures are preferred over chemical or surgical pleurodesis. While few studies have detailed the impact of pleural procedures on transplant outcomes, many centers have found that prior pleural procedures increase the complexity of recipient pneumonectomy and pleural bleeding. In one large single-center report, Meachery and colleagues reported on outcomes for 176 individuals with CF who underwent lung or heart–lung transplantation from 1989 to 2007. For the 12% who had prior pneumothorax (including 6 patients with medical or surgical pleurodesis), outcomes were no worse in individuals with prior pneumothoraces and pleurodesis compared with the larger cohort.[32] Thus, individuals with prior pneumothoraces, including those treated by pleurodesis, can, in the care of an experienced transplant team, have comparable outcomes. Similarly, prior lobectomy or pneumonectomy is not a contraindication to lung transplant in some programs.

Cystic Fibrosis Bacterial Pathogens

Some transplant centers consider pretransplant colonization with pan-resistant strains of *Pseudomonas aeruginosa* or *Burkholderia cepacia* as predictive of poor posttransplant outcomes and therefore, a contraindication to transplantation. Beginning with studies in 1997, there had been some controversy over the impact of pan-resistant bacteria other than *B cepacia* on outcomes from lung transplantation for CF. While patients with sensitive *Pseudomonas* appear to have better outcomes than other transplant recipients,

Box 3
Criteria for listing for lung transplantation for cystic fibrosis

- FEV$_1$ <30% predicted or rapidly declining lung function
- Frequent exacerbations requiring antimicrobial therapy
- Recent exacerbation requiring mechanical ventilation
- Increasing oxygen requirements
- Recurrent hemoptysis despite embolization procedures
- Refractory or recurrent pneumothorax
- Baseline hypercapnia (pCO$_2$ >50 mm Hg)
- Pulmonary hypertension
- Ongoing weight loss despite aggressive nutritional supplementation

outcomes in the pan-resistant group were comparable to those in the US registry. Both groups had very good outcomes, leading to the conclusion that patients with more resistant *Pseudomonas* species should not be excluded from consideration for transplantation.[33] A more recent registry analysis confirmed this conclusion.[34]

There remains considerable debate regarding whether patients infected with *Burkholderia* species are appropriate candidates for lung transplantation. Studies in the 1990s indicated that individuals infected with *B. cepacia* had a high risk of posttransplant mortality, and over time, fewer and fewer transplant centers have offered transplant evaluation and listing for patients infected with *B cepacia*.[35] Over the last decade or more, LiPuma and colleagues have contributed immensely to understanding the microbiology of *Burkholderia*, first by distinguishing this group of pathogens from *Pseudomonas*, then more recently by identifying genotypically distinct species that seem to impact differently on transplant outcomes. Using 2 large databases [the CF Foundation patient registry, and the Scientific Registry of Transplant Recipients (SRTR)] to identify cohorts of over 1000 transplant candidates and more than 500 recipients, and the data available from the *Burkholderia* Research Laboratory and Repository, Murray *and colleagues* were able to assess the mortality risk of different *Burkholderia* species.[36] *Burkholderia* infection significantly impacted post-transplant survival in several ways: 1) patients infected with *Burkholderia gladioli* had a significantly higher posttransplant mortality than uninfected recipients

and recipients infected with *Burkholderia multivorans*; 2) recipients infected with *B. multivorans* before transplant had no appreciable difference in mortality compared with uninfected patients; 3) overall, transplant recipients infected with *Burkholderia cenocepacia* (n = 31) before transplant did not have an overall worse one- and 5-year survival compared with uninfected patients; 4) in contrast, subgroup analysis revealed that patients infected with nonepidemic *B. cenocepacia* strains (eg, strains other than the 2 epidemic strains in this dataset—the Midwest clone and PHDC) before transplant had a significantly higher risk of mortality compared with uninfected recipients or recipients infected with *B multivorans*. Notably, the excess mortality associated with *B gladioli* and nonepidemic strains of *B. cenocepacia* occurred in the first 6 months after transplant and were typically attributable to recurrent infection. Similar observations were reported in individuals with CF infected before transplant with *Burkholderia dolosa*.[37]

Other investigators have reported comparative analyses of transplant outcomes for individuals infected with *B cepacia* complex (Bcc) transplanted between 1990 and 2006. Survival rates for patients infected with *B. cenocepacia* were significantly lower than for those infected with other species, and patients with *B. cenocepacia* were six times more likely to die in the first year after transplantation (one year survival 89%–92% for non-*Burkholderia* and Bcc species other than *cenocepacia* vs 29% for *B. cenocepacia* infected).[38] Similarly, in a study from France, individuals infected with *B. cenocepacia* before transplant had higher mortality rates than those infected with other *Burkholderia* species, while patients infected with strains other than *cenocepacia* did not have a statistically higher mortality risk compared with those not infected with Bcc species. Three of the six deaths in patients with *cenocepacia* occurred in the postoperative period and were directly attributable to *cenocepacia* infection.[39] A recent meta-analysis of risk factors for posttransplant mortality confirmed risk associated with *cenocepacia*.[40] These cumulative data suggested that more aggressive, or alternative, antibiotic regimens targeted at preventing early infection are necessary to improve outcomes for individuals with *B. cenocepacia*. Anecdotally, newer carbapenem or cephalosporin/lactamase inhibitors have reduced early posttransplant infection with *B. cenocepacia*. In addition, further correlation of molecularly characterized species with outcomes are needed to fully resolve subtype differences and to determine definitively whether it is ethically appropriate to exclude all patients with *B. cenocepacia* from lung transplantation.

Reasonable outcomes in at least one transplant center[41] support a recommendation to refer individuals with CF and *Burkholderia spp.* and allow the transplant program to determine candidacy, rather than a common practice to not refer[10] and deny the individual an opportunity to be considered.

The impact of other less frequent Gram-negative CF pathogens is not well defined. *Stenotrophomonas* and *Achromobacter* species do not appear to pose an increased risk for early mortality.[42] Several studies have demonstrated a negative impact of infection with Methicillin-resistant *Staphylococcus aureus* (MRSA) on survival with CF,[43] but the impact of pre-transplant MRSA on post-transplant outcomes is unclear.

Fungal Pathogens

Aspergillus and other fungi are found in respiratory cultures from a significant fraction of adults with CF, but with few exceptions, do not appear to adversely impact transplant outcomes. Up to 70% of adults with CF harbor *Aspergillus fumigatus*, and Allergic Bronchopulmonary Aspergillosis may occur in up to 10% of patients over the course of their disease. Mycetomas are much less common, and true invasive aspergillosis has rarely been reported. In one recent single-center study, 70% of patients transplanted for CF had Aspergillus before transplant, and almost 40% had fungus in explanted lung cultures. The risk of invasive aspergillus after transplant was high (22%), and often temporally related to treatment of acute cellular rejection; however, preoperative aspergillus did not appreciably increase the risk for early mortality after transplant.[44] Particularly with the availability of newer azole antifungals and experience with inhaled amphotericin,[45] *Aspergillus spp.* are not considered a contraindication to lung transplant. Other fungal pathogens such as *Scedosporium spp.* are seen much less frequently and should be considered carefully given case reports of early mortality attributable to these fungi.[46]

Nontuberculous Mycobacteria

Nontuberculous mycobacteria (NTM) seem to be an increasing challenge in CF and significantly impact lung transplant candidacy. Prevalence studies at a large number of US CF Centers over a decade ago demonstrated that approximately 13% over the age of 10 had respiratory cultures with NTM, with 72% being *Mycobacterium avium* and 16% *Mycobacterium abscessus*.[47] While a decline in lung function was not appreciably different between those with and without NTM, a subset with multiple positive cultures had serial CT changes suggestive of progressive disease.[48] Differentiating colonization from infection is often difficult; however, what is clear is that individuals with *M. abscessus* who undergo transplantation are at risk for localized infections (eg, at wounds or in pleural space), and rarely, disseminated infection. Consequently, potential transplant candidates with CF and NTM colonization or infection are often deemed to be unsuitable for transplant due to the risk of infectious complications. However, data to support any NTM as an absolute contraindication for transplant are lacking, and data for the more virulent and antibiotic-resistant *M. abscessus* are generally poor, but most single center and small case series support lung transplantation in this CF population.

In one study, almost 20% of transplant referrals with CF had a history of NTM, and of the 18 patients who had NTM before transplant, 7 were culture positive after transplant.[49] However, only 4 of these had NTM disease, including 2 wound infections among 8 patients who had *M. abscessus* before transplant. Six of 8 patients with pretransplant *M. abscessus* had negative airway cultures after transplant. There were no deaths attributable to NTM and median survival among the NTM positive and negative cohorts was not appreciably different. An update reported 6 patients with *M. abscessus* disease before transplant, with 3 posttransplant mycobacterial infections, all of which were controlled with therapy and were not associated with worse survival.[50] Similar conclusions resulted from a review of 4 individuals with pretransplant *M. abscessus*; 3 developed wound infections or cutaneous abscesses and all resolved with debridement and prolonged mycobacterial therapy.[51] A similarly high frequency of postoperative infections in recipients with pretransplant *M. abscessus* was reported by others, supporting the notion that pretransplant *M. abscessus* increases posttransplant infectious risk and morbidity, without excess mortality.[52] Most recently, two centers reported acceptable outcomes in individuals with pretransplant *M. abscessus*, including those with positive cultures at time of transplant.[12,13] With the emergence of alternative agents for NTM, including clofazimine,[14] bedaquiline and bacteriophages,[15] most transplant centers and infectious disease clinicians currently take a conservative approach that potentially pathogenic NTM, particularly *M. abscessus*, be controlled with a tolerable NTM regimen before transplantation to minimize the posttransplant risk. Infection with NTM should not preclude transplant referral; however, during the transplant evaluation, individuals with CF should be educated in detail about the risk and burden of prolonged post-transplant NTM therapy when NTM are isolated within the year before transplant.

Gastrointestinal Comorbidities

A number of GI manifestations of CF potentially impact transplant candidacy and outcomes, including liver dysfunction, exocrine pancreatic insufficiency, and malnutrition. Early autopsy studies reported almost uniform focal biliary cirrhosis among adults with CF, while more recent reviews report cholestasis by laboratory testing in over a quarter of adults with CF. A very small proportion of individuals with CF (<5%), manifest cirrhosis and portal hypertension, with the majority recognized before adulthood. While the natural history of cirrhosis in CF seems to be relatively indolent, perhaps due to aggressive use of ursodeoxycholic acid for cholestasis in CF, most individuals with cirrhosis complicating CF can be managed medically and/or endoscopically, and do not require liver transplantation.[16–18] A number of adults with CF are known to have cirrhosis and/or portal hypertension before referral for lung transplantation or are found to have varying degrees of liver dysfunction during the evaluation process. Patients with liver disease limited to cholestasis are generally deemed low risk for perioperative liver decompensation. However, patients with cirrhosis are more controversial, as many are prematurely deemed unsuitable for isolated lung transplantation.

Data on the impact of cirrhosis are limited to small case series, making evidence-based decisions regarding lung transplantation with CF liver disease difficult. A recent case-control series strongly suggested that selected patients with CF and advanced liver disease can undergo uneventful lung transplantation without concomitant liver transplantation. Six patients with CF and liver cirrhosis, defined as esophageal varices, imaging evidence of cirrhosis, and/or splenomegaly or diagnostic histology, underwent isolated lung transplantation, with no appreciable difference in perioperative complications or survival compared with a matched control group.[18] Notably, none of the 6 patients with cirrhosis, with Model for End-stage Liver Disease (MELD) scores ranging from 27 to 34 and Child-Pugh scores of 5 to 8, exhibited decompensation of liver disease in the first 4 years after lung transplantation.[18] This single-center experience at a high volume lung transplant program demonstrates the feasibility of isolated lung transplant with CF and cirrhosis. Experience at the authors' institution is similar. For 16 patients with CF and Child's A or B cirrhosis who underwent isolated lung transplantation, there were no perioperative mortalities. The published and anecdotal experiences at high-volume transplant centers indicate that concomitant lung liver transplant is likely only necessary when there is significant synthetic hepatocellular dysfunction and uncontrolled complications of CF liver disease. Therefore, most individuals with CF and mild cirrhosis should not be declined for lung transplant due to liver disease. Because it is often challenging to obtain lung and liver *en bloc* in the US, it is critical to better define the severity of CF liver disease that precludes isolated lung transplantation. For the few individuals who require combined lung liver transplant, survival seems comparable to lung only transplant recipients.[19]

Pancreatic insufficiency and malnutrition are more common GI complications of CF. Pancreatic insufficiency affects > 85% of adults with CF, thus lung transplantation in individuals with CF who are pancreatic sufficient is relatively uncommon. Surprisingly, one recent review demonstrated that pancreatic sufficient transplant recipients have a higher risk of mortality than those who are pancreatic insufficient, and malnutrition (BMI <18.5) was not associated with worse outcomes.[41] The latter contradicts the conclusion of an earlier study using a larger registry cohort which demonstrated an approximately 10% lower 5-year survival for patients with CF who were had a BMI <18.5 compared with a cohort with normal pretransplant BMI.[20] However, even individuals with a BMI <17 were recently demonstrated to have comparable survival to recipients with pulmonary fibrosis,[21] suggesting that mild malnutrition in itself should not preclude lung transplant referral and listing. Further studies that examine both nutritional status as assessed by BMI, and by markers of protein and fat-soluble vitamin deficiency, are necessary, as are studies of Vitamin D deficiency and transplant outcomes.[22] While many US transplant centers will not offer lung transplant to patients with BMI <18, most view this marker as at most a relative contraindication and often modifiable risk factor for poorer outcomes after lung transplantation. Highly effective CFTR modulators are likely to significantly reduce the incidence of malnutrition in CF, including those with advanced lung disease.

Sinus Disease

Sinus disease, manifesting as chronic sinusitis with or without nasal polyposis, is nearly ubiquitous in CF, particularly those with advanced lung disease. Very few studies have attempted to determine the impact of CF sinus disease on transplant outcomes. It is assumed that the sinuses in patients with CF provide a reservoir for bacterial pathogens that predisposes patients to lower airway colonization or infection and may contribute to allograft dysfunction and worse post-transplant outcomes. In a recent study, cultures of the sinuses of lung recipients with CF after transplantation were compared with lower airway cultures; there was significant concordance in isolates from sinus aspirates and bronchoscopic cultures,[53,54] which is consistent with the reservoir hypothesis. Moreover, patients who underwent sinus surgery followed by routine nasal douches had a higher incidence of negative sinus and lower airway Pseudomonas colonization after transplantation, and improved survival and freedom from higher-grade bronchiolitis obliterans syndrome/chronic rejection. These findings corroborate earlier reports that lung recipients with CF and Pseudomonas colonization after transplantation had worse outcomes compared with a Pseudomonas-negative cohort.[55,56] These findings suggest that outcomes after transplant in patients with CF may be improved by preventive measures against lower airway infection, particularly with the management of sinus disease, and perhaps routine mucosal antibiotics to prevent lower airway colonization and infection, and judicious endoscopic sinus surgery.[56–60]

Osteoporosis

Osteoporosis is common in advanced lung disease, and osteoporosis with fractures has long been considered a relative contraindication to lung transplantation. In adults with CF, osteoporosis is very common, with mean average bone mineral densities two standard deviations below an age-matched control population.[61] Individuals with CF had increased fracture rates, particularly vertebral-compression and rib fractures, and a surprisingly high incidence of kyphosis associated with loss of height. While the possible mechanisms for this high rate of severe bone disease in a young population are not fully defined, vitamin D deficiency, malnutrition, early puberty, glucocorticoid exposure, and chronic inflammation are favored mechanisms. The implication of these potential risk factors for osteoporosis for transplantation is that the fracture risk is often high before transplant and may increase further with the required immunosuppressive regimen following transplantation. Some studies have demonstrated safety and efficacy for bisphosphonates in conjunction with vitamin D and calcium supplementation to improve bone mineral density in adults with CF.[62,63] Thus, for most transplant centers, osteoporosis is perceived as a remediable comorbidity, and only

uncontrolled pain related to fractures is considered a contraindication to lung transplantation.

Diabetes

Cystic fibrosis-related diabetes (CFRD) is the most common comorbidity in individuals with CF, occurring in approximately 20% of adolescents and 40% to 50% of adults.[64] CFRD is associated with worse lung function, more chest infections, overall poorer nutrition, and increased mortality irrespective of lung transplantation.[65] New onset diabetes occurs in approximately 38% of patients without pre-existing CFRD following lung transplantation. Potential candidates with CF should be counseled about the risk of developing diabetes following transplantation. In one study, both *de novo* and pre-existing diabetes were associated with an increased risk of death following transplantation.[66] However, a more recent analysis did not demonstrate an impact of diabetes on transplant outcomes for recipients with CF.[41] Poorly controlled diabetes is considered by many to be a relative contraindication for lung transplantation, as this poor control may be a surrogate for adherence with medical therapies. Aggressive treatment of diabetes is strongly recommended before, and following lung transplantation. However, further studies evaluating the impact that tight glycemic control has on overall survival after transplant are warranted.

Listing for Lung Transplantation

From the provider perspective, the decision to recommend that an individual with CF and advanced lung disease be listed for transplant is complex and should consider the rate of decline in pulmonary function, frequency of exacerbations, complications such as pneumothorax and hemoptysis, troublesome pathogens, and the development of awake hypercapnia, hypoxemia, and/or pulmonary hypertension. Current recommendations from the International Society of Heart and Lung Transplantation are based on small studies and expert opinion consensus [23] (see **Box 3**).

Listing for lung transplantation should be considered when survival from respiratory-related complications from CF is anticipated to be less than survival after lung transplantation. The decision on when to list is best a mutual one based on the informed and detailed discussion between the individual with CF, the CF physician, and the transplant team. Limitations in predicting 1-year survival without a transplant preclude data-driven decision-making to identify the time point at which survival with a transplant exceeds survival with CF. Compounding this problem is the unpredictability of waiting time once placed on the lung transplant list. Wait times vary from days to months to years, and while the Lung Allocation System (LAS) in the US attempts to prioritize organs for individuals with the highest risk of 1-year mortality, up to 15% of individuals with CF die while waiting for transplant. Ideally, transplant should occur before the onset of respiratory failure and the need for mechanical ventilation or extracorporeal support, to reduce morbidity and maximize transplant survival. Lastly, the decision of when to list is challenged by the increasing experience of individuals with CF and advanced lung disease suffering rapid decline to respiratory failure when seemingly stable clinically. In some instances, there is a clear precipitant to the acute decline, such as an infectious exacerbation or pneumonia, hemoptysis, pneumothorax or viral infection, pulmonary embolism; however, in others, a clear precipitant cannot be identified. Ultimately, the decision to list and proceed with transplant must be mutual and consider access to and response to highly effective CFTR modulator, anticipated survival, quality of life, patient preferences, and transplant program experience with transplanting individuals with respiratory failure.

Transplant Waitlist and Lung Allocation

The time from transplant listing to transplant is highly variable; however, changes in the allocation of lungs since 2005 have attempted to minimize waiting time for the sickest transplant candidates to reduce the chances of death while awaiting transplant.[67–70] Unfortunately, the LAS remains limited in its ability to identify patients most likely to benefit from transplantation. Waitlist time currently varies from days to 1 to 2 years, with lung candidates with smaller chest cavities waiting longer, and those with severe hypoxemia and acute respiratory failure waiting shorter times. Most individuals with CF require supplemental oxygen and have advanced pulmonary impairment before achieving a sufficiently high LAS to receive donor lungs, and based on practices at most transplant centers, individuals with CF undergo transplant in the several weeks to months after listing.

Given the variable waiting, after addition to the UNOS lung transplant waitlist, transplant candidates are assessed regularly by the lung transplant program and undergo updated testing approximately every 3 months, in parallel with maximizing conditioning and medical therapy for their underlying medical problems. Most transplant programs

require regular exercise or pulmonary rehabilitation. Also, maintenance of optimal nutrition and good control of extrapulmonary manifestations of CF, including sinusitis and diabetes, is important to transplant candidates achieving optimal transplant outcomes with low morbidity. Communication between the CF team and transplant team, on a regular basis and more acutely with changes in clinical status, is critical to ensuring that lung transplant candidates remain candidates for transplant and enjoy good outcomes.

Mechanical Support as a Bridge to Lung Transplantation

Historically, the requirement of mechanical ventilation had been considered to be a relative contraindication to lung transplantation as mechanical ventilation before lung transplantation was associated with an increased risk of mortality in the first year after lung transplantation. However, in individuals with CF, the risk attributed to mechanical ventilation has been controversial, with some reports, suggesting that mechanical ventilation may be associated with a longer intensive care unit stay, and longer need for mechanical ventilation postlung transplantation without a significant change in overall survival.[71,72] Noninvasive ventilation is useful to control respiratory acidosis and has been helpful to support patients with advanced lung disease while waiting for lung transplantation. Noninvasive ventilation in patients with CF before lung transplantation is not associated with any adverse outcomes postlung transplant.[73,74] In recent years, accumulating experience indicates that extracorporeal membrane oxygenation (ECMO) is useful as a bridge to lung transplantation with comparable postlung transplantation short, and mid-term outcomes, as well as low mortality.[75,76] Newer ECMO strategies, including the use of a dual-lumen single cannula which allows for ambulatory veno-venous ECMO, can be conducted in awake, spontaneously breathing patients, and allow for oral intake and participation in physical therapy.[77] In general, mechanical support can be efficacious as a bridge to lung transplantation, and perhaps as a bridge to recovery, in experienced centers with adequate resources.

Survival and Quality of Life Concerns

Survival in CF is determined by multiple interactive factors involving the respiratory system and lung transplantation is widely accepted as an appropriate option for many individuals with CF who have a high risk of short-term mortality since there is a clear survival benefit.[78–81]

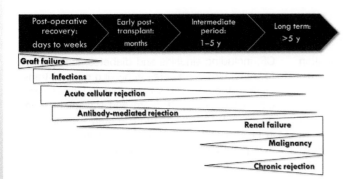

Fig. 2. Complications of lung transplant.

The median survival from lung transplantation in the international registry for individuals with CF is approaching 10 years, which is significantly better than patients who were transplanted in earlier eras, or for other diseases such as chronic obstructive pulmonary disease and pulmonary fibrosis.[1] Patients with CF who survive beyond the first year have a median survival of well more than 10 years.[1] This may reflect the overall younger age and less cardiac and renal comorbidity of CF recipients, in comparison to other lung transplant recipients. The major causes of death within the first year following lung transplantation, irrespective of pretransplant lung disease, involve technical problems, primary graft dysfunction resulting, ultimately, in graft failure, and acute infections. Infections account for approximately 35% of deaths between 1 month and 1 year following lung transplantation. After the first year, bronchiolitis obliterans syndrome, the major form of chronic lung allograft dysfunction (CLAD), and noncytomegalovirus infections account for most of the deaths.[1]

Prior studies have documented worsening health-related quality of life in patients with CF as lung function declines.[82,83] Patients with CF are younger, spend more days on the waiting list, and are more likely to be working or going to school in comparison to other patients on the lung transplant waiting list.[84] However, in comparison to other patients with other end-stage lung diseases, patients with CF waiting for lung transplantation have lower levels of anxiety, higher levels of social support, and use more functional coping strategies.[85] Following lung transplantation, patients with CF report better quality of life, including physical and social functioning, treatment burden, and chest symptoms.[86,87] In addition, energy level and sleep quality are also significantly improved following lung transplantation.[84] In general, patients with CF have the same improvements in overall quality of life in comparison to patients with other solid organ transplants.[88]

Complications of Lung Transplant

Most individuals who undergo transplants have one or more complications, ranging from the time of transplant to many years later. **Fig. 2** provides a high-level overview of the more common complications and their relative time line. Surgical complications from the transplant itself include bleeding from pleural adhesions and coagulopathy from platelet and coagulation factor consumption that may require significant transfusions, distributive shock from the release of endotoxin during the manipulation of the recipient lungs, acute kidney injury, and primary graft dysfunction (PGD). Progress in surgical techniques and the use of extracorporeal membrane oxygenation (ECMO) in lieu of cardiopulmonary bypass has the potential to reduce these early complications. With improved techniques to identify recipient antibodies against HLA antigens and avoidance of these antigens (referred to as a 'virtual crossmatch'), hyperacute rejection caused by antibody deposition and complement-mediated lung injury is exceedingly rare. In contrast, PGD, defined as hypoxemia related to capillary leak and inflammatory changes,[89–93] occurs in more than 50% of lung transplants, but severe PGD is uncommon. With supportive measures that may include postoperative ECMO, PGD typically resolves over a period of days to weeks, and many transplant recipients who had significant PGD at the time of transplant recover to long-term survival.[90] Airway ischemia-reperfusion injury (IRI) occurs to varying degrees[94] and results from poor perfusion of the airway associated with loss of the bronchial circulation. The airway wall and mucosa typically heal, however, airway IRI may lead to bronchial stenosis that requires balloon dilatation and/or endobronchial stents. Given these potential complications, the duration of mechanical ventilation and need for tracheostomy varies widely, but most lung transplant recipients require < 3 to 5 days of ventilator support and < 10% require posttransplant tracheostomy to provide support as PGD resolves.[95]

Infections are a common complication after lung transplant and may occur at any time. Donor-derived and early postoperative pneumonia and empyema are uncommon with antibiotic prophylaxis, despite many recipients with CF having multi-drug or pan-resistant bacterial pathogens in the native airways. Avoiding early bacterial infections with inhaled antibiotics and typically a several week course of intravenous antibiotics has made early post-transplant pneumonia uncommon. After the initial transplant, the lung allograft is susceptible to a broad range of infections, including viral (opportunistic such as CMV to community-acquired viruses such as coronaviruses, influenza, parainfluenza, and Respiratory Syncytial Virus), bacterial (in CF, often typical CF pathogens that are likely related to residual bacteria in the sinuses), mycobacterial (*M. avium intracellulare* and *M. abscessus* in particular), and opportunistic (fungi such as *Aspergillus fumigatus* and *S spp.*, *Nocardia spp.*, *Pneumocystis jiroveci*, and others). Extrapulmonary infections may be more frequent after lung transplant; particularly in CF, acute and chronic sinusitis that may prove difficult to manage. A variety of systemic viral infections may occur after transplant, including reactivation or primary infection with Epstein Barr Virus that may lead to posttransplant lymphoproliferative disorder (PTLD), and CMV in the retina or GI tract with or without pneumonitis. Thus, infection remains a significant cause of morbidity and mortality after lung transplant.

Acute cellular rejection (ACR) is relatively common complication of lung transplant, as ~40% of recipients require augmented immunosuppression to resolve cellular rejection and potentially reduce the risk of more chronic rejection. The standard for preventing ACR is maintenance immunosuppression that typically consists of a calcineurin inhibitor (tacrolimus or cyclosporine), an antimetabolite (mycophenolate or azathioprine), and a corticosteroid (prednisone). Less commonly, a mTOR inhibitor such as everolimus or sirolimus is a component of maintenance immunosuppression. Despite broad immunosuppression, ACR is common in the first few years after transplant. ACR may manifest as respiratory or systemic symptoms, such as cough, fever, malaise, shortness of breath, and decline in lung function, or ACR may be asymptomatic. Consequently, most lung transplant programs perform surveillance transbronchial biopsy at defined intervals after transplant to detect ACR. Antibody-mediated rejection, caused by recipient antibodies against donor HLA or other antigens, occurs less commonly than cellular rejection and may require antibody depletion with plasmapheresis and therapies such as rituximab, bortezomib, or carfilzomib to deplete antibody-producing B and plasma cells. As donor-specific antibodies increase the risk of chronic rejection and are associated with shortened survival, techniques to detect and deplete donor-directed antibodies may improve posttransplant survival.

The primary cause of longer-term death after lung transplant is chronic rejection, recently recategorized within the broad term, Chronic Lung Allograft Dysfunction (CLAD). Based on current consensus among lung transplant experts,[100,101] CLAD consists of chronic fibrosis involving either or both compartments of the lung: 1) fibrosis of the airways- Bronchiolitis Obliterans Syndrome, BOS—known pathologically as Obliterative Bronchiolitis and physiologically as progressive airway obstruction, and/or 2) fibrosis involving the lung parenchyma— restrictive allograft syndrome (RAS)—causing restrictive physiology and manifest as subpleural fibrotic changes in imaging. The pathophysiology of CLAD remains to be defined; however, the current paradigm is that CLAD results from recipient immune cells or antibodies injuring the allograft airway or alveolar compartments to cause loss of lung function. While new techniques to identify early CLAD with blood or bronchoalveolar lavage or bronchial brush molecular signatures [119] or imaging, such as Parametric Response Monitoring (PRM) are in progress,[96] much work remains to define pathogenesis and optimal treatments. Azithromycin,[97] and perhaps montelukast[98] appear to be useful adjuncts to maintenance immunosuppression; however, augmenting immunosuppression often leads to infections and the role of steroids and other immunosuppressive agents in the treatment of CLAD is unclear. New therapies for the treatment of CLAD are in clinical trials, including inhaled cyclosporine and extracorporeal photopheresis. Survival after the development of CLAD remains highly variable, from a few months to many years with a median of 3 to 4 years for double lung recipients,[99] and many individuals with CLAD after transplant for CF succumb to respiratory failure or require retransplantation.

Opportunities for Improved Transplant Outcomes

Despite improvements in surgical techniques that have reduced early mortality after lung transplantation, long-term survival remains poor relative to other solid organ transplants, with 5 and 10-year survivals estimated at 65% and 50%, respectively, based on registries.[1,41] Improvements in 1-year survival have not translated to improved long-term survival due to the high frequency of CLAD that is most commonly manifest as bronchiolitis obliterans pathologically and progressive obstructive lung disease physiologically. Potential explanations for the lack of progress in preventing this common complication are infrequent patient follow-up with physicians trained in transplantation, resulting in the late recognition of chronic rejection; lack of available biomarkers for early allograft dysfunction; wide variability in transplant center experience with transplant for CF; poor insight to the pathophysiology of chronic rejection; and lack of defined optimal immunosuppressive regimens to prevent chronic rejection. The observation that there are differences in transplant outcomes between US centers[1] and across national boundaries[41,103,104] suggest that benchmarking to identify best practices for posttransplant monitoring and care, and comanagement of the individual with CF after lung transplantation may be productive. Also, the creation of a detailed registry of transplant outcomes, akin to the CF patient registry that has facilitated comparative effectiveness research and helped transform routine CF care, may provide critical observations that could improve the quality of posttransplant care, establish standard therapies that will facilitate multi-center clinical trials of new interventions, and ultimately improve the long-term survival for lung transplant recipients with CF.

Routine Care of the Posttransplant Patient by the Cystic Fibrosis Team

After lung transplant, longitudinal care of the individual with CF who has undergone a transplant is optimal when the transplant and CF teams collaborate. Concensus statements on care of the individual with CF after lung transplant were recently published [117]. Unless the lung transplant physician is also a CF provider, routine visits to both transplant and CF centers are encouraged to capitalize on the complementary areas of expertise. Establishing mutual expectations and maintaining regular communication are important to seamless posttransplant care. The transplant team should make all decisions regarding pulmonary care, including immunosuppression management, prophylactic antibiotics, and treatment of acute infections. Typically, the CF team manages nonpulmonary manifestations of CF, including sinus disease, nutrition, bone disease, and in the absence of an endocrinologist with experience in CF, diabetes. CF lung transplant recipients monitor lung function at home and/or in the pulmonary function laboratory at regular intervals to assess allograft function, and typically are assigned a lung transplant coordinator for all communications on transplant-related issues and hospitalizations. The lung recipient or CF team should inform the transplant team of any acute illnesses, hospitalizations, and medication changes to avoid unwanted drug interactions and decide whether transfer to the transplant hospital is appropriate in lieu of local care; the transplant team should provide regular communication to the CF team on recipient progress and complications. Lastly, other members of the CF and transplant teams, such as social workers, mental health providers, and dieticians, often benefit from communication with one another on problems to optimize care plans.

Use of Cystic Fibrosis Transmembrane Conductance Regulator Modulators After Lung Transplant

A difficult decision is whether and when to resume highly effective CFTR modulators after transplant. Most individuals with CF have improved nutrition after transplant without the use of a CFTR modulator, and there are drug interactions with azoles and calcineurin inhibitors that make use of IVA or ETI after transplant complex and are potentially risky. Since the recipient's lungs are genetically normal, the potential indications for resuming IVA or ETI after transplant are for improved nutrition, sinus disease refractory to medical and surgical therapy, and in rare circumstances, glycemic control. Experience thus far suggests that the initiation of ETI is associated with modest weight gain[116]. Notably, early experience suggests that ETI is not tolerated in up to a third of lung transplant recipients[116], in marked contrast to use before transplant whereby the intolerance rate is < 5%. Additional registry data are necessary to better define the use of IVA or ETI after lung transplant. In the interim, this author recommends that ivacaftor or ETI be used after lung transplant only for extra-pulmonary manifestations that are refractory to other medical and surgical interventions. Examples are severe sinus disease contributing to lung allograft function or poor quality of life and malnutrition. Modulators should be prescribed only after discussion between the CF and transplant providers, with the consideration of risk/benefit and important drug–drug interactions such as those occurring through the cytochrome P450 system (eg, calcineurin inhibitors, azoles, and CFTR modulators).

SUMMARY

Lung transplantation is a viable option for individuals with CF and end-stage lung disease. Despite comorbidities including infections with multi-drug resistant organisms, diabetes, and gastrointestinal complications, adults with CF clearly benefit from lung transplantation in terms of quantity and quality of life. Further studies are needed to optimize referral, candidate selection, lung allocation,[102] and posttransplant management to further improve outcomes following lung transplantation. Additional opportunities for research and discussion include mechanisms to prevent allograft colonization with CF pathogens, immune responses of transplant recipients with CF, and the effect that socioeconomic status and health care systems influence access to lung transplantation and outcomes.[5,41,103,104]

CLINICS CARE POINTS

- Despite significant advances in treatments for CF, lung disease in CF is generally progressive and leads to premature death

- Predicting survival for individuals with advanced CF lung disease, defined as $FEV_1 < 40\%$ predicted, is difficult so discussion of all treatment options is critical

- Lung transplant is a treatment option for many individuals with CF who suffer from severe lung disease, with median survival after transplant now approaching 10 years

- Determination of who is an acceptable lung transplant candidate varies among transplant centers and decisions on candidacy are best deferred to transplant centers rather than determined by CF care teams

- Early referral for transplant is critical to optimize the chance of having a successful transplant before dying of CF lung disease

- Optimal care of individuals with CF after lung transplant is achieved through collaboration between a transplant team and CF team

DISCLOSURE

The author has nothing to disclose.

REFERENCES

1. Chambers DC, Perch M, Zuckerman A, et al. The International Thoracic Organ Transplant Registry of the International Society for Heart and Lung Transplantation: Thirty-eighth adult lung transplantation report - 2021; Focus on recipient characteristics. J Heart Lung Transpl 2021; 40(10):1060–72.

2. MacKenzie T, Gifford AH, Sabadosa KA, et al. Longevity of patients with cystic fibrosis in 2000 to 2010 and beyond: survival analysis of the Cystic Fibrosis Foundation patient registry. Ann Intern Med 2014;161:233–41.

3. Valapour M, Lehr CJ, Skeans MA, et al. OPTN/ SRTR 2017 annual data report: lung. Am J Transpl 2019 Feb;19(Suppl 2):404–84.

4. Kerem E, Reisman J, Corey M, et al. Prediction of mortality in patients with cystic fibrosis. New Engl J Med 1992;326:1187–91.

5. Ramos KJ, Quon BS, Heltshe SL, et al. Heterogeneity in survival in adult patients with cystic fibrosis with $FEV_1 < 30\%$ of predicted in the United States. Chest 2017;151(6):1320–8.

6. Middleton PG, Mall MA, Dřevínek P, et al. VX17-445-102 Study Group. Elexacaftor-Tezacaftor-Ivacaftor for Cystic Fibrosis with a Single Phe508del Allele. N Engl J Med 2019;381(19): 1809–19.

7. Heijerman HGM, McKone EF, Downey DG, et al. VX17-445-103 Trial Group. Efficacy and safety of the elexacaftor plus tezacaftor plus ivacaftor combination regimen in people with cystic fibrosis homozygous for the F508del mutation: a double-blind, randomised, phase 3 trial. Lancet 2019 pii; S0140-6736(19):32597–8.

8. Mayer-Hamblett N, Rosenfeld M, Emerson J, et al. Developing cystic fibrosis lung transplant referral criteria using predictors of 2-year mortality. Am J Respir Crit Care Med 2002;166: 1550–5.

9. Augarten A, Akons H, Aviram M, et al. Prediction of mortality and timing of referral for lung transplantation in cystic fibrosis patients. Pediatr Transplant 2001;5:339–42.

10. Ramos KJ, Somayaji R, Lease ED, et al. Cystic fibrosis physicians' perspectives on the timing of referral for lung transplant evaluation: a survey of physicians in the United States. BMC Pulm Med 2017 Jan 19;17(1):21. https://doi.org/10.1186/s12890-017-0367-9.

11. Ramos KJ, Smith PJ, McKone EF, et al. CF lung transplant referral guidelines committee. Lung transplant referral for individuals with cystic fibrosis: cystic fibrosis foundation consensus guidelines. J Cyst Fibros 2019;18(3):321–33.

12. Perez AA, Singer JP, Schwartz BS, et al. Management and clinical outcomes after lung transplantation in patients with pre-transplant Mycobacterium abscessus infection: a single center experience. Transpl Infect Dis. 2019;21(3):e13084

13. Raats D, Lorent N, Saegeman V, et al. Successful lung transplantation for chronic Mycobacterium

abscessus infection in advanced cystic fibrosis, a case series. Transpl Infect Dis. 2019;21(2):e13046.

14. Hamad Y, Pilewski JM, Morrell M, et al. Outcomes in lung transplant recipients with Mycobacterium abscessus infection: a 15-year experience from a large Tertiary care center. Transpl Proc. 2019; 51(6):2035-2042.

15. Dedrick RM, Guerrero-Bustamante CA, Garlena RA, et al. Engineered bacteriophages for treatment of a patient with a disseminated drug-resistant Mycobacterium abscessus. Nat Med. 2019;25(5): 730-733.

16. Nash KL, Allison ME, McKeon D, et al. A single centre experience of liver disease in adults with cystic fibrosis 1995-2006. J cystic fibrosis : official J Eur Cystic Fibrosis Soc 2008;7:252-257.

17. Rowland M, Gallagher CG, O'Laoide R, et al. Outcome in cystic fibrosis liver disease. Am J Gastroenterol 2011;106:104-109.

18. Nash EF, Volling C, Gutierrez CA, et al. Outcomes of patients with cystic fibrosis undergoing lung transplantation with and without cystic fibrosis-associated liver cirrhosis. Clin Transplant 2012;26: 34-41.

19. Salman J, Grannas G, Ius F, et al. The liver-first approach for combined lung and liver transplantation. Eur J Cardiothorac Surg. 2018;54(6):1122-1127

20. Lederer DJ, Wilt JS, D'Ovidio F, et al. Obesity and underweight are associated with an increased risk of death after lung transplantation. Am J Respir Crit Care Med 2009;180:887-895.

21. Ramos KJ, Kapnadak SG, Bradford MC, et al. Underweight patients with cystic fibrosis are suitable candidates for lung transplantation. Chest 2020; 157:898-906.

22. Lowery EM, Bemiss B, Cascino T, et al. Low vitamin D levels are associated with increased rejection and infections after lung transplantation. J Heart Lung Transplant 2012;31:700-7.

23. Leard LE, Holm AM, Valapour M, et al. Consensus document for the selection of lung transplant candidates: An update from the International Society for Heart and Lung Transplantation. J Heart Lung Transplant 2021;40:1349-79.

24. Mendeloff EN, Huddleston CB, Mallory GB, et al. Pediatric and adult lung transplantation for cystic fibrosis. J Thorac Cardiovasc Surg 1998;115: 404-13. ; discussion 13-4.

25. Shennib H, Noirclerc M, Ernst P, et al. Double-lung transplantation for cystic fibrosis. The cystic fibrosis transplant study group. Ann Thorac Surg 1992;54:27-31.

26. Venuta F, Diso D, Anile M, et al. Evolving techniques and perspectives in lung transplantation. Transplant Proc 2005;37:2682-3.

27. Meyers BF, Sundaresan RS, Guthrie T, et al. Bilateral sequential lung transplantation without sternal division eliminates posttransplantation sternal complications. The J Thorac Cardiovasc Surg 1999; 117:358-64.

28. Cohen RG, Barr ML, Schenkel FA, et al. Living-related donor lobectomy for bilateral lobar transplantation in patients with cystic fibrosis. Ann Thorac Surg 1994;57:1423-7. ; discussion 8.

29. Date H, Sato M, Aoyama A, et al. Living-donor lobar lung transplantation provides similar survival to cadaveric lung transplantation even for very ill patients. Eur J cardio-thoracic Surg : official J Eur Assoc Cardio-thoracic Surg 2015;47: 967-73.

30. Battafarano RJ, Anderson RC, Meyers BF, et al. Perioperative complications after living donor lobectomy. J Thorac Cardiovasc Surg 2000;120: 909-15.

31. Flume PA, Strange C, Ye X, et al. Pneumothorax in cystic fibrosis. Chest 2005;128:720-8.

32. Meachery G, De Soyza A, Nicholson A, et al. Outcomes of lung transplantation for cystic fibrosis in a large UK cohort. Thorax 2008;63:725-731.

33. Hadjiliadis D, Steele MP, Chaparro C, et al. Survival of lung transplant patients with cystic fibrosis harboring panresistant bacteria other than Burkholderia cepacia, compared with patients harboring sensitive bacteria. J Heart Lung Transplant : official Publ Int Soc Heart Transplant 2007;26:834-838.

34. Lay C, Law N, Holm AM, et al. Outcomes in cystic fibrosis lung transplant recipients infected with organisms labeled as pan-resistant: an ISHLT Registry-based analysis. J Heart Lung Transpl 2019 May;38(5):545-52.

35. Aris RM, Gilligan PH, Neuringer IP, et al. The effects of panresistant bacteria in cystic fibrosis patients on lung transplant outcome. Am J Respir Crit Care Med 1997;155:1699-704.

36. Murray S, Charbeneau J, Marshall BC, et al. Impact of burkholderia infection on lung transplantation in cystic fibrosis. Am J Respir Crit Care Med 2008; 178:363-71.

37. Wang R, Welsh SK, Budev M, et al. Survival after lung transplantation of cystic fibrosis patients infected with Burkholderia dolosa (genomovar VI). Clin Transpl 2018 May;32(5):e13236.

38. Alexander BD, Petzold EW, Reller LB, et al. Survival after lung transplantation of cystic fibrosis patients infected with Burkholderia cepacia complex. Am J Transplant 2008;8:1025-30.

39. Boussaud V, Guillemain R, Grenet D, et al. Clinical outcome following lung transplantation in patients with cystic fibrosis colonised with Burkholderia cepacia complex: results from two French centres. Thorax 2008;63:732-737.

40. Koutsokera A, Varughese RA, Sykes J, et al. Pretransplant factors associated with mortality after

lung transplantation in cystic fibrosis: a systematic review and meta-analysis. J Cyst Fibros 2019 May; 18(3):407–15.

41. Stephenson AL, Sykes J, Berthiaume Y, et al. Clinical and demographic factors associated with post-lung transplantation survival in individuals with cystic fibrosis. J Heart Lung Transpl 2015 Sep; 34(9):1139–45.

42. Lobo LJ, Tulu Z, Aris RM, et al. Pan-resistant achromobacter xylosoxidans and Stenotrophomonas maltophilia infection in cystic fibrosis does not reduce survival after lung transplantation. Transplantation 2015;99(10):2196–202.

43. Dasenbrook EC, Checkley W, Merlo CA, et al. Association between respiratory tract methicillin-resistant Staphylococcus aureus and survival in cystic fibrosis. JAMA 2010;303:2386–92.

44. Luong ML, Chaparro C, Stephenson A, et al. Pre-transplant Aspergillus colonization of cystic fibrosis patients and the incidence of post-lung transplant invasive aspergillosis. Transplantation 2014;97:351–7.

45. Peghin M, Monforte V, Martin-Gomez MT, et al. 10 years of prophylaxis with nebulized liposomal amphotericin B and the changing epidemiology of Aspergillus spp. infection in lung transplantation. Transpl Int 2016 Jan;29(1):51–62.

46. Symoens F, Knoop C, Schrooyen M, et al. Disseminated Scedosporium apiospermum infection in a cystic fibrosis patient after double-lung transplantation. J Heart Lung Transplant : official Publ Int Soc Heart Transplant 2006;25:603–7.

47. Olivier KN, Weber DJ, Wallace RJ Jr, et al. Nontuberculous mycobacteria. I: multicenter prevalence study in cystic fibrosis. Am J Respir Crit Care Med 2003;167:828–34.

48. Olivier KN, Weber DJ, Lee JH, et al. Nontuberculous mycobacteria. II: nested-cohort study of impact on cystic fibrosis lung disease. Am J Crit Care Med 2003;167:835–40.

49. Chalermskulrat W, Sood N, Neuringer IP, et al. Nontuberculous mycobacteria in end stage cystic fibrosis: implications for lung transplantation. Thorax 2006;61:507–13.

50. Lobo LJ, Chang LC, Esther CR Jr, et al. Lung transplant outcomes in cystic fibrosis patients with pre-operative Mycobacterium abscessus respiratory infections. Clin Transplant 2013;27:523–9.

51. Gilljam M, Scherstén H, Silverborn M, et al. Lung transplantation in patients with cystic fibrosis and Mycobacterium abscessus infection. J cystic fibrosis 2010;9:272–6.

52. Qvist T, Pressler T, Thomsen VO, et al. Nontuberculous mycobacterial disease is not a contraindication to lung transplantation in patients with cystic fibrosis: a retrospective analysis in a Danish patient population. Transplant Proc 2013;45:342–5.

53. Vital D, Hofer M, Benden C, et al. Impact of sinus surgery on pseudomonal airway colonization, bronchiolitis obliterans syndrome and survival in cystic fibrosis lung transplant recipients. Respiration; Int Rev Thorac Dis 2013;86:25–31.

54. Vos R, Vanaudenaerde BM, Geudens N, et al. Pseudomonal airway colonisation: risk factor for bronchiolitis obliterans syndrome after lung transplantation? The Eur Respir J 2008;31:1037–45.

55. Botha P, Archer L, Anderson RL, et al. Pseudomonas aeruginosa colonization of the allograft after lung transplantation and the risk of bronchiolitis obliterans syndrome. Transplantation 2008;85:771–4.

56. Vital D, Hofer M, Boehler A, et al. Posttransplant sinus surgery in lung transplant recipients with cystic fibrosis: a single institutional experience. Eur Arch Otorhinolaryngol 2013;270:135–9.

57. Aanaes K, von Buchwald C, Hjuler T, et al. The effect of sinus surgery with intensive follow-up on pathogenic sinus bacteria in patients with cystic fibrosis. Am J Rhinol Allergy 2013;27:e1–4.

58. Virgin FW, Rowe SM, Wade MB, et al. Extensive surgical and comprehensive postoperative medical management for cystic fibrosis chronic rhinosinusitis. Am J Rhinol Allergy 2012;26:70–5.

59. Liang J, Higgins T, Ishman SL, et al. Medical management of chronic rhinosinusitis in cystic fibrosis: a systematic review. Laryngoscope 2014;124:1308–13.

60. Alanin MC, Aanaes K, Høiby N, et al. Sinus surgery postpones chronic Gram-negative lung infection: cohort study of 106 patients with cystic fibrosis. Rhinology 2016;54:206–13.

61. Aris RM, Renner JB, Winders AD, et al. Increased rate of fractures and severe kyphosis: sequelae of living into adulthood with cystic fibrosis. Ann Intern Med 1998;128:186–93.

62. Aris RM, Lester GE, Renner JB, et al. Efficacy of pamidronate for osteoporosis in patients with cystic fibrosis following lung transplantation. Am J Respir Crit Care Med 2000;162:941–6.

63. Aris RM, Lester GE, Caminiti M, et al. Efficacy of alendronate in adults with cystic fibrosis with low bone density. Am J Respir Crit Care Med 2004;169:77–82.

64. Moran A, Dunitz J, Nathan B, et al. Cystic fibrosis-related diabetes: current trends in prevalence, incidence, and mortality. Diabetes care 2009;32:1626–31.

65. Brennan AL, Geddes DM, Gyi KM, et al. Clinical importance of cystic fibrosis-related diabetes. J cystic fibrosis : official J Eur Cystic Fibrosis Soc 2004;3:209–22.

66. Hackman KL, Bailey MJ, Snell GI, et al. Diabetes is a major risk factor for mortality after lung

transplantation. Am J Transplant : official J Am Soc Transplant Am Soc Transpl Surgeons 2014; 14:438–45.

67. Egan TM, Murray S, Bustami RT, et al. Development of the new lung allocation system in the United States. Am J Transpl 2006;6(5 Pt 2): 1212–27.

68. Egan TM, Edwards LB. Effect of the lung allocation score on lung transplantation in the United States. J Heart Lung Transpl 2016; 35(4):433–9.

69. Glazier A. The lung lawsuit: a case study in organ allocation policy and administrative law. J Health Biomed 2018;XIV:139–48.

70. Mooney JJ, Bhattacharya J, Dhillon GS. Effect of broader geographic sharing of donor lungs on lung transplant waitlist outcomes. J Heart Lung Transpl 2019;38:136–44.

71. Bartz RR, Love RB, Leverson GE, et al. Pre-transplant mechanical ventilation and outcome in patients with cystic fibrosis. J Heart Lung Transplant 2003;22:433–8.

72. Vermeijden JW, Zijlstra JG, Erasmus ME, et al. Lung transplantation for ventilator-dependent respiratory failure. J Heart Lung Transplant 2009;28: 347–51.

73. Spahr JE, Love RB, Francois M, et al. Lung transplantation for cystic fibrosis: current concepts and one center's experience. J cystic fibrosis 2007;6:334–50.

74. Moran F, Bradley JM, Piper AJ. Non-invasive ventilation for cystic fibrosis. Cochrane database Syst Rev 2013;4:CD002769.

75. Bermudez CA, Rocha RV, Zaldonis D, et al. Extracorporeal membrane oxygenation as a bridge to lung transplant: midterm outcomes. Ann Thorac Surg 2011;92:1226–31. ; discussion 31-2.

76. Toyoda Y, Bhama JK, Shigemura N, et al. Efficacy of extracorporeal membrane oxygenation as a bridge to lung transplantation. J Thorac Cardiovasc Surg 2013;145:1065–70. ; discussion 70-1.

77. Hayes D Jr, Kukreja J, Tobias JD, et al. Ambulatory venovenous extracorporeal respiratory support as a bridge for cystic fibrosis patients to emergent lung transplantation. J cystic fibrosis 2012;11:40–5.

78. Liou TG, Adler FR, Huang D. Use of lung transplantation survival models to refine patient selection in cystic fibrosis. Am J Respir Crit Care Med 2005; 171:1053–9.

79. Liou TG, Adler FR, Cox DR, et al. Lung transplantation and survival in children with cystic fibrosis. New Engl J Med 2007;357:2143–52.

80. Sweet SC, Aurora P, Benden C, et al. Lung transplantation and survival in children with cystic fibrosis: solid statistics–flawed interpretation. Pediatr Transplant 2008;12:129–36.

81. Thabut G, Christie JD, Mal H, et al. Survival benefit of lung transplant for cystic fibrosis since lung allocation score implementation. Am J Respir Crit Care Med 2013;187:1335–40.

82. Gee L, Abbott J, Conway SP, et al. Validation of the SF-36 for the assessment of quality of life in adolescents and adults with cystic fibrosis. J cystic fibrosis 2002;1:137–45.

83. Gee L, Abbott J, Conway SP, et al. Quality of life in cystic fibrosis: the impact of gender, general health perceptions and disease severity. J cystic fibrosis 2003;2:206–13.

84. Vermeulen KM, van der Bij W, Erasmus ME, et al. Improved quality of life after lung transplantation in individuals with cystic fibrosis. Pediatr pulmonology 2004;37:419–26.

85. Burker EJ, Carels RA, Thompson LF, et al. Quality of life in patients awaiting lung transplant: cystic fibrosis versus other end-stage lung diseases. Pediatr pulmonology 2000;30:453-460.

86. Gee L, Abbott J, Hart A, et al. Associations between clinical variables and quality of life in adults with cystic fibrosis. J cystic fibrosis 2005; 4:59–66.

87. Singer LG, Chowdhury NA, Faughnan ME, et al. Effects of recipient age and diagnosis on health-related quality of life benefit of lung transplantation. Am J Respir Crit Care Med 2015;192:965–73. https://doi.org/10.1164/rccm.201501-0126OC.

88. Busschbach JJ, Horikx PE, van den Bosch JM, et al. Measuring the quality of life before and after bilateral lung transplantation in patients with cystic fibrosis. Chest 1994;105:911–7.

89. Snell GI, Yusen RD, Weill D, et al. Report of the ISHLT working group on primary lung graft dysfunction, part I: definition and grading-A 2016 consensus group statement of the international Society for heart and lung transplantation. J Heart Lung Transpl 2017;36:1097–103.

90. Diamond JM, Arcasoy S, Kennedy CC, et al. Report of the international Society for heart and lung transplantation working group on primary lung graft dysfunction, part II: epidemiology, risk factors, and outcomes-A 2016 consensus group statement of the international Society for heart and lung transplantation. J Heart Lung Transpl 2017;36:1104–13.

91. Gelman AE, Fisher AJ, Huang HJ, et al. Report of the ISHLT working group on primary lung graft dysfunction Part III: mechanisms: A 2016 consensus group statement of the international Society for heart and lung transplantation. J Heart Lung Transpl 2017;36:1114–20.

92. Van Raemdonck D, Hartwig MG, Hertz MI, et al. Report of the ISHLT working group on primary lung graft dysfunction Part IV: prevention and treatment: a 2016 consensus group statement of the

international Society for heart and lung transplantation. J Heart Lung Transpl 2017;36:1121–36.

93. Cantu E, Diamond JM, Suzuki Y, et al. Lung transplant outcomes group. Quantitative evidence for revising the definition of primary graft dysfunction after lung transplant. Am J Respir Crit Care Med 2018;197:235–43.

94. Crespo MM, McCarthy DP, Hopkins PM, et al. ISHLT Consensus Statement on adult and pediatric airway complications after lung transplantation: definitions, grading system, and therapeutics. J Heart Lung Transpl 2018;37:548–63.

95. Eberlein M, Arnaoutakis GJ, Yarmus L, et al. The effect of lung size mismatch on complications and resource utilization after bilateral lung transplantation. J Heart Lung Transpl 2012;31:492–500.

96. Belloli EA, Degtiar I, Wang X, et al. Parametric response mapping as an imaging biomarker in lung transplant recipients. Am J Respir Crit Care Med 2017;195:942–52.

97. Ruttens D, Verleden SE, Vandermeulen E, et al. Prophylactic azithromycin therapy after lung transplantation: post hoc analysis of a randomized controlled trial. Am J Transpl 2016;16:254–61.

98. Vos R, Eynde RV, Ruttens D, et al, Leuven Lung Transplant Group. Montelukast in chronic lung allograft dysfunction after lung transplantation. J Heart Lung Transpl 2019;38:516–27.

99. Kulkarni HS, Cherikh WS, Chambers DC, et al. Bronchiolitis obliterans syndrome-free survival after lung transplantation: an international Society for heart and lung transplantation thoracic transplant registry analysis. J Heart Lung Transpl 2019;38:5–16.

100. Glanville AR, Verleden GM, Todd JL, et al. Chronic lung allograft dysfunction: Definition and update of restrictive allograft syndrome-A consensus report from the Pulmonary Council of the ISHLT. J Heart Lung Transplant 2019;38:483–92.

101. Verleden GM, Glanville AR, Lease ED, et al. Chronic lung allograft dysfunction: Definition, diagnostic criteria, and approaches to treatment-A consensus report from the Pulmonary Council of the ISHLT. J Heart Lung Transplant 2019;38:493–503.

102. Lehr CJ, Skeans M, Dasenbrook EC, et al. Effect of including important clinical variables on accuracy of the lung allocation score for cystic fibrosis and chronic obstructive pulmonary disease. Am J Respir Crit Care Med 2019 Jun;14. https://doi.org/10.1164/rccm.201902-0252OC.

103. Quon BS, Psoter K, Mayer-Hamblett N, et al. Disparities in access to lung transplantation for patients with cystic fibrosis by socioeconomic status. Am J Respir Crit Care Med 2012;186:1008-1013.

104. Merlo CA, Clark SC, Arnaoutakis GJ, et al. National healthcare delivery systems influence lung transplant outcomes for cystic fibrosis. Am J Transplant 2015;15:1948–57.

105. Ramsey BW, Davies J, McElvaney NG, et al. A CFTR potentiator in patients with cystic fibrosis and the G551D mutation. N Engl J Med 2011;365(18):1663–72.

106. Barry PJ, Plant BJ, Nair A, et al. Effects of ivacaftor in patients with cystic fibrosis who carry the G551D mutation and have severe lung disease. Chest 2014;146(1):152–8.

107. Polenakovik HM, Sanville B. The use of ivacaftor in an adult with severe lung disease due to cystic fibrosis (DeltaF508/G551D). J Cyst Fibros 2013;12(5):530–1.

108. Taylor-Cousar J, Niknian M, Gilmartin G, et al. Effect of ivacaftor in patients with advanced cystic fibrosis and a G551D-CFTR mutation: safety and efficacy in an expanded access program in the United States. J Cyst Fibros 2016;15(1):116–22.

109. Salvatore D, Terlizzi V, Francalanci M, et al. Ivacaftor improves lung disease in patients with advanced CF carrying CFTR mutations that confer residual function. Respir Med 2020;171:106073.

110. Keating D, Marigowda G, Burr L, et al. VX-445-Tezacaftor-Ivacaftor in Patients with Cystic Fibrosis and One or Two Phe508del Alleles. N Engl J Med 2018;379(17):1612–20.

111. Middleton PG, Mall MA, Drevinek P, et al. Elexacaftor-Tezacaftor-Ivacaftor for Cystic Fibrosis with a Single Phe508del Allele. N Engl J Med 2019;381(19):1809–19.

112. Heijerman HGM, McKone EF, Downey DG, et al. Efficacy and safety of the elexacaftor plus tezacaftor plus ivacaftor combination regimen in people with cystic fibrosis homozygous for the F508del mutation: a double-blind, randomised, phase 3 trial. Lancet 2019;394(10212):1940–8.

113. Burgel PR, Durieu I, Chiron R, et al. Rapid improvement after Starting elexacaftor-tezacaftor-ivacaftor in patients with cystic fibrosis and advanced pulmonary disease. Am J Respir Crit Care Med 2021;204(1):64–73.

114. Volkova N, Moy K, Evans J, et al. Disease progression in patients with cystic fibrosis treated with ivacaftor: data from national US and UK registries. J Cyst Fibros 2020;19(1):68–79.

115. Trimble AT, Donaldson SH. Ivacaftor withdrawal syndrome in cystic fibrosis patients with the G551D mutation. J Cyst Fibros 2018;17(2):e13–6.

116. Ramos KJ, Guimbellot JS, Valapour M, et al, CFLTC Study Group. Use of elexacaftor/tezacaftor/ivacaftor among cystic fibrosis lung transplant recipients. J Cyst Fibros 2022;21:745–52.

117. Shah P, Lowery E, Chapparo C, et al. Cystic fibrosis foundation consensus statements for the care of cystic fibrosis lung transplant recipients. J Heart Lung Transplant 2021;40(7):539–56.

118. Martin C, Reynaud-Gaubert M, Hamidfar R, et al. Sustained effectiveness of elexacaftor-tezacaftor-ivacaftor in lung transplant candidates with cystic fibrosis. J Cyst Fibros 2022;21(3): 489–96.

119. Iasella CJ, Hoji A, Popescu I, et al. Type-1 immunity and endogenous immune regulators predominate in the airway transcriptome during chronic lung allograft dysfunction. Am J Transplant 2021;21(6): 2145–60.

UNITED STATES POSTAL SERVICE ® — Statement of Ownership, Management, and Circulation
(All Periodicals Publications Except Requester Publications)

1. Publication Title
CLINICS IN CHEST MEDICINE

2. Publication Number
000 – 706

3. Filing Date
9/18/2022

4. Issue Frequency
MAR, JUN, SEP, DEC

5. Number of Issues Published Annually
4

6. Annual Subscription Price
$408.00

7. Complete Mailing Address of Known Office of Publication (Not printer) (Street, city, county, state, and ZIP+4®)
ELSEVIER INC.
230 Park Avenue, Suite 800
New York, NY 10169

Contact Person
Malathi Samayan

Telephone (Include area code)
91-44-4299-4507

8. Complete Mailing Address of Headquarters or General Business Office of Publisher (Not printer)
ELSEVIER INC.
230 Park Avenue, Suite 800
New York, NY 10169

9. Full Names and Complete Mailing Addresses of Publisher, Editor, and Managing Editor (Do not leave blank)

Publisher (Name and complete mailing address)
DOLORES MELONI ELSEVIER INC.
1600 JOHN F KENNEDY BLVD. SUITE 1800
PHILADELPHIA, PA 19103-2899

Editor (Name and complete mailing address)
Joanna Collett, ELSEVIER INC.
1600 JOHN F KENNEDY BLVD. SUITE 1800
PHILADELPHIA, PA 19103-2899

Managing Editor (Name and complete mailing address)
PATRICK MANLEY, ELSEVIER INC.
1600 JOHN F KENNEDY BLVD. SUITE 1800
PHILADELPHIA, PA 19103-2899

10. Owner (Do not leave blank. If the publication is owned by a corporation, give the name and address of the corporation immediately followed by the names and addresses of all stockholders owning or holding 1 percent or more of the total amount of stock. If not owned by a corporation, give the names and addresses of the individual owners. If owned by a partnership or other unincorporated firm, give its name and address as well as those of each individual owner. If the publication is published by a nonprofit organization, give its name and address.)

Full Name	Complete Mailing Address
WHOLLY OWNED SUBSIDIARY OF REED/ELSEVIER, US HOLDINGS	1600 JOHN F KENNEDY BLVD. SUITE 1800 PHILADELPHIA, PA 19103-2899

11. Known Bondholders, Mortgagees, and Other Security Holders Owning or Holding 1 Percent or More of Total Amount of Bonds, Mortgages, or Other Securities. If none, check box ► ☐ None

Full Name	Complete Mailing Address
N/A	

12. Tax Status (For completion by nonprofit organizations authorized to mail at nonprofit rates) (Check one)
The purpose, function, and nonprofit status of this organization and the exempt status for federal income tax purposes:
☒ Has Not Changed During Preceding 12 Months
☐ Has Changed During Preceding 12 Months (Publisher must submit explanation of change with this statement)

PS Form 3526, July 2014 [Page 1 of 4 (see instructions page 4)] PSN: 7530-01-000-9931   PRIVACY NOTICE: See our privacy policy on www.usps.com.

---

13. Publication Title
CLINICS IN CHEST MEDICINE

14. Issue Date for Circulation Data Below
JUNE 2022

15. Extent and Nature of Circulation

		Average No. Copies Each Issue During Preceding 12 Months	No. Copies of Single Issue Published Nearest to Filing Date
a. Total Number of Copies (Net press run)		391	338
b. Paid Circulation (By Mail and Outside the Mail)	(1) Mailed Outside-County Paid Subscriptions Stated on PS Form 3541 (Include paid distribution above nominal rate, advertiser's proof copies, and exchange copies)	228	208
	(2) Mailed In-County Paid Subscriptions Stated on PS Form 3541 (Include paid distribution above nominal rate, advertiser's proof copies, and exchange copies)	0	0
	(3) Paid Distribution Outside the Mails Including Sales Through Dealers and Carriers, Street Vendors, Counter Sales, and Other Paid Distribution Outside USPS®	117	92
	(4) Paid Distribution by Other Classes of Mail Through the USPS (e.g. First-Class Mail®)	0	0
c. Total Paid Distribution (Sum of 15b (1), (2), (3), and (4)) ►		345	300
d. Free or Nominal Rate Distribution (By Mail and Outside the Mail)	(1) Free or Nominal Rate Outside-County Copies included on PS Form 3541	26	20
	(2) Free or Nominal Rate In-County Copies Included on PS Form 3541	0	0
	(3) Free or Nominal Rate Copies Mailed at Other Classes Through the USPS (e.g. First-Class Mail)	0	0
	(4) Free or Nominal Rate Distribution Outside the Mail (Carriers or other means)	26	20
e. Total Free or Nominal Rate Distribution (Sum of 15d (1), (2), (3) and (4)) ►		26	20
f. Total Distribution (Sum of 15c and 15e) ►		371	320
g. Copies not Distributed (See Instructions to Publishers #4 (page #3)) ►		20	18
h. Total (Sum of 15f and g) ►		391	338
i. Percent Paid (15c divided by 15f times 100) ►		92.99%	93.75%

* If you are claiming electronic copies, go to line 16 on page 3. If you are not claiming electronic copies, skip to line 17 on page 3.

16. Electronic Copy Circulation

	Average No. Copies Each Issue During Preceding 12 Months	No. Copies of Single Issue Published Nearest to Filing Date
a. Paid Electronic Copies ►		
b. Total Paid Print Copies (Line 15c) + Paid Electronic Copies (Line 16a) ►		
c. Total Print Distribution (Line 15f) + Paid Electronic Copies (Line 16a) ►		
d. Percent Paid (Both Print & Electronic Copies) (16b divided by 16c × 100) ►		

☒ I certify that 50% of all my distributed copies (electronic and print) are paid above a nominal price.

17. Publication of Statement of Ownership
☒ If the publication is a general publication, publication of this statement is required. Will be printed in the DECEMBER 2022 issue of this publication.   ☐ Publication not required.

18. Signature and Title of Editor, Publisher, Business Manager, or Owner

Malathi Samayan

Malathi Samayan - Distribution Controller

Date 9/18/2022

I certify that all information furnished on this form is true and complete. I understand that anyone who furnishes false or misleading information on this form or who omits material or information requested on the form may be subject to criminal sanctions (including fines and imprisonment) and/or civil sanctions (including civil penalties).

PS Form 3526, July 2014 (Page 3 of 4)   PRIVACY NOTICE: See our privacy policy on www.usps.com

Printed and bound by CPI Group (UK) Ltd, Croydon, CR0 4YY

08/05/2025

01864704-0010